DATE DUE

THE SUBTLE BODY

THE SUBTLE BODY

THE STORY OF YOGA IN AMERICA

STEFANIE SYMAN

FARRAR, STRAUS AND GIROUX

NEW YORK

Farrar, Straus and Giroux
18 West 18th Street, New York 10011

Copyright © 2010 by Stefanie Syman
All rights reserved
Distributed in Canada by D&M Publishers, Inc.
Printed in the United States of America
First edition, 2010

Library of Congress Cataloging-in-Publication Data
Syman, Stefanie.
    The subtle body : the story of yoga in America / Stefanie Syman.—
1st ed.
        p.   cm.
    Includes bibliographical references and index.
    ISBN 978-0-374-23676-2 (hardcover : alk. paper)
    1. Yoga.   2. United States—Religion.   3. Leisure—Economic aspects—
United States.   4. Big Business—United States.   I. Title.

B132.Y6S96   2010
204'.360973—dc22

                                                        2010002358

Designed by Jonathan D. Lippincott

www.fsgbooks.com

1   3   5   7   9   10   8   6   4   2

TO ALL OF MY TEACHERS

CONTENTS

THE SUBTLE BODY

INTRODUCTION

The day after Easter, thousands of families gathered on the White House grounds for the annual Easter Egg Roll.

The event was as choreographed as any other presidential ceremony. Secret Service men mingled in the crowd; television reporters stood in pools of artificial light, describing the day's goings-on; and anyone who was admitted abided by the usual prohibitions (no duffel bags, no food or drink of any kind, no aerosols, no real or simulated weapons, etc.).[1]

At 10:25 a.m., the first family appeared on the White House balcony, emerging from the inner sanctum like regal miniatures in a cuckoo clock.

President Obama made a few remarks and then ceded the microphone to the First Lady, the day's hostess.

"Welcome, everybody. I don't have much to say," she demurred. "Our goal today is just to have fun. We want to focus on activity, healthy eating. We've got yoga, we've got dancing, we've got storytelling, we've got Easter-egg decorating."[2]

The yoga sessions had started at dawn. Wearing winter jackets, sweatpants or jeans, and sneakers, children—from toddlers to teens—had taken their places on brightly colored yoga mats in bunches of fifty. The teachers had come from studios as far as Sacramento and as near as D.C.'s downtown to walk each set through a half-hour sequence of Hatha Yoga poses.

With the White House in the background, the kids attempted "airplane" pose (Vīrabhadrāsana III), teetering on one foot, one arm touching the ground, the other reaching into the sky, while trying to keep their back leg parallel to the lawn, which was lumpier than you might have wished if you had been doing the balancing.

They learned "crow" pose (Bakasana)—you balance on your forearms, knees tucked into your armpits, rear lifted in the air; "mountain" pose

(Tāḍāsana)—you stand feet planted into the ground, heels touching, arms at your side; and a few other postures. Then the instructors planted their hands on the ground, pressed their heels into the grass, with about three feet in between, forming a tunnel of "downward dogs," and the kids crawled through.[3]

The scene, as presented in news stories and on the official White House blog, was wholesome and productive. Yoga, it was tacitly agreed, was a great form of exercise that, like basketball, soccer, or dance, might help stem the tide of childhood obesity.

Everyone was fairly sure that this was the first time yoga had been practiced on the White House lawn, save the run-through the day before. (A reporter on Sunday press-pool duty had glimpsed several instructors "stretching and doing both handstands and headstands" not far from the south driveway.)[4]

There certainly was no better proof that Americans had assimilated this spiritual discipline. We had turned a technique for God realization that had, at various points in time, enjoined its adherents to reduce their diet to rice, milk, and a few vegetables, fix their minds on a set of, to us, incomprehensible syllables, and self-administer daily enemas (without the benefit of equipment), to name just a few of its prerequisites, into an activity suitable for children. Though yoga has no coherent tradition in India, being preserved instead by thousands of gurus and hundreds of lineages, each of which makes a unique claim to authenticity, we had managed to turn it into a singular thing: a way to stay healthy and relaxed. How that happened, and what it all means, is the subject of this book.

But a few things are worth noting here.

The yoga on display that April day had been extracted and distilled, like some homeopathic remedy, from centuries-old Hindu, Hatha Yoga scriptures. These taught the spiritual aspirant how to conquer death and, more to the point, how to reach states of bliss so engulfing and powerful they were beyond description. The best the texts could do was to state what these lacked, which was any sense of suffering or time or boundedness.[5]

Hatha Yoga scriptures are far more precise about how you transit from one state to the other, how you turn mere human flesh into a vehicle for the divine.

Put simply, to do this, you need to gain control of the subtle body.

Now the term *the subtle body*, or *sūkṣma-śarīra*, like the word *yoga* itself, has several related but distinct meanings.[6]

In Hatha Yoga, the subtle body describes a network of channels (nadis) and wheel-like vortices (chakras). These are invisible to the naked eye and even the microscope; the subtle body is distinct from the gross or physical body, though manipulating one necessarily affects the other.

The purpose of practicing Hatha Yoga, including the postures as well as internal cleansing practices and breathing exercises, is to raise Kundalini, a powerful energy, which is typically lodged in the bottom chakra at the base of your spine, to the crown of your head, the top chakra.

You'd be hard-pressed to see the connection between this Hatha Yoga and the yoga those youngsters learned on the White House lawn.

But many of those aspects of yoga—the ecstatic, the transcendent, the overtly Hindu, the possibly subversive, and even the seemingly bizarre—that you couldn't see on the White House grounds that day and that you won't find in most yoga classes persist, right here in America.

Like some sort of collective id, they're half-buried. You can find them at the Burning Man festival in Nevada's Black Rock Desert or at solstice celebrations in the high mountains of New Mexico or deep in its forests. There yoga is a sacred ritual that directly, overtly, and insistently relates sex to God, bodies to transcendence. It's not so much a way to stay healthy as it is a method for disrupting ordinary waking consciousness in order to see a deeper, divinized reality. At places such as the Rainbow Gathering of the Tribes, yoga is one way to blow your mind.

Usually thousands come to the annual, weeklong Fourth of July Rainbow Gathering of the Tribes. This year, they came by plane, by car, and by foot to the Parque Venado in the Santa Fe National Forest. Most wore their hair dreadlocked or shaven clean off. Clothes, when they were wearing them at all, were tie-dyed and loose. Delicate, hennaed patterns of flowers and leaves snaked up one woman's torso and circled her bare breasts. Many had pierced navels and noses and eyebrows. A few of the men wore Native American shawls and feathers.

Some mornings you'd see a circle of tattooed young men and women vigorously inhaling and exhaling, as if hyperventilating, but clearly they did so intentionally, at specific intervals for a set period. And then they too would do some yoga poses.

They were practicing Kundalini Yoga, which is what it sounds like.

The techniques—the breathing exercises, meditation, chanting, and postures—are designed to raise Kundalini through the subtle body.

The scene was a reprise on a much smaller scale of one that had taken
place forty years earlier. The summer of 1969 on Yasgur's farm in Bethel,
New York, a fierce blond, ponytailed young man taught "the breath of
fire." From the stage, he led hundreds of thousands of young people, one
hand pinching his nostril, the other muscled arm raised up high so people
could see him, and he taught a much smaller group of shirtless men and
long-haired women sprawled on the grass, dogs barking in confusion and
a towheaded toddler placidly looking on.

As the group panted in loud, rhythmic bursts, he told them, "These
are all beginning exercises of Kundalini Yoga. *Yoga* means 'union.' It's the
same energy that drugs give you, force a rush on, right. It's the same channels, only drugs do it for you, and this way you can do it yourself."[7]

The Rainbow Tribe is made up of the spiritual heirs and heiresses of
the Woodstock hippies, and it gathers every year to promote world peace,
ecology, and tolerance. And like their forebears, members of the Rainbow
Tribe, or nonmembers as they like to call themselves, are dedicated to
altering their consciousness, by most any means necessary.

If the yoga on the White House lawn was sanitized, sanctioned, and
family-friendly, the yoga in the New Mexico forest was not. It was spiritual and tied up in a subculture that sees hallucinogens as agents of divine
revelation. And it was sexual. As one attendee put it, there's a "very fine
line between Kirtan, chanting, and dancing and erotic spiritual massage."[8]

This yoga is just as much a product of American culture as the Hatha
Yoga taught at the White House Easter Egg Roll and, at least as practiced
by Rainbow Tribe nonmembers, it leaves just as much out, namely the
ethical precepts and strictures that traditionally applied to aspirants, in
even the most outré forms of yoga.

In a country as vast and as diverse as ours, yoga has had this going for it:
it's not a unified system, nor even a tree with many branches. It might be
three or five trees of different species, each with many branches. Or it's a
city, it's New York or Bombay, where the contrasts between neighbor-
hoods are sharp, where you can get lost in its vastness, and which changes
anyone who stays but not in the same way or for the same reasons.

Yoga is so massive and complicated, so contradictory and baroque, that American society has been able to assimilate any number of versions of it, more or less simultaneously.

The process hasn't been smooth or continuous. It has got caught up around a number of issues, often the same ones, over and over, as several generations of Americans have tried to make sense of yoga and put it to use in their lives.

The biggest stumbling block has always been the difficulty of defining yoga. Is it religion? A religious practice that might be severed from the whole the way you can take a battery out of a clock and use it to power a blow-dryer? Is it exercise? Does it produce scientifically measurable changes in your heart rate, respiration, or cognition?

How Americans have defined yoga has had profound implications, especially since those who see yoga as a religion, or irrevocably part of one, are more apt to see in it a full-blown critique of American culture.

How Americans have defined yoga has also been tied up with their understanding of the subtle body, a difficult, even confounding, concept. It's not physical but it describes a kind of spiritual physics. And yet it's not exactly a metaphor either, since once you learn to control its energies, you should feel specific effects. So the subtle body has a strange ontological status—not physical and yet not wholly imagined.

How yoga teachers have talked about the subtle body, or whether they have talked about it at all, is a good index of their intentions, particularly in the first half of this story.

Perhaps the most vexing issue Americans have had to confront has been the nature of the guru. Is he a monk who can teach us how to transcend the beastliness and boredom of human existence? A magician who can unlock the mysteries of the occult? A charlatan or a God-man? A healer of bodies or of souls?

Any given guru might appear to be both monk and magician, charlatan and God-man, depending on your perspective, and yoga quickly found adherents and critics in America in almost equal numbers.

To tell the story of yoga here is to negotiate between the conflicting claims of devotees and skeptics.

One thing, though, is clear: when Americans first learned about yoga, in the nineteenth century, they learned that it required "annihilating . . . the body and the world" and that it perverted one's moral sense. They

learned that yoga corrupted body and soul. It was about as useful as ma-
laria or consumption but far easier to avoid.[9]

Over about a hundred years, Americans' understanding of yoga
changed dramatically, from bewilderment and hostility to a foreign—even
heathen—practice to widespread admiration and acceptance. But unlike
the turning of homely caterpillar to butterfly, this process was not foreordained, not coded into the discipline itself. Indian swamis and their
American disciples, American yoga teachers and students and fellow travelers, slowly and deliberately chipped away at the bigotry, fear, and misin-
formation that encased yoga, that at first made this spiritual discipline
seem like a very bad idea indeed.

To do this, they used a variety of tools and tactics. One was careful
editing. The earliest Indian purveyors of yoga in America, people such as
Swami Vivekananda, felt Americans would abuse certain elements of the
practice and its philosophy, so they were highly selective in teaching the
discipline. Like Hollywood directors skilled at making older stars look
young, they'd show yoga only from certain angles, in soft, radiant light.
Such subtractions and elisions continue to this day.

Another common tactic has been to couple yoga to some other cause
or movement with a lot of energy and momentum, such as the alternative
health movement or psychedelics.

At the time, this move often feels disastrously misguided, and its immediate consequences are unclear. Yet, for yoga, such couplings have had
several useful effects: because these mongrel movements, however contentious, have the country's attention, Americans end up talking about
yoga, even negatively or dismissively, more than they would otherwise
have; famous and sometimes even esteemed individuals associate themselves with the practice, which adds to its currency; and finally, yoga benefits from the energy behind these other ideas, as their advocates make
great efforts to legitimize themselves and to root their ephemeral practices in something more substantial.

Of course, there's much more to this process than a few rhetorical
tricks and savvy PR. Mostly, yoga has become a very good thing, good
enough for the first family to include in their Easter celebrations, because
thousands of people—Henry David Thoreau, Pierre A. Bernard, Margaret Woodrow Wilson, Christopher Isherwood, and Sally Kempton among
them—have devoted themselves to the discipline, often in defiance of
prevailing mores.

This book tells the stories of some of these people. Needless to say, the teachers, students, and sympathizers who have contributed to the assimilation of yoga are beyond numbering. No author could do justice to them all. So this book sets out to show how and why certain forms of yoga took hold in particular eras. It also shows how yoga has forced Americans to reckon with a whole host of assumptions about themselves and the nature of reality. The discipline almost immediately challenged Americans' belief that the physical wasn't sacred, as well as the Cartesian split between mind and body. You could say yoga has given us a way out of these maddening dualities.

Yoga has also been the aspect of Asian culture most readily and widely assimilated (outside of food), though Buddhism was taken up with just as much interest at first. Yoga then is one of the first and most successful products of globalization, and it has augured a truly post-Christian, spiritually polyglot country.

Finally, yoga has been a sort of multiplier, increasing the number of divine interlocutors. No longer is this a role reserved for a few long-dead prophets. Your guru might well be a channel for the divine, and the discipline promises that you might be too. It's this possibility—of turning yourself into the very thing you worship, call it God, superconsciousness, Brahman, Krishna, Kali, Shiva, the Self—that animates this story.

1

BRAHMA?

In the fall of 1857, a new magazine went into the U.S. mails. Its design was emphatically plain. Its title, *The Atlantic Monthly. A Magazine of Literature, Art, and Politics*, was printed in black type on paper the color of pine boards. Inside, two long, tight columns ran down its pages. There weren't any illustrations, except, on the cover, a small engraving of John Winthrop, Puritan founder of Massachusetts Bay Colony, in a ruffled collar and thick goatee. Whether Winthrop was the magazine's patron saint or muse, you couldn't mistake the *Atlantic*'s lineage. It had strong ties to the eastern seaboard in general, and Boston in particular.[1]

Contributors, or "literary persons," were listed on the inside front cover, but the essays and poems that filled the magazine were unsigned, as was then customary. No reader was confused for long, though, about who had written a set of verses titled "Brahma," on page 48, because the *Atlantic*'s publisher had leaked the byline to a Boston newspaper. The author was Ralph Waldo Emerson—poet, philosopher, prophet, Sphinx—and his presence in the magazine was one of its selling points.[2]

Emerson, along with several other New England luminaries, had helped Francis H. Underwood launch the *Atlantic*. Underwood saw the magazine as an intellectual platform; his employer, book publisher Moses Dresser Phillips, saw it as a way to boost book sales.

Happily, Phillips's business interests intersected with Emerson's self-interest. At the time, it was nearly impossible for him to make a living as an author, and the *Atlantic* promised a wider readership as well as a much appreciated source of additional income.

But the literary persons behind the *Atlantic*—a group that included Oliver Wendell Holmes, Harriet Beecher Stowe, Henry Wadsworth Longfellow, and James R. Lowell—were nothing if not high-minded, and the pecuniary reasons for starting a new magazine paled beside their self-appointed mission, which was to free American belles lettres from European condescension once and for all. The *Atlantic* would provide this badly needed aesthetic leadership. It would be a place where quality trumped popular taste, and American, rather than English or French, authors reigned.

The new magazine had one other purpose: to denounce, in a "scholarly and gentleman like" tone, the most egregious social injustice of the day—slavery.

The founders had their differences (Holmes, for one, was notoriously impatient with Emerson's "Oriental" meanderings), but they agreed on three things: American writers must be supported, slavery must be abolished, and at times readers must be damned. And so, the author of "American Scholar" gave voice to "Brahma":[3]

> *If the red slayer think he slays,*
> *Or if the slain think he is slain,*
> *They know not well the subtle ways*
> *I keep, and pass, and turn again.*

> *Far or forgot to me is near,*
> *Shadow and sunlight are the same,*
> *The vanished gods to me appear,*
> *And one to me are shame and fame.*

> *They reckon ill who leave me out;*
> *When me they fly, I am the wings;*
> *I am the doubter and the doubt,*
> *I am the hymn the Brahmin sings.*

> *The strong gods pine for my abode,*
> *And pine in vain the sacred Seven;*
> *But thou, meek lover of the good!*
> *Find me, and turn thy back on heaven.*

In the *Atlantic* number 1, this pithy celebration of nonduality—"shadow and sunlight are the same"—followed three other poems, all Emerson's, and it stands out from the group for its austerity. "Brahma" eschews the exoticism of "The Romany Girl" (which is about a Gypsy beauty) and "Days" (where time marches like "barefoot dervishes") for simple declarative sentences. In it, Emerson managed to compress Brahman, the Absolute, or Supreme Being, whose names, qualities, and powers clutter India's most sacred texts, into four adamantine verses.

"Brahma" is not so much a poem as a paean to a divinity that more closely resembles gravity, an impersonal, immutable force, than it does the God of the Bible.

Yet if Emerson was making some sort of declaration of his heterodoxy, it was probably lost on readers. Most had no idea who or what Brahma was, didn't recognize him as part of the Hindu pantheon at all, and, if they did, could justifiably have been confused about his exact identity since, in Emerson's day, transliterated spellings of certain Sanskrit words were even less standardized than they are today.

The word *Brahma* sometimes referred to the concept Brahman (as it's now commonly spelled), the Absolute or Supreme Being "behind and above all the various deities . . . beings, and worlds." Other times, nearly the same word designated the creator god, who is part of the classic Hindu triad along with Vishnu, the preserver, and Shiva, the destroyer.[4]

The New York Times immediately deemed the poem an "exquisite piece of meaningless versification." Soon friends and sympathizers came to Emerson's aid. In mid-November, Walt Whitman published a concise piece in the *Brooklyn Daily Times* reminding readers of Brahma's identity (an Indian deity, etc.) and defending the poem. Not long after, the *Brooklyn Eagle* quoted an obscure periodical that had excerpted "a passage from the *Mahabharata*, similar both in thought and in phrasing," to "Brahma."[5]

But even after Brahma's identity was revealed—Emerson's poem clearly referenced the Absolute—newspapers and magazines across the country continued to mercilessly deride it. Twenty-six parodies were written in just the first month after the poem's publication, and these were frequently reprinted over the next year.[6]

It hardly mattered to Emerson. His repudiations of "sacraments, supernaturalism, biblical authority, and of Christianity," in the words of one of his most ardent followers, had electrified audiences from Maine to Minneapolis for two decades. Irreverence was his stock-in-trade, and it had made him famous. By the time "Brahma" appeared, he was an icon of independent thinking in a country proud of its independence. In Emerson's hands, "Brahma" was American.[7]

Whitman once said of Emerson, "Even when he falls on stony ground he somehow eventuates in a harvest."[8]

Since its appearance in 1857, "Brahma" has helped spur a century-and-a-half-long engagement with Hinduism. The yield has been plentiful and varied: American translations of Sanskrit texts, the philosophy of William James, new academic specialties, and, more to the point, an American yoga.

That Emerson himself was indifferent to yoga makes him no less central to its assimilation here. Yoga is connected to a host of philosophies as well as competing and even contradictory metaphysics; it encompasses varied practices and is technically a part of three "world religions": Hinduism, Buddhism, and Jainism. Steered by his own family toward Hinduism, Emerson steered Americans toward a specific understanding of yoga even though the discipline didn't really interest him. Just as the computer scientists who built ARPANET created the conditions for Google without ever having anticipated it, Emerson created the conditions for an American yoga.

Like many Boston Unitarians and intellectuals of his era, Emerson's father, the Reverend William Emerson, was an armchair Orientalist (an eighteenth-century term applied to anyone who studied or wrote about Oriental cultures).

William Emerson was one of the founders of the *Monthly Anthology*, which published Sir William Jones's translation of a famous Hindu play—*Sacontalá; or, The Fatal Ring*—in 1805. When William Emerson died six years later, he left his wife and three young sons (Ralph, Edward, and Charles) a library that included several major works on India and its religious culture.[9]

Together, the Emerson family would read J. Priestly's *Heathen Philosophy* or Elizabeth Hamilton's *Translation of the Letters of a Hindoo Rajah: Written Previous to, and during the period of his residence in England*, an evening's fireside entertainment and edification.[10]

These were groundbreaking books. As late as 1785, Western research into Indian religion was, in the words of the infamous Warren Hastings, then governor-general of Bengal, still very much "a wide and unexplored field of fruitful knowledge."

Colonial administrators and British missionaries were among the first to sally forth into this intellectual wilderness. But they were hobbled by the usual barriers that confront anyone trying to translate elements of one culture into another. There was the problem of language, of course. There was also the presumption, shared by clergymen and colonizers alike, that the Enlightenment had left India behind.

For those who could find ways around the first two, more slippery problems awaited them. The first was the temptation to refer to a wide variety of practices and beliefs as a coherent, defined religion. Many missionaries succumbed, and most described what they saw as either heathenism or, more respectfully, Brahmanism or Hinduism.[11]

Another problem, related to this, was the belief that if you could rightly point to something called Brahmanism, it would function much like Christianity and Judaism did in Western society: it was textually based, was geared toward salvation, and made claims to universal truth.

This was an understandable but grave error.

To assimilate something is to conform it to your own worldview.

To see the varied beliefs and practices of India through the prism of "world religion" was to assimilate these activities before even describing them.[12]

As for yoga, early interlocutors who considered it at all tended to dismiss it as uncouth.

Take the Reverend William Ward. Unlike most of his peers, he did extensive firsthand research in addition to consulting with native pundits and English Sanskritists. He refrained from using the word *heathenism* or *heathens* to describe his subject.

Still, he was dismissive of their practices.[13]

"A most singular ceremony, called yogŭ," he writes in the introduction to his widely read, three-volume exposition of the history, literature, and mythology of the Hindus, "is said to have been practiced by ascetics to prepare them for absorption" into Brahman. Several pages later he added, "The absurdity and impiety of the opinions upon which the practices of these yogēēs are founded, need not be exposed: the doctrine which destroys all accountability to the Creator, and removes all that is criminal in immortality, must be condemned by every good man."[14]

•

When they read books about the Orient, the Emersons favored travel tales or extracts from Orientalist tracts. As a boy, Ralph Waldo Emerson also read translations of "Hindoo" scriptures, pressed upon him by his aunt Mary Moody Emerson.

Mary Moody, the Reverend William Emerson's sister, was a voracious and intrepid reader, who took the Emerson brothers' education seriously. Emerson considered her something of a visionary.[15]

She directed him to Rammohun Roy's translation of the *Ishopanishad* and indulged his early dismissals of Roy and his religion.[16]

At Harvard, Emerson also read a variety of Oriental texts. No professorships in Sanskrit or Asian religions existed yet in America, but the output of European Orientalists, most famously the philologists William Jones, H. T. Colebrooke, and Charles Wilkins, had substantially increased since the turn of the nineteenth century. These experts, who lived in India and by day worked as British civil servants, had a more sympathetic relationship to the country and its traditions—textual, spiritual, ritual—than the missionaries had. They strived to present Indian thought in context, and to do so, they learned to read Sanskrit (which, at least in Jones's case, they'd translate into Latin before rendering it into English). They quickly disseminated their knowledge via the Asiatic Society of Bengal.[17]

Emerson read Sir William Jones's memoirs as well as scores of articles on Indian culture and history in journals such as the *Edinburgh Review*. One was a review of William Ward's book, which struck Emerson with its descriptions of India's "immense 'goddery'" and the "squalid and desperate ignorance" of Asians, as he remarked in his journal. He also rather viciously denigrated "Yoguees of Hindostan" in these pages. Having never encountered one, he deemed them morally and mentally diseased and unrivaled "in their extravagancies and practices of self-torture."[18]

After graduation, Emerson's journal entries related to Hinduism multiplied, and his reading list on the subject slowly grew. Eventually, Emerson, who was by then going by the name Waldo, warmed up to some of the books that had fascinated his aunt, including Roy's translation of the *Ishopanishad*.

Rammohun Roy, a Bengali of Brahmin caste, was one of the few Indians publishing works in English in the early nineteenth century, but he was hardly a dispassionate translator; he was deeply troubled by "Hindoo idolatry" as well as the temples built and ceremonies performed to propitiate "innumerable gods and goddesses" and believed his countrymen had lost sight of the true meaning of the Vedas, the scriptural bedrock of "Hinduism."

He was also probably the first "Hindu" to have used the word *Hinduism* (in 1816), and the term gained in popularity over the nineteenth century. Like *Brahmanism, Hinduism* elides all sorts of philosophical, theological, and metaphysical disputes, not to mention diverse rituals. As noted above, that Hinduism might be encapsulated in its scriptures is already an imposition of Western conceptions of religion.[19]

This approach served Roy's broader argument that the *Upanishads*, which together constitute Vedanta, espoused a gospel of monotheism. Roy assigned himself the task of demonstrating this to the world, which made him popular with New England's liberal Christians. (He also helped set up the first Unitarian Mission in Calcutta, in 1821; this and his pamphlet "The Principles of Jesus, the Guide to Peace and Happiness" incited controversy amid India's Trinitarians, which further endeared him to American Unitarians.)[20]

The *Ishopanishad*, in Roy's view, was a particularly powerful counterweight to descriptions such as Ward's, which detailed the objects of Hindu worship: besides 333 million gods and goddesses, there were "beings in strange shapes," "beasts," "birds," "rivers," and "a log of wood."[21]

The bulk of the *Ishopanishad* circles around the Supreme Spirit, heaping adjectives and qualities upon him even though he supposedly defies apprehension. "He pervades the internal and external parts of the whole universe"; and he is "one unchangeable" who seems "to move everywhere, although he in reality has no motion. . . . He overspreads all creatures. . . . He is pure, perfect, omniscient, the ruler of the intellect, omnipresent, and the self-existent."[22]

This is Brahman, a God transcendent—it's both everything at once and yet completely independent of all that it's supposed to be.

With any idea of the divine as one and unified, questions arise: If everything is God and it's all the same *stuff*, why do we see the world as made up of all sorts of different objects and beings? To which Vedanta answers, the world isn't really separate and distinct. We just see it that way. Vast cataracts of ignorance cloud our vision. Ultimately, there is no difference between the pitch pine and the sumac, the rhododendron and the bulrushes, the copperhead and the pickerel, your neighbor and yourself. All mask the infinite, eternal, immutable soul of the universe. As for Jesus Christ, he also partakes of the Supreme Being; however, to say that the Supreme Being was a man, even a divine one, and not everything else at the same time would be to limit the infinite, which is like trying to pour the ocean into a cup.

The *Katha Upanishad* (at least as translated by Roy) expresses a similar unitary conception of the divine: "As fire, although one in essence, on becoming visible in the world appears in various forms and shapes, according to its different locations, so God, the soul of the universe, though one, appears in various modes . . . and *like space*, extends over all."[23]

Call it pantheism or the philosophy of identity or a brand of idealism, Emerson's church-bred convictions didn't stop him from absorbing, and later transmitting, this idea. At the time, it moved him so much he added a fragment from Sir William Jones's "A Hymn to Narayena" to the end of several pages of musings on God:

> . . . *"Of dew-bespangled leaves and blossoms bright*
> *Hence! vanish from my sight,*
> *Delusive pictures; unsubstantial shews!*
> *My soul absorbed, one only Being knows,*
> *Of all perceptions, one abundant source,*
> *Hence every object, every moment flows,*
> *Suns hence drive their force,*
> *Hence planets learn their course;*
> *But suns and fading worlds I view no more,*
> *God only I perceive, God only I adore!"*[24]

Most of Emerson's contemporaries wouldn't have recognized the God who appears in the "fine pagan strains" he cribbed from Sir William Jones's poem. Gone was the stern Father of the Universe, gone was the loving son who suffered for our sins. Gone too was God as "an all communicating Parent" (in the words of one Unitarian minister). Gone also were flowers and leaves, the earth itself. The remnants? An absorbing force that hurtles us forward.[25]

Emerson quoted the "Hymn" in 1821. Similar ideas surfaced in his work, but slowly, like mountains arising from the movement of tectonic plates, after nearly another twenty years of reading and writing. And it would be another decade after that before Emerson celebrated Indian thought overtly.

In 1842, John Pickering, William Jenks, J. J. Dixwell, and a few others founded the American Oriental Society. The three main founders were Harvard alumni, and the society was based in Boston.[26]

The AOS, an exemplar of the American impulse to form associations, as Tocqueville had so recently put it, particularly when they wished "to advance some truth," defined the "Orient" expansively: it encompassed Egypt, Iran, Africa, Asia Minor, India, Indonesia, Malaysia, China, and Japan as well as several Pacific islands. By studying these varied places and cultures, the AOS sought to "furnish some useful additions . . . for the complete ethnography of the globe." Language was the key to its whole project.[27]

The founders, and certainly Pickering, also thought America had an edge. A lawyer and philologist, Pickering had turned down two professorships, the Hancock Professor of Hebrew and Other Oriental Languages and the Eliot Professorship of Greek Literature, both at Harvard. He considered the English only middling linguists and ethnographers, and he was convinced the Americans, whose missions were particularly active when it came to native language and literature, could do better.[28]

Despite its broad definition of the Orient, the AOS spent a disproportionate amount of its energies on India and Hinduism, especially in relation to other Asian countries, and made deciphering Sanskrit scriptures one of its first orders of business.[29]

As was often still the case when it came to this subject, New England missionaries, clergymen, and theologians were most committed to the organization and its goals. They formed the bulk of the society's membership, dominated its leadership, and contributed nearly half of the articles published in its journal until after the Civil War. Through the American Oriental Society, these men (and they were all men) brought Hinduism—and yoga—that much closer to the rest of the country.[30]

Emerson too was delving ever deeper into Indian thought. Since leaving his pastorate at the Second Church in 1832, he had become a successful lecturer, published two books to good reviews, and had, with Margaret Fuller and others, founded The Dial in 1840. In its brief life span, the small literary periodical ran American translations of several Buddhist and Hindu scriptures. *The Dial* was the Transcendentalists' house organ, and it reflected the group's fascination with Oriental literature.

Around this time, Emerson read the *Vishnu Puruna* and the *Sankhya Karika*. And he owned one of the only editions in the Boston area of Sir Charles Wilkins's translation of the *Bhagavad-Gita*.[31]

With increasing frequency and conviction, Emerson began to insert Hindu ideas and images from his reading into his essays and poetry.[32]

Today, thanks to the assiduous work of scholars and Emersonians, you can trace how a translation of a particular text wended its way into American literature. In the case of the *Bhagavad-Gita*, you can almost see assimilation as it happened.

Emerson acquired the Wilkins *Bhagavad-Gita* in 1843. That June he wrote Miss Elizabeth Hoar, "The only other event is the arrival in Concord of the Bhagavat Gītā, the much renowned book of Buddhism, extracts from which I have often admired, but never before held the book in my hands." (It was not a Buddhist book, and his confusion shows just how new this field of knowledge was in America.)[33]

The Wilkins translation he had got his hands on was first published in 1785 and remains one of the most well-known products of the entire Orientalist enterprise, which was, whatever its shortcomings, to make Asian texts and culture accessible to Westerners.

Wilkins began his career as a writer for the East India Company in 1770 and mastered Sanskrit in his spare time. However, when he decided to translate the *Bhagavad-Gita*, he quickly realized language alone wouldn't be enough to pry open this scripture.[34]

One of the most formidable obstacles he faced in putting the *Gita's* more than seven hundred verses into fairly lucid English was its subject, which is "highly metaphysical."

In fact, the *Bhagavad-Gita* is only one small part of the *Mahabharata*, an epic poem that's often compared to the *Iliad*.

This part of the story, which is difficult to date but was probably composed between the fifth and fourth century B.C.E. and added to later, takes place on the dusty plains of Kuru, where warring factions are poised to fight.[35]

After years of exile, the five Pandava brothers, led by the mighty bowman Arjuna, have come to win back their rightful throne; their enemies are cousins, teachers, and kinsmen. This troubles Arjuna, who stalls mid-battlefield. Krishna, his charioteer and teacher, berates him and exhorts him to enter the fray, to no avail. Horses snort and strain at their reins, stray arrows whistle across the front lines, but Arjuna doesn't budge until after the last of the *Gita*'s verses is spoken.

Though Wilkins called the text "Dialogues of Krĕĕshnă and Ărjŏŏn," the literal translation of *Bhagavad-Gita* is "Lord's song." Historically, it had been sung. But to any American who got hold of it, Wilkins's *Gita*, rendered in prose, not verse, read more like a divine monologue, in which Krishna expounds a metaphysics and philosophy, a spiritual rationale if you will, for action in this world, even violent action. Arjuna's dilemma— lives are quite literally at stake, he is pausing on the battlefield!—charges Krishna's highly abstract exposition with drama and emotion.

Krishna's message is this: Know me. With this knowledge, you can murder without sinning. Without it, worship will pin you to the wheel of existence.

Some consider the *Bhagavad-Gita* the first full-fledged yoga scripture. Krishna doesn't just tell Arjuna he must know him; he tells him how to do this, and the method he offers is yoga. The *Gita* is an elaboration of yoga as a route to divine knowledge, to God figured as Krishna. In the short postscripts that close each chapter, the text refers to itself as a yoga *shāstra* (yogic teaching) as well as an *Upanishad*.[36]

Whether or not it's the first, the *Gita* is certainly more preoccupied with yoga than most works that preceded it.[37]

But in it, yoga is not any single practice; Krishna describes several types. There's meditation, and there's the yoga of devotion (Bhakti Yoga) and of selfless action (Karma Yoga), among others. All lead to Brahman's "supreme abode."[38]

To further complicate matters, the term *yoga* confounded Wilkins, and when he was first confronted by it in the *Bhagavad-Gita*, he threw up his hands. "*Yog.*—There is no word in the *Sanskrēēt* language that will bear so many interpretations as this," Wilkins writes in a long footnote. "It's first significance is *junction* or *union*. It is also used for bodily or mental application; but in this work it is generally used as a theological term, to express the application of mind in spiritual things, and the performance of religious ceremonies."[39]

Wilkins goes on to say that *devotion* will be a serviceable synonym and enthusiastically purges *yog* from much of the rest of the text, which is quite a feat.

About two years after he finally got hold of Wilkins's translation, Emerson wrote what would become the first lines of "Brahma" in his journal. They were a direct response, nearly phrase for phrase, to Wilkins's *Gita*. In Lecture II, when Krishna is trying to convince Arjuna to fight, he explains, "The man who believeth that it is the soul which killeth, and he who thinketh that the soul may be destroyed, are both alike deceived; for it neither killeth, nor is it killed."[40] Emerson wrote:

> *What creature slayeth or is slain?*
> *What creature saves or {is} saved is?* ↑ *{brings or reaches*
>   *bliss?}* ↓
> *{Each loses or}* ↓
> *His life {each}* ↑ *will either* ↓ *lose{s} or gain{s},*
> *As he* ↑ *shall* ↓ *follow{s} {good}harm or {evil}bliss.*[41]

A decade later, in 1855, the rest of the poem came to him. "Brahma" appears as an exhalation of verse between long paragraphs copied out of the *Upanishads*. (And it's here that Emerson makes it clear to whom, or what, he's referring. He writes, quoting the *Katha Upanishad*, "The word is *Om*. This sound means Brahma, means the supreme.")[42]

These later verses also riff on passages in the *Gita*. "I am the sacrifice; I am the worship . . . ," sings Krishna, and "he also is my beloved servant . . . to whom praise and blame are one."

"And one to me are shame and fame," wrote Emerson. ". . . I am the hymn the Brahmin sings."

Around the time he completed "Brahma," Emerson had created a mini-dictionary of Sanskrit terms in his *Notebook Orientalist*, one of several topical notebooks he had begun in the 1850s. Emerson primarily used this particular notebook for translations of Persian poetry and for final drafts of a handful of poems that may or may not have had an Oriental theme.[43]

The brief Sanskrit glossary Emerson transcribed begins with the word *Avatar*, which he defines as "Manifestation." Farther down the page, *Yoga* is defined simply as "the effort to unite with the Deity. Concentration. See *Roer, p. 117.*"

Several other references to yoga are in the *Notebook*, clumped together a few pages later, which add little to this initial definition and again refer to Roer, a well-known Indologist and member of the Asiatic Society of Bengal, who translated numerous *Upanishads* and other works from Sanskrit.[44]

Roer touched on yoga in several places. Yoga, he averred, is a technique, or "appliances," which include "keeping the body erect, taking and exhaling breath according to certain rules, selection of a quiet place, &c., &c." The aim is to subjugate the senses and the mind, necessary preconditions for receiving the "highest knowledge."

In May 1857, two months after the Supreme Court decided Dred Scott was neither a citizen nor a free man, a newly enthusiastic Moses D. Phillips convened the dinner now celebrated as the birthday of the *Atlantic*.[45]

Emerson was there, along with Oliver Wendell Holmes, James R. Lowell, Henry Wadsworth Longfellow, and a few others.[46]

Lowell accepted the editorship of the new magazine, and at a later dinner Holmes christened it. The name suggested trade between the New and Old Worlds, and, as Phillips had noted, each of the founding contributors "was known alike on both sides of the Atlantic."[47]

But another name had been ventured, this one by an employee of Phillips, Sampson and Company's—*The Orient*.[48]

For Emerson, the word was laden with significance. Upon reading Walt Whitman's *Leaves of Grass* for the first time in 1855, an awed Emerson noted that he found the book "so extraordinary for its oriental largeness of generalization."[49]

Emerson also ascribed frivolity and excess to the "Orient" and "Asia," the way a parent might describe her child as defiant, a defiance of which she is secretly proud. "Mine Asia" was the nickname Emerson gave to his second wife, Lydia Jackson, explaining, "No New Englander that he knew had ever possessed such a depth of feeling that was continually called out on such trivial occasions."[50]

In Emerson's imagination, the Orient recalibrated the particulars of reality, deepening, intensifying, and expanding these until they became another order of thing.

Although Holmes's more patriotic name won the day, Emerson hoped the *Atlantic* would possess a "largeness of generalization." He saw it as nothing less than a new type of bible.[51]

Emerson's optimism was rewarded. The *Atlantic*'s first few issues, which cost twenty-five cents or three dollars for a year's subscription, sold out printings of twenty thousand. And by 1859, more than half of its circulation was "foreign," which meant these issues were mailed out of state; many were distributed in the Midwest, to small towns in Ohio and smaller ones in Minnesota. There, the *Atlantic* became a badge of cosmopolitanism.[52]

"Brahma," though, was considered something of a joke, at best.[53]

"His poetry is called transcendental," Mohammed Pacha wrote huffily in the *Boston Daily Advertiser* in 1859, "because it transcends the comprehension of everybody except the men and women of Boston."

Emerson was more amused than dismayed by readers' confusion; at the time, he suggested they substitute the word *Jehovah* for Brahma.[54]

Even Lowell, Emerson's good friend and editor, and the man responsible for "Brahma"'s public debut, was mildly chagrined by the poem. "What the deuse have we to do with Brahma?" he wondered aloud a few years after its publication, in a review of Emerson's *Conduct of Life*. "We will only say that we have found grandeur and consolation in a starlit night without caring to ask what it meant . . . and as for Brahma, why, he can take care of himself and won't bite us at any rate."[55]

Others saw in "Brahma" a deft articulation of key ideas in Indian philosophy and a succinct description of yoga and, in making this case, coupled yoga more firmly to Hinduism, at least in American literature.

William T. Harris, a renowned educator and philosopher, concluded a lengthy disquisition, "Oriental Philosophy and the Bhagavad Gita," which appeared in *The Western*, by noting, "The substance of all of these [quotations from the *Gita* and *Sankhya Karika*] and much more can be found in Emerson's 'Brahma,' a poem that condenses the Yoga doctrine into four short verses, and furnishes a surprising contrast to the tedious recapitulation in oriental literature."[56]

For a while, Emerson's reputation as an assimilator of Oriental thought was still in play.

The American Oriental Society honored Emerson, who had become a Corporate member in 1860 and had passed away the month before, at their May 24, 1882, meeting, noting, "We were permitted and called upon to bear our part, along with all America and the whole civilized world, in homage to the genius and illustrious character Emerson."[57]

Many Indian thinkers had an equally exalted view of the man, claiming a sort of spiritual brotherhood. Protap Chunder Mozoomdar, head of the Brahmo Samaj, an offshoot of the reform organization founded by Rammohun Roy, described Brahmanism as "a state of being rather than a creed" and deemed Emerson "the best of Brahmins." (Mozoomdar exaggerated. Brahmanism would have been as antithetical to Emerson's "original relation to the universe" as Christianity since he believed adopting any faith or doctrine to be akin to spiritual suicide.)[58]

At the same time, Oliver Wendell Holmes, doctor, professor at Harvard Medical School, and author, worked hard to promote the image of Emerson as a prototypical American intellectual, reassuring readers that his dear friend was Yankee at the core and his interest in the Orient purely aesthetic.

Lest "Brahma" had fooled anyone, Holmes insisted in his 1885 biography, *Ralph Waldo Emerson*, the poem was one of Emerson's "spiritual divertissements" and not to be taken too seriously.[59]

That view didn't hold up over time. Later students of Emerson's Oriental influences (a subspecies of Emersonians) combed through the historical record and found it impossible to rescue the poet-philosopher from his Hindu preoccupations.

In the most famous of these efforts, *The Orient in American Transcendentalism*, published in 1932, Arthur Christy reconstructed an exhaustive chronology of every book from or about Asia and the Middle East Emerson ever read based on his journals, letters, book collection, and borrowing records from Harvard College Library and the Boston Athenaeum. Christy's labors weren't in vain. His book marshaled enough evidence to counter any claim that Emerson had brought back only trinkets and cloud castles from his mental journeys to India.

2

THOREAU'S EXPERIMENT

Moncure Conway, an antislavery activist, disaffected Unitarian minister who had given up entirely on God, and author, then based in London, wrote an homage to his friend Henry David Thoreau. "Like the pious Yógi of the East one, so long motionless whilst gazing on the sun that knotty plants encircled his neck and the cast snake-skin his loins, and the birds built their nests upon his shoulders," he effused in *Fraser's Magazine*, a British periodical, a year after the Civil War had ended, "this seer and naturalist seemed by an equal consecration to have become a part of the field and forest amid which he dwelt."[1]

Conway had long admired the Transcendentalists and was himself an enthusiastic Orientalist. But Thoreau as he saw him wasn't just an onlooker, reading Oriental literature or studying Indian culture or even consulting with its wise men, as Conway eventually did. Thoreau lived these books, he imbibed them so deeply he could enact them. He could make "the smallest, most ordinary facts attain a mystic significance."[2]

As Conway suggested, Thoreau practiced yoga, or tried to, and recorded some success in doing so.

The groundwork was laid for his experiments when Ellen Sewall refused Thoreau's proposal of marriage in 1840, not six months after she had declined his brother, John. Though Thoreau might have found another mate, he didn't. This proved a boon in at least one sense: with no wife and no children to feed, Thoreau was at liberty to do as he pleased.

Over the next five years, Thoreau had a hard time wringing much out of his freedom. He had more success improving the production process at his family's pencil factory than getting his writing published.

The Dial, then edited by Emerson, was the only venue willing to take a risk on him, and it shut down in the spring of 1844.

Soon after, out on a fishing expedition near Fairhaven Bay, not far from Concord, Thoreau and a friend accidentally set a fire that burned more than three hundred acres.[3]

The following spring Thoreau built a cabin on a tract of land Emerson had recently bought, and on July 4, he moved into the simple structure, where he intended to "live deliberately." He was about to turn twenty-eight years old.[4]

Thoreau lived at Walden for a little more than two years (he left on September 6, 1847). At the time, some of his neighbors considered him a misanthropic hermit. Later, when his chronicle of the episode came out, one observer dubbed him a "Yankee Diogenes," suggesting that there was more theater to his renunciations than Thoreau might have admitted.[5]

Others glorified Thoreau's retreat. To them, Thoreau was a forest sage and the first American Yogi.

I initially resisted this view of Thoreau, put forth metaphorically by Conway, then elaborated by Arthur Christy in the early 1930s, and reaffirmed by Frank MacShane three decades later in his essay "Walden and Yoga."[6]

Henry David Thoreau, the pencil maker who turned his resistance to capitalism, industrialism, and slavery into poetry, who drew up close to nature and disencumbered himself not only of things, but of the ambitions most of us labor under—to make him first in a lineage of American Yogis seemed like a highly self-congratulatory bit of mythologizing. If Thoreau was first, he elevates the rest of us as we attempt a difficult pose in a city yoga studio, beside thirty other similarly toiling students.

Then too, the image of Thoreau entwined by vines and snake skins would probably have irritated the man himself; he clearly disdained those Brahmins who made such severe penance.

And of course it's dangerous to reduce a man of such complexity and knowledge to a single noun. Whether Thoreau was or wasn't a Yogi, he was certainly a lot of other things and was influenced by many streams of thought from his native Unitarianism to Confucius to classical thinkers such as Sophocles, Homer, and Ovid.[7]

Yet, the more I returned to the sources of Thoreau's yoga, the more convinced I became that Thoreau was in fact practicing yoga as he understood it and that the greatest challenge to the idea of Thoreau as a Yogi is not in his methods, but in his aims.

•

Before I lay out all the reasons Thoreau deserves this moniker, the term itself bears investigating.

A fair bit of information about yoga and the Yogi(n) was available during Thoreau's lifetime—including H. H. Wilson's *Religious Sects of the Hindus* (first published in 1828 and 1832). According to Wilson, yoga was both a practice engaged in by numerous Hindu sects as well as its own school, "the Yoga or Patanjala school of philosophy." Wilson's description of this type of yoga rings surprisingly familiar, despite his tone:

> The practices consist chiefly of long continued suppressions of respiration; of inhaling and exhaling the breath in a particular manner; of sitting in eighty-four different attitudes; of fixing the eyes on the top of the nose, and endeavouring, by the force of mental abstraction, to effect a union between the portion of vital spirit residing in the body and that which pervades all nature, and is identical with SIVA, considered as the supreme being and source and essence of all creation. When this mystic union is effected, the Yogi is liberated in his living body from the clog of material incumbrance, and acquires an entire command over all worldly substance.

Wilson later adds that this yoga is unsuitable for "modern times" and that the Yogis are more like magicians, who seek merely "the superhuman powers which the performance of the Yoga is supposed to confer."

The status of the Yogi in India was even worse, in Wilson's view (and recent scholarship has borne this out). Compared with his fellow sannyasis and other "mendicant characters," the Yogi was seen as the greatest "mountebank" of them all, one who frequently performed "low mummeries," "juggling tricks," and even levitation.[8]

Like the American Indian during the nineteenth century, the Yogi as described by the Orientalists, particularly the most sympathetic students of Indian culture among them, was untrustworthy and uncultivated but not entirely beyond redemption.

In fact, the two figures had much in common. The American Indian was alternately sentimentalized, by such people as Washington Irving and

James Fenimore Cooper, and demonized, by English missionaries and, later, Mark Twain.

The analogy can be stretched even further, since Thoreau himself was fascinated by these indigenous Americans, producing more writing on the subject than on any other (though little of it was published in his lifetime).[9]

The main difference between the American Indian and the Yogi for Thoreau was that he could meet and talk to and even become mildly disillusioned with the former, while the latter remained fixed in his imagination.

Thoreau was a Yogi, in part, because he tried to be one. This idea, that he could practice yoga and thereby apprehend the divine, came from books.

Much as his aunt had pressed certain works on him, Emerson urged Thoreau to read a number of Asian books, beginning in the late 1830s. A few years later, when Thoreau was living with the Emersons, he plundered his friends' library. The *Laws of Manu* particularly moved him. "I cannot read a sentence in the book of the Hindoos," he confided during this period, "without being elevated as upon the table land of the Ghauts."[10]

Unlike Emerson, Thoreau read these Indian books—and particularly a handful of Hindu ones—as instruction manuals. And some scholars, including Christy and MacShane, have linked his decision to go to Walden directly to his reading of Hindu literature.[11]

Thoreau himself made the connection obliquely in *A Week on the Concord and Merrimack Rivers*, which he completed at Walden. In the "Monday" chapter, Thoreau dilates briefly on "contemplation," underrated, in his view, by Europeans, and the "wonderful power of abstraction" Brahmins attained through spiritual discipline. He doesn't stop there. Perhaps to prove a point he fears, rightly, he must defend, Thoreau stacks quotes from the *Bhagavad-Gita*, like cordwood, and recommends it as highly as the Bible.[12]

Another piece of evidence that Thoreau was a Yogi was his asceticism, which defined his life at Walden and bore strong traces of his reading of Indic literature. There, on summer mornings, he would bathe in the pond. (This ritual ablution made Thoreau cleaner than most of his neighbors; in

1845 Boston went so far as to forbid bathing except on specific medical advice.) He lived in solitude in a house ten feet wide by fifteen feet long. He reduced his diet to mostly vegetables and cereals. After a while he dispensed with yeast, baking unleavened bread over his fire, and even gave up bread altogether for more than two months. He drank nothing but water.

He saved money by eating this way, but the reasons for his dietary austerities were not wholly, or even primarily, economic. "I believe that every man who has ever been earnest to preserve his high or poetic faculties in the best condition," he noted in *Walden*, "has been particularly inclined to abstain from animal food, and from much food of any kind."[13]

Thoreau also advocated chastity, something Krishna promotes in the *Gita*, most explicitly in his discussion of meditation.

These were his purifications, and quoting Rammohun Roy, Thoreau noted their necessity in "the mind's approximation of God." He added that if he knew of a wise man who had attained to purity, "I would go to seek him forthwith."[14]

Thoreau hadn't merely simplified his life. He saw his own asceticism through the prism of Indian thought and yoga, which make purifying one's mind and body a precondition for spiritual practice.

That said, Thoreau's asceticism has been somewhat exaggerated.

His cabin at Walden was five hundred yards from train tracks, not exactly a deep-forest ashram, and he didn't enjoy complete solitude. Thoreau would receive the occasional visitor. Sometimes he walked into the village, and in the second year of his retreat, he hosted the antislavery society's annual meeting.[15]

Nor was he much more extreme in his diet than other vegetarians (who were part of a growing trend in alternative health, one soon to have its own magazines). In this, Thoreau, who occasionally ate fish, was actually less strict than some of his friends, particularly Amos Bronson Alcott, who wouldn't eat any animal products and even swore off vegetables, such as carrots, that grew downward rather than "aspiring" upward.[16]

That Thoreau was more moderate in his habits than some have imagined hardly disqualifies him as a Yogi. If the *Bhagavad-Gita* is your sourcebook, it makes him a truer one, for that text was clearly written as an argument against self-abnegation and extreme forms of renunciation. ("This divine discipline," Krishna explains to Arjuna, "is not to be attained by him who eateth more than enough, or less than enough; neither by him

who hath a habit of sleeping much, nor by him who sleepeth not at all.")
Above all, the yoga of the *Gita* belongs to the man who is "moderate" and
devout.[17]

Thoreau subscribed to this idea. In *Walden,* to make the point that his
neighbors in Concord—mostly clerks, merchants, and farmers—are un-
consciously enslaved, Thoreau equates them with Brahmins "sitting in
four fires and looking in the face of the sun; or hanging suspended with
their heads downward, over flames." Both labor in vain, the Brahmins no
more or less so than the clerks, unable to pluck "the finer fruits" of life.[18]

On some summer mornings, after his bath in the pond, Thoreau sat in
the doorway of his cabin "rapt in revery, amid the pines and hickories
and summachs, in undisturbed solitude and stillness." In terms of the
Bhagavad-Gita, Thoreau was practicing devotion, or "Yōg," which Krishna
explains at great length in Lecture VI of Wilkins's translation. Confus-
ingly, Yog, or yoga, is both the state of union one achieves and the method
for achieving it. Here, Krishna is discussing a particular kind of yoga, one
that demands subduing the senses and fixing your mind on "one object
alone"—Krishna. Put simply, Thoreau was meditating.

Thoreau claimed he'd sit thus absorbed from sunrise to noon, returning to normal consciousness only when the sun fell in his west window or
when he heard a traveler's wagon in the distance.

These were no daydreams. Thoreau was deliberate and self-conscious
about his reveries and understood them as an attempt at meditation. The
hours that passed while rapt was not "time subtracted from my life," wrote
Thoreau, "but so much over and above my usual allowance. I realized
what the Orientals mean by contemplation and the forsaking of works."[19]

That Thoreau's experience might have been at some remove from
meditation as conducted by Indian Yogis is inevitable since he got his
ideas about Oriental contemplation entirely from books. There was no
other way, since Thoreau didn't travel abroad, and during his lifetime the
vast majority of immigrants came from Great Britain and Northern Europe and a relatively few from India.[20]

However, the instructions for meditation these books supplied were
not always detailed and were somewhat contradictory.

In Lecture VI of the *Bhagavad-Gita,* Krishna describes yoga as a private and constant exercise of the spirit, in which the Yogi sits on a grass mat covered in a skin or cloth and, "keeping his head, his neck, and body, steady, without motion, his eyes fixed on the point of his nose," fastens his mind on "one object alone"—on Krishna. This is clearly a form of meditation. Anticipating one of the main impediments the novice confronts, Krishna advises, "Wheresoever the unsteady mind roameth, he should subdue it, bring it back, place it in his own breath."[21]

The *Vishnu Puruna* also recommends mental concentration (Pratyā-hāra); it's the fifth of the eight "divisions" of Patanjali Yoga, following on moral and religious restraint (yama), the five obligations (niyama), taking a seated posture and engaging in contemplation (asana), and controlling the vital airs (pranayama). But the book doesn't detail any specific techniques for mental concentration, or contemplation, for that matter.

A few pages later, the text instructs the aspirant to meditate upon Vishnu in a variety of manifestations ("as the winds, Daityas, all the gods and their progenitors, men, animals, mountains, oceans, rivers, trees"). The advanced sage will then mediate on Vishnu as "that imperceptible, shapeless form of Brahma, which is called by the wise, 'That which is,' and in which all the before described reside."[22]

Such passages are a great place to begin. Still, books are kind but imperfect teachers. They ignore your failures *and* your successes. Nor can they steer you in the right direction when you first begin to go off course.

There's no evidence that Thoreau practiced specific breathing exercises (pranayama), a sort of prerequisite for meditation according to the *Vishnu Puruna*, or that he used his breath as an anchor to steady his mind if it roamed, as Krishna advises in the *Gita*.

Given that he lacked these tools as well as a teacher, Thoreau's success at contemplation is debatable.

He couldn't quite quell his senses. His brain teemed with sights and sounds, and he was sometimes overwhelmed by stimuli he could neither escape nor harmonize. "I have the habit of attention to such excess," Thoreau wrote some years after his stay at Walden, "that my senses get no rest, but suffer from a constant strain." This shows up in his writing as a sort of logorrhea. Once he begins a description of an object—a ditch, a tree, a school of fish—he can't let it go until he's enumerated every possible detail and given approximate measurements when these are possible.[23]

His meditations were also somewhat irregular and tinged with anxiety; he feared that if he ever did communicate with the gods, he'd be insane.[24]

Once at Walden, when he got as close to "being resolved into the essence of things" as he ever had in his life, a friend interrupted him to see if he wanted to go fishing. Thoreau fretted about being able to pick up the thread of meditation for a minute, then off they went to the Concord River.[25]

So the question remains, did his meditations work? Did he have one true vision?

Thoreau says publicly that these did. He said Walden transformed him. He lived freer, intuited "new, universal, and more liberal laws," and saw that "solitude will not be solitude, nor poverty, poverty, nor weakness, weakness." Next to that deep, clear pond, he pierced the stark and arbitrary divisions between good and bad, he *experienced* the idea that "Brahma" articulated.[26]

The more honest answer to the question is the one he gave in an 1849 letter to his friend and disciple H.G.O. Blake: "Rude and careless as I am, I would fain practice the *yoga* faithfully." A few lines later, Thoreau reiterated the point: "To some extent, and at rare intervals, even I am, a yogin."[27]

What of this Yogin Thoreau imagines himself to be at rare intervals? Where did he come from? What does he look like?

In the letter, Thoreau supplied a few details: "The yogin breathes a divine perfume, he hears wonderful things. Divine forms traverse him without tearing him, and, united to nature which is proper to him, he goes, he acts as animating original matter."[28]

He was clearly quoting the *Harivamsa*, an appendix to the *Mahabharata* composed during the second or third century C.E. that describes the lineage of Vishnu (Hari). Thoreau copied the exact same passage into his journals a year and a half later, and he inserted several lines from the *Harivamsa* into *Walden*, particularly the chapter "Where I Lived, and What I Lived For."[29]

Fluent in several languages, Thoreau relied on Langlois's French version of the original Sanskrit, which he'd then translate into English.[30]

It's a striking image and slightly different from those Thoreau would have come across in the *Bhagavad-Gita*. There, you'll find several iterations of the Yogi. In one, Krishna lays the emphasis on the Yogi's steadiness and indifference to his circumstance: "The Yōgēē of a subdued mind, thus employed in the exercise of his devotion, is compared to a lamp, standing in a place without wind, which waveth not." This Yogi, Krishna adds, "is not moved by the severest pain."[31]

Interestingly, in that same letter to Blake, Thoreau evinces just this sort of equanimity. He tells his friend he's "subsisting on certain wild flowers . . . which unaccountably sustain me, and make my apparently poor life rich." These are not mere metaphors. Thoreau's post-Walden life had not worked out as planned, largely because the first book he managed to publish, at his own expense, *A Week on the Concord and Merrimack Rivers*, hadn't been well received. The book's failure had sent Thoreau into a debt of nearly three hundred dollars, an average American's yearly salary at the time. He was forced to return to his family's pencil factory, working long hours there and even selling some of the finished product.[32]

Whether Thoreau mastered such equipoise in the face of calamity or just wished Blake to believe that he had, he strove for something else altogether.

The Yogi of the *Harivamsa* retains his subjectivity. He hears, smells, and sees amazing things. In this he looks more like another Yogi of the *Gita*, the one who sees Krishna in all things (and not incidentally, this is the one Krishna favors above all).[33]

Thoreau celebrates the Yogi of the *Harivamsa* because he didn't really want to unite with Brahman. The idea of subsuming his subjectivity into a singular consciousness, no matter how pleasurable, was mildly repugnant to him. (He even denied in one letter to Blake he had any designs on God at all.)[34]

His reasons were quite plain. As he saw it, the end, for the Yogi, "is an immense consolation; eternal absorption in Brahma." But the price of this consolation—infinite stagnation and everlasting moral drudgery—was too high for him.[35]

The Yogi he aspired to, the Yogi who "breathes a divine perfume" and "hears wonderful things," the Yogi who might value "buoyancy, freedom, flexibility, variety, [and] possibility," looks more like Joe Polis, the Penobscot Indian guide Thoreau memorialized in *The Maine Woods*.[36]

Polis was a devout Protestant and lived in a two-story, white house surrounded by a garden and fruit trees. By the time Thoreau met him,

Polis was fairly assimilated to American manners, so much so, he was particularly disappointed that the small party would be traveling on the Sabbath. But, in Thoreau's estimation and despite their conflicts, Polis had retained his essential Indianness. He was far closer to nature than Thoreau was, and he was able to read its every utterance. ("The Indian, who can find his way so wonderfully in the woods," wrote Thoreau to Blake in 1857, "possesses so much intelligence which the white man does not,—and it increases my own capacity, as well as faith, to observe it.")[37]

Thoreau learned some of Joe's tricks before they had even met. In his eulogy for the *Atlantic* in 1862, Emerson wrote that Thoreau "saw as with a microscope, heard as with an ear-trumpet," and that "his memory was a photographic register of all he saw and heard."[38]

There was more to Joe's vision than that, though. He and his brethren taught Thoreau that the woods weren't "tenantless," but rather "chokefull of honest spirits as good as myself any day."[39]

Joe Polis expanded Thoreau's native pantheism, he helped him hear those divine sounds, which some have read as a form of Bhakti Yoga.[40]

For Thoreau, the aim of yoga was creation, not dissolution, and at Walden another feature of Thoreau's yoga took shape: he transmuted his work into an act of devotion, he made a religion of writing. Thoreau attuned his senses to the forest and its spirits and strove for the supersensory awareness of the Yogi because he was an artist, and nature was his medium.

Thoreau was famous for his dogged, trudging writing process, his refusal to heed literary convention, and his stubbornness. During his lifetime, many saw him as an eccentric, talentless crank. Lowell thought he was an egotistical romantic (and published him in the *Atlantic* anyway).[41]

Thoreau saw it differently.

"If it is surely the means to the highest end we know, can any work be humble or disgusting?" asked Thoreau in a letter to Blake. "Will it not rather be elevating as a ladder, the means by which we are translated?" Only some Brahmins, he pointed out in that same letter, "can work on their navels."[42]

To sanctify his labors with the broader public, Thoreau inserted a self-portrait, disguised as a Hindu parable, into *Walden*.

In his conclusion, he tells the story of the artist of Kouroo, who possessed a rare and complete single-pointed concentration and set out to carve a perfect wooden staff. When he finished, eons had passed and he had, by his simple devotion to his task, made "the fairest of all the creations of Brahma. He had made a new system in making a staff."[43]

Thoreau clearly means this to be yoga, which he later defined as "an exercise of penance or extreme devotion," and, in locating the artist in Kouroo, clearly connects this parable to the *Gita*.[44]

The yogic elements of this story are even stronger if you look at one likely, though not Hindu, source—a Taoist parable, which puts much more emphasis on the conditions necessary to create and the days the artist spent reducing his "mind to absolute quiescence," before he began to carve.[45]

Either way, what results is not the prize Krishna offers in the *Gita*; it's a pure and wonderful thing—and a new mode of production.

Thoreau's yoga not only preserved individual genius, since the artist is never subsumed in Brahman; his yoga exalted it.

Turning an individual into a channel for the divine was an idea that Thoreau articulated repeatedly, in all sorts of ways. He told Blake in one letter that God is here, and all we need to do is "to bow before him in profound submission in every moment, and He will fill our souls with his presence." And you could say Thoreau's yoga simply reiterates this fundamental principle, that through devotion the individual is divinized.[46]

But you can also detect in Thoreau's adaptation of yoga a peculiarly American cussedness. Much as he stood against convention, Thoreau lived as a citizen in a nation still recently liberated from British dominion and emphatic about its toleration of difference (even if this wasn't always practiced).

Is it any wonder he retreated from that final act of the Yogi, the merging into a formless, boundless, all-pervading force?

Americans "are the Romans of the modern world," quipped one of Oliver Wendell Holmes's characters in the inaugural issue of the *Atlantic*, "the great assimilating people."

Thoreau was the first to assimilate yoga.

3

THE GURU ARRIVES

In the summer of 1894, two imaginative and independent-minded women turned Green Acre, a hotel located on the grassy banks of the Piscataqua River in southern Maine, into a spiritual retreat.

The hotel, built on a ten-acre parcel of riverfront property and conveniently located a few miles from the train station, could accommodate forty guests, had river views, and was surrounded on three sides by verdant fields.

From a business perspective, turning Green Acre into a spiritual retreat was a sound move; that summer the place was filled to capacity, as were several cottages in the surrounding town of Eliot.

Eliot residents welcomed the tourists. Some rented rooms in their homes to accommodate the surfeit of visitors.[1]

At the same time, the locals were horrified by a number of the activities that went on at the resort. They were particularly appalled by the younger guests who traversed Green Acre's well-tended lawns at daybreak—barefoot. Farmers would hide behind walls to watch the ladies, their dresses hiked scandalously to their knees, as they paraded around in the damp grass.

Strange as their morning ritual must have seemed, there was nothing mystical about it. The "dew walkers," as they came to be known, strolled for their health on the advice of a German priest, who also recommended tenting and cold baths.[2]

There were other unusual rites. Every morning a turbaned young Indian would lead a handful of men and women across the fields beyond the hotel and into the woods. They'd disappear for an hour or so and return much the same way, the swami in front, the others bunched behind.

There were no secrets in Eliot, and soon enough the purpose of these excursions was revealed. Local papers reported that each morning

"Vivekananda, the Hindoo monk from India," would sit cross-legged under a tall pine about three-quarters of a mile up from the river and discourse "of the things of the soul."[3]

Josephine Locke, one of the women present, jotted down some of his
more striking points. Under thick, spreading branches, the swami talked
about the nature of God and worship, the morality of Unity, and exhorted
his listeners to love God for love's sake, not for health or money.

From Locke's notes it's also clear the young swami began to teach the
small group yoga.[4]

Yoke, he said, is a derivation of the word *yoga*, which "means joining
ourselves with God. Joining me with my real self."

From there his instruction got quite specific, if never altogether clear.
According to Locke's notes, the first step was to make automatic actions
voluntary, and "bring them into consciousness." To do this, you have to
first "get hold of the air, then the nervous system, then the mind, then the
atma or spirit."

Yoga, in Vivekananda's presentation, involved pushing one's "nerve
force" through the spinal column. He also told the students, who sat, or
rested on crooked elbows, or even lay on their backs staring at the sky,
that the pineal gland in the center of the brain was the seat of potential
energy. Somehow this energy connected to God.

The swami also mentioned "Kundaline" in these talks, but no definition or elaboration survives.[5]

Vivekananda said nothing, or at least nothing that Locke or another
student, the famous vocalist Emma Thursby, recorded, about swinging
from hooks or staring into a fire. He did talk quite a bit about concentration and meditation, telling his students, "The highest meditation is to
think of nothing. If you can remain one moment without thought, great
power will come."[6]

Born in Bengal in 1863, Swami Vivekananda, whose given name was Nar-
endranath Datta, had arrived in the United States in the spring of 1893. A
sense of national pride, and duty, propelled him those thousands of miles
from his native Calcutta to America. The swami was no traditionalist—he
had a Western education and had been a member of the Brahmo Samaj
reform movement as a youth—but he took offense at the Christian missionaries and their efforts in India.

If India was to be saved, Indians had to do it. He saw his visit as the best way to begin. "With a bleeding heart," he wrote to a fellow monk, "I have crossed half the world to this strange land seeking help."

Like many before and after him, Vivekananda was lured by America's wealth. He came to raise funds for the downtrodden Indian masses and thereby regenerate his homeland.[7]

Upon his arrival in the United States, Vivekananda quickly realized he had his work cut out for him.

Besides a financial panic and depression, Vivekananda met a more basic problem. He had to convince his audiences that starving Indians hadn't brought their misery upon themselves by worshipping false gods. The missionaries were doing a thorough job of demonizing Hindus and had drowned out Thoreau and Emerson, whose effusions didn't apply to contemporary Hindus, anyway.

We need look no further than the Reverend William Ward's influential, prejudiced, and massive treatise to see why Americans might find Hinduism suspect. Of Krishna, the revered avatar and teacher of yoga, he says, "Krishnŭ resembles Apollo in his licentious intrigues. . . . Krishnŭ's image is that of a black man, with a flute in his hand. His colour points out, that he fills the mind with sensual desires, and the flute designates him as the author of musical sounds."

Krishna devotees, in Ward's hands, are perhaps even more repugnant. They sometimes lick the dust where celebrations of Krishna have taken place or "fall to the ground while singing," exhibiting "all the symptoms of superstitious frenzy."[8]

It was left to travel writers such as Caleb Wright, who visited India in the 1840s, to fill out this picture after the Civil War.[9]

In a revised edition of his immensely popular book, *Historic Incidents and Life in India*, published to slake interest in India fanned partly by the 1857 rebellion, Wright relates the myth that Krishna "married sixteen thousand wives" and notes that many of the girls who dance in Krishna temples are "united in wedlock" to their "senseless idol," which dooms them to a life of "vice and infamy."[10]

James Freeman Clarke's 1871 book, *Ten Great Religions* (parts of which appeared in the *Atlantic*), probably did more than any other single book to acquaint Americans with Hinduism. Yet he said little about Hindu deities or the millions of modern-day devotees. Like the Transcendentalists and Indian reformers such as Rammohun Roy, Clarke wanted to present a sympathetic picture of Asian religions, and given the context, such details might have undermined his whole project.[11]

As a result, by the end of the century, American missionaries were still providing some of the most specific information about Indian religious practice. Their literature was filled with lurid descriptions of various Hindu deities and the rites and rituals they were said to inspire among their devotees. Unlike the Transcendentalists, the missionaries based their observations on popular Hinduism, which they encountered in streets and temples, rather than in books. If these men, typically young Americans who had grown up on farms and never traveled, got some of the details right—many devout Hindus *did* die during the annual Jagannath ceremonies in Orissa; crowds pushed unlucky worshippers under the wheels of the cart that drew the massive statue of the deity, and others were simply trampled—their steadfast belief that "the gods of India . . . are of the basest character" necessarily affected their reporting.[12]

These portrayals were quite effective recruitment tools. The number of American missionaries in India increased from 394 in 1892 to 1,025 in 1903.[13]

Now Vivekananda had to answer these misconceptions. He had unwittingly shouldered an immense task. He had to demonstrate that Hinduism was a suitable religion for *Indians*.

The possibility of teaching anything of lasting spiritual import to Americans didn't even dawn on him until he had been here for more than a year.[14]

The World Parliament of Religions, convened as part of the World's Columbian Exposition in 1893 in Chicago, seemed the ideal place for Vivekananda to begin his fund-raising campaign. Though he had no official invitation, he traveled to the United States with the expectation of participating.

The stated purpose of the exposition was to celebrate the quatercentenary of Columbus's discovery; its tacit one was to outdo the French, whose extravagant Exposition Universelle four years before had astonished the world.[15]

A congressional committee report, issued before the great fair opened, deemed it unique "in all history" and unsurpassed in "its scope and magnificence."[16]

It certainly cost more than other similar enterprises—over $35 million (more than $7 billion in today's dollars), a sum that would comfortably have built two Brooklyn Bridges. In the closing months of construction on the Jackson Park site, nearly twenty thousand men were employed plastering, planting, setting up concession stands, and repairing roofs damaged by a steady spring rain.

By May 1893, when the fair opened, more than two hundred buildings were set amid a network of canals. The largest among them formed a central court pierced by the Grand Basin. In record time, Frederick L. Olmsted had turned a marshy spit of land into a garden paradise.[17]

All the structures were painted white, and this ended up unifying the sprawling complex. In the early mornings, the first rays of light turned the buildings a pale blue; as the sun dipped toward the horizon, they were tinted ocher and veiled in a fine orange dust. Then hundreds of thousands of electric lights came on. As one fairgoer put it later, "Having seen nothing but kerosene lamps for illumination, this was like getting a sudden vision of heaven."[18]

The Parliament of Religions opened on September 11, 1893. Of all the attractions, the parliament seemed, on the face of it, the least in the spirit of things.

The exposition was an affirmation, on a gargantuan scale, of American science and industry. The millions of visitors from all over the country were treated to "marvels of modern architecture," such as the hall of Manufactures and Liberal Arts, which enclosed more than forty acres of exhibiting space. Electric launches ferried people along the exposition's canals. The grand halls displayed countless exhibitions of the latest inventions.[19]

According to *The Book of the Fair*, an illustrated record of the exposition, the contents of the Palace of Mechanic Arts, or "Machinery Hall," alone "represented almost every mechanical device fashioned by the ingenuity of man." Electric, hydraulic, and steam engines, a collection of fire extinguishers, Jacquard looms weaving silk portraits of General Grant and exposition badges, and a display of printing and typesetting machines, among others, vied for fairgoers' attention. The Agricultural building, the hall of Electricity, the hall of Mines and Mining, and the Transportation building mounted similarly impressive exhibits.[20]

For fifty cents (twenty-five for children) visitors could also ride the world's first Ferris wheel.

Against this backdrop of technical progress, the organizers of the Parliament of Religions set out to achieve ten objectives; besides bringing together "leading representatives of the great Historic Religions of the world," these boiled down to finding common ground among the various faiths represented and ascertaining what religion had to offer vis-à-vis pressing social problems, especially "Temperance, Labor, Education, Wealth, and Poverty." A more sober gathering, outside of a church, is hard to imagine.[21]

And yet the parliament attracted more than 150,000 attendees over seventeen days and was the most popular of the all the auxiliary congresses. A reporter for *Cosmopolitan* observed, "The Columbian Exposition which accentuated the material glories of modern civilization, needed the Parliament of Religions to bring back to the human mind the greater world of the Spirit."[22]

In truth the organizers of the parliament were no less invested in American triumphalism than their counterparts at the exposition. Led by the Presbyterian minister Dr. John H. Barrows, they invited Brahmans, Buddhists, Jews, Muslims, and a Jain, but favored Christian delegates, confident that these pious men would demonstrate Christianity's superiority to "millions in Oriental lands."[23]

Their conviction on this point was as implacable as it was ill-founded, and the strategy nearly backfired before the parliament began. It wasn't the non-Christian delegates who objected, though. The archbishop of Canterbury believed the parliament would create the impression that other religions were equal to Christianity, which was, in the words of a Hong Kong minister, "treason against Christ."[24]

Held in what's now the Art Institute of Chicago and was then not even completed (and was not part of the fairgrounds), the parliament opened its doors in the morning and closed them late in the evenings. The delegates spoke from a stage almost devoid of decoration, in the hall of Columbus.

The audience was largely female—according to one newspaper report, there were "ladies, ladies packing every place—filling every corner"—partly because sessions were held during the day on working days. Though they had yet to make great strides toward equality (the religious representatives who addressed this largely female gathering were almost uniformly male), women's *liberty* had noticeably expanded since the Civil War.[25]

Besides Vivekananda, B. B. Nagarkar and Protap Mozoomdar of the

Brahmo Samaj, Narasimha Acarya, representing Hinduism, and Angarika Dharmapala, representing Buddhism, participated. Shinto priests, Confucians, and Zoroastrians contributed papers. But of the roughly two hundred major papers delivered, more than three-quarters came from representatives of some form of Christianity.[26]

This nearly cost the organizers their audience. The Jain delegate recalled that "at least a third and sometimes two-thirds of the great audience . . . would make a rush for the exits when a fine orator from India had closed his speech."

Soon thereafter, the organizers slated these Asian delegates toward the end of each session's program and gave them top billing on the bulletin board. This maneuver had the intended effect; the Christian delegates had a respectable audience, and on the fourth day, the crowd swelled so much it briefly overtook a second hall.[27]

Like his Asian colleagues, Vivekananda was a draw. According to the *Chicago Inter Ocean*, "Great crowds of people, the most of whom were women, pressed around the doors leading to the hall of Columbus, an hour before the time stated for opening the afternoon session, for it had been announced that Swami Vivekananda, the popular Hindu Monk, who looks so much like McCullough's Othello, was to speak."[28]

Over seventeen days, the young swami addressed the parliament nearly a dozen times. Keenly aware of the organizers' real aims—he once described the parliament as a "'heathen show' before the world"—in his speeches he returned again and again to the idea of tolerance. "The Hindu may have failed to carry out his plans. But if there is ever to be a universal religion," Vivekananda implored, "it must be one which will have no location in place and time . . . and whose sun will shine upon the followers of Krishna and Christ."[29]

Vivekananda and the other Asian delegates may justifiably have felt more kinship with the men and women inhabiting the exotic model villages set up on the Midway Plaisance. *The Book of the Fair* made no real distinction between these two groups and lavished attention on the ersatz "Chinese joss-house, with its multitudinous idols and graven images," as a supreme example of the saying "the religion of God is one, but the religions of man are many."[30]

Vivekananda uttered almost exactly the same words. Yet, had they listened closely, attendees might have been surprised by the subtext of his pleas for nonsectarianism. Vivekananda didn't merely make a case for Hinduism as a religion on par with Christianity, he subtly argued for its primacy.

Of all the faiths, in his view, Hinduism was the only one predicated on inclusiveness, a point he made in his introductory remarks. (He said he was proud to be from a religion that "taught the world both tolerance and universal acceptance.") Vivekananda expanded on the theme in his longest discourse. To the Hindu, he said, "the whole world of religions is only a traveling . . . through various conditions and circumstances, to the same goal."[31]

Although he was as much of a religious chauvinist as the parliament's organizers, Vivekananda was careful to reassure the audience. "Do I wish that the Christian become Hindu?" he asked himself rhetorically in his final address, and answered reassuringly, "God forbid."

This blend of ethnic pride and liberality moved his listeners, yet nothing in his speeches accounts for the power and depth of the young swami's appeal, which would reverberate through America. Nor do the usual explanations—his charisma, his rhetorical genius, his good looks—satisfy.

The real secret of Vivekananda's fame was that he simultaneously fulfilled and debunked Orientalist stereotypes, allowing his audiences to romanticize him and India without abandoning too many of their cherished ideals.

This began with his appearance. For the parliament, Vivekananda donned scarlet or orange robes and a pale yellow turban. He wasn't the most flamboyant figure onstage; he sat alongside a Shinto priest in flowing, rainbow-colored raiment and a Greek archbishop swaddled in purple and black, set off by a waist-length veil and glittering gold chains. However, news reports almost never fail to mention Vivekananda's outfit. Mozoomdar (who represented the Brahmo Samaj and had so admired Emerson), on the other hand, wore "black clothes hardly to be distinguished from European dress."[32]

Having made such a lasting impression, the swami didn't readily give up his Indian clothes. Though he was eventually outfitted in a brown suit, Vivekananda continued to wear his "flaming red robe" when he lectured, and in most photographs taken in America, he wears a turban. These articles were not incidental to his image. Vivekananda presented himself as a Hindu monk, and he looked the part.

To the surprise of his American hosts, he didn't always comport himself like one, or at least how Americans imagined an Indian monk should.

Vivekananda ate meat and ice cream, smoked, and even used snuff, which he apparently expectorated profusely on the floors when no spittoon was available.[33]

Other aspects of his presentation also worked against type. He spoke fluent, sonorous English. "His voice," wrote Harriet Monroe, the founder of *Poetry* magazine, who attended the parliament, was "as rich as a bronze bell." He was short, at five and a half feet, and had long, curly, black locks, but had a sturdy build (he called himself fat). He had none of the "passive immobility," in Thoreau's words, of the yogi. On the lecture platform he'd gesture, at times wildly, to great effect.

Most important, Vivekananda defied the feminine quality often ascribed to Asians. The swami had a fierce, some said leonine, presence, and one observer compared him to Napoléon. This was no accident; he fashioned himself a warrior and claimed he was of the Kshatriya caste, like the mighty bowman Arjuna, though it's likely he wasn't.[34]

Vivekananda was also rhetorically nimble—in defending some feature of Hinduism noxious to Americans, he'd marshal the most sacred principles of Western thought.

He studiously avoided the word *yoga*, though his colleague Mozoomdar mentioned it. Instead, when speaking about attaining perfection or union with Brahma, which many Christians saw as akin to becoming "a stock or stone," Vivekananda played his trump card. The unity sought by the Hindu, he explained, was the same unity science had uncovered.

In his defense of "those that are called idolaters," he asked the assembled, "Why is the Cross holy? Why are there so many images in the Catholic Church?" When he spoke of Krishna, he described his doctrine as a "message of love," emphasizing the most Christian dimension of his philosophy.[35]

Yet, while Vivekananda invoked Christianity and science, he never ceded ground to them, preferring to keep Hindu rituals and metaphysics intact.

Mozoomdar, on the other hand, had already capitulated to Christianity, or at least a version of it, by the time of the parliament. In his book *The Oriental Christ*, published in 1883 to wide acclaim, he repudiated "crumbling systems of Hindu error and superstition" and even went so far as to embrace the Trinity.[36]

At the parliament itself, Mozoomdar denounced "the din and clash of polytheism and strange worship," which rent the stillness of the Indian sky, and closed his speech saying, "Representatives of all religions, may all your religions merge into the Fatherhood of God and in the brotherhood of man, that Christ's prophecy might be fulfilled, and mankind become one in the kingdom of God, our Father."[37]

Mozoomdar, in effect, turned Christ into an Indian and then accepted Him as his savior; Vivekananda reanimated Hindu pride by making Krishna seem more masculine and more Christian, up to a point.

The message resonated enough to get write-ups in New England papers. ("The four thousand fanning people in the Hall of Columbus would sit smiling and expectant, waiting for an hour or two of other men's speeches," reported the *Boston Evening Transcript*, "to listen to Vivekananda for fifteen minutes.")[38]

Not long after the parliament closed, Vivekananda signed up with the Slayton Lecture Bureau of Chicago. He saw profits in his newfound notoriety.[39]

Within a few months it became clear that the Slayton Bureau was cheating Vivekananda; he wasn't making much money and certainly not enough to fulfill his dream of saving his own country. Plus, he wouldn't always accept funds when they were offered. In the end, he wasn't a good fundraiser.[40]

But he was a persuasive spiritual teacher. During the summer of 1894, two New England women—Sara Chapman Bull and Sarah Jane Farmer—launched this phase of his career in the United States.

Unfortunately, considering how pivotal their roles, no authoritative biography has been written about either Sarah Farmer or Sara Bull; the only published accounts of their lives are official histories, put out by the National Spiritual Assembly of the Bahá'ís of the United States, which took over Green Acre in 1926, and the Sri Sarada Math (part of the Ramakrishna Sarada Mission, founded by Vivekananda), respectively. The rest of the story is in their letters and effects, which, in Sara Bull's case, are scattered across the country.

Of the two women, Sarah Farmer provided the critical infrastructure for Green Acre—she owned the hotel and had a unique vision for it.

There was always something seraphic, something pure, unsullied, and beneficent, about Farmer. Her friends used words like *tranquillity, chastity,* and *gentleness* to describe her. She had pale skin, brown eyes, and brown hair, and in photographs she looks calm but determined.

Farmer was the daughter of civic-minded Transcendentalists. Her parents, Moses and Hannah Farmer, gave away thousands of dollars to various causes and opened their home in Dover, New Hampshire, as a way station on the Underground Railroad.

Like her parents, Sarah sought to serve others. On her fortieth birthday, John Greenleaf Whittier, a family friend, wrote of Farmer:

> *God's angel we rank her!*
> *If vainly we thank her*
> *For all she has given,*
> *The years of right living,*
> *Of blessing and giving,*
> *Are counted in Heaven.*[41]

In the mid-1880s, the Farmers had moved to Eliot, a farming town that bordered the Piscataqua River, sixty-six miles north of Boston. Sarah was in her late thirties and unmarried when the family relocated, and, as ever, "indefatigable." After successfully reviving the Eliot Library Association, she entered into a partnership to build a resort on the river. The Eliot Hotel opened the summer of 1890, and during this first season Whittier rechristened the inn Green Acre.[42]

Farmer claims the vision for Green Acre as a summer spiritual retreat came to her in June 1892. Listening to a lecture, "The Abundant Life," in a stuffy Boston lecture hall, she realized "how much more receptive the mind and heart would be if the body were in such a cool and healthy environment" as Eliot, Maine.[43]

Death brought Sarah Farmer and Sara Bull together. Farmer's father died in May 1893, just weeks after Bull's mother had passed away. At the time, Bull was in her early forties. She had been born and raised in Madison, Wisconsin, daughter of a wealthy businessman who became a state senator. Her mother, Amelia Thorp, had been a skilled hostess and an active leader in the early women's rights movement.[44]

Like Amelia, Sara Chapman Thorp was ambitious and impatient with the status quo. At the age of twenty, Sara, a petite woman with masses of chestnut brown hair and searing light eyes, married the world-renowned Norwegian violinist Ole Bull, a man forty years her senior. Ole Bull had six children from a previous marriage; together they had one daughter, Olea.

After a stormy early marriage, the couple settled in Cambridge, Massachusetts, where they socialized with Whittier, the Lowells, the Fields, the Longfellows, and the writer Sarah Orne Jewett and spent summers at their villa on Lysoen, an island off the coast of Norway.

By the time Amelia Thorp passed away, Sara Bull's daughter, Olea, had decided to pursue a career on the stage, and her husband, Ole, had been dead for more than a decade.[45]

After her mother's burial, Bull was free to do as she liked. She and Sarah Farmer, who had been a friend of Amelia's, decided to sail for Europe.[46]

The two women had much in common. Besides their affection for Amelia, both were interested in the Parliament of Religions; they discussed the event incessantly, on their Atlantic crossing, in Norway, and back in Cambridge.

Though she missed the parliament itself, Farmer went to Chicago in October 1893. There, at various social gatherings connected to the fair, she met Swami Vivekananda and Angarika Dharmapala, among others, and renewed her acquaintance with Dr. Bonney, the president of the Parliament of Religions.[47]

Upon her return to Eliot, she and Sara Bull put their plan for a spiritual summer camp at Green Acre into motion, slating the metamorphosis of the resort for the following July.

The difficulty of traveling between the United States and Asia (the trip to India took about three weeks) worked to their advantage. Like Vivekananda, many of the other Asian delegates stayed on in the United States. Farmer and Bull sent out formal letters of invitation; many accepted.

Under a big white tent on July 3, 1894, Sarah Farmer opened the first ever Green Acre Conferences; Sara Bull delivered the welcoming address and organized the music program.[48]

Farmer offered the conferences for free and charged only for lodging. Younger, less prosperous guests who couldn't afford rooms in the main inn set up tents on a broad shelf of grass west of the hotel, known as Sunrise Camp.[49]

Even when camping, Green Acreites didn't completely abandon Victorian formality. The women's skirts fell comfortably below their ankles, and their high collars admitted no summer breezes. (However, they wouldn't hesitate to wear gowns cut suggestively low in the bodice on formal occasions.) The men dressed in three-piece suits and ties; straw hats seemed to have been their only concession to the season. Vivekananda found such notions of decorum perplexing. "Women sometimes are not embarrassed to expose their bodies above the waist," he wrote to a Bengali friend, "but they say that to go bare-foot is as bad as being naked."[50]

The program of events at Green Acre lasted until the end of August. Formal lectures took place in the great tent, and smaller classes were held throughout the day. Speakers came from far and wide and filled the eight weeks with discussions on topics intended "to quicken and energize the spiritual, mental, and moral natures." Some, such as "The Scientific and Economic Preparation of Food" and "How to Make the Christ Life Practical," aimed to instruct; some, such as Miss Emily Morgan's talk, "Vacation Homes," to entertain. Many addressed the confluence of science and spirituality. "The Material Expressions of the Spiritual Age," "Divine Healing," and "Christian Scientific Methods in Biology" fell into this latter category. There were also talks on Spiritualism and Theosophy.

This eclecticism cut both ways though. Swami Vivekananda found some of the offerings, by "mystics" who dragged "the spiritual into the material plane," dubious and the attendees either too cerebral or credulous, going "after faith cure, table turning, witchcraft, etc., etc."[51]

At Green Acre, Vivekananda taught incessantly on a variety of topics.

Of his lessons on yoga, little remains save Josephine Locke's and Emma Thursby's notes. According to these, Vivekananda described concentrating nerve force in different plexuses (or lotuses) up until the pineal gland, which he described as "the seat of conservation and potential energy, the source of both activity and passivity."

These ideas must have spurred a host of questions—where are the lotuses? Can you see them? Are they all physical, like the pineal gland, or purely symbolic? How do you concentrate the nerve force exactly?—but neither these nor his answers survive.

Vivekananda spent as much if not more time teaching on subjects such as the nature of God, which he used freely as a translation for Brahman. To American ears, the swami's descriptions would have sounded distinctly Emersonian; his was a formless, boundless, immutable divinity. It was the basis of the universe, "Bliss Absolute."

Vivekananda drew on a number of Sanskrit texts to elucidate his idea of God, including the *Avadhuta Gita* and some of the sage Shankara's verses. Like "Brahma," these fragments present an uncompromisingly monist view and seem to leave no room for yoga. "Why go seeking God here and there?" Vivekananda asked his students. "Seek not and that is God. Be your own self."[52]

Reactions to the conferences were mixed; country folk registered their disgust even as they profited from the increased traffic to Eliot. To attend one of Vivekananda's classes in the woods, was, in local parlance, to go "a-niggerin' in the pines."[53]

Correspondents from the *Portsmouth Daily Chronicle* and the *Boston Evening Transcript* were more sympathetic. One mused, "Emerson and Bronson Alcott and all of the old Concord set would have enjoyed sitting out under the stars at Greenacre."[54]

It's hard to overstate the continuity between the Transcendentalists and Green Acre. Bull and Farmer were part of the literary milieu Emerson and Alcott had fostered, and *The Atlantic Monthly* had consolidated. Bull had known Emerson through her husband and was related to Longfellow by marriage (her brother had married his youngest daughter).

Emerson once said of Ole Bull, "He played as a man who found a violin in his hand, & so was bent to make much of that; but if he had found a chisel or a sword or a spyglass or a troop of boys, would have made much of them. It was a beautiful spectacle. I have not seen an artist with manners so pleasing."[55]

When Sara's parents moved from Madison, Wisconsin, to Cambridge to be closer to Sara and Ole, they rented J. R. Lowell's house.[56]

In time, these friends encouraged Sara to venture beyond her inherited Protestantism. (Though her grandfather was a Presbyterian minister, Sara's Christianity was less clearly defined; her father was focused on politics, and her mother advocated both social and spiritual freedom.)[57]

Then, as now, circles were small and tight. When someone thought she had stumbled on a particularly gifted medium or efficacious spiritual technique, she'd enthusiastically pass this information along to her friends, just as she would offer up the name of a good dressmaker.

Not long after Ole Bull's death, Celia Thaxter, a poet and regular contributor to the *Atlantic*, acquainted Sara Bull with Spiritualism. Then Thaxter tired of Spiritualism and turned to Theosophy. She wrote to Bull, "It is the <u>only</u> thing I have ever found that explains & satisfies."[58]

Thaxter also introduced Sara to Mohini Mohan Chatterjee, whose Vedantic interpretations of the New Testament renewed Sara's faith in Christianity.[59]

And so it was that Bull met Vivekananda. Two friends, Emma Thursby and Sarah Farmer, admired the swami. At Green Acre, Bull had the chance to get to know him.

Their relationship was one of the most important products of the Green Acre Conferences.

At the end of July, the *Portsmouth Daily Chronicle* reported that Vivekananda "by his simplicity and earnest devotion has won to himself some very warm friends."[60]

Buoyed by the enthusiastic responses to the Green Acre Conferences, Sara Bull and Sarah Farmer decided to extend them into the fall. Bull took the reins and quickly organized an Annex, which came to be known as the Cambridge Conferences.

Sara Bull, whose activities were frequently and admiringly reported in the local papers, was determined to confer intellectual bona fides upon Vivekananda, and she crafted the Annex carefully.

She also began to actively, if discreetly, distance herself from Sarah Farmer. Bull believed associations with the "occult side" had tainted her friend and collaborator.

Through her summer conferences, Farmer had tried to restore the integrity of Spiritualism and psychic phenomena by promoting the most worthy practitioners—experts she felt were beyond reproach. Bull became convinced this was a fool's errand and enlisted Dr. Lewis Janes, professor of political science and president of the Brooklyn Ethical Association, to organize the Annex.

Janes had a reputation for being able to harmonize discordant thinkers and ideas; he was knowledgeable, well connected, politically deft, and highly regarded by other religious liberals.[61]

"Mediumship that depletes the body and weakens the individual fibre seems to me too great a cost, and a very *material* thing," Bull wrote in a long letter to Janes outlining her views on the matter. ". . . I dare not ever for my own duties' sake, stand behind Miss Farmer in the pursuit of this kind of thing."[62]

Held in December 1894 in a Cambridge house not far from Bull's own on Brattle Street, the Annex presented seven lectures over two weeks. Vivekananda gave two of these, "The Vedanta Philosophy" and "The Rajpoot Women and Ideals of Motherhood in India." Female speakers and their concerns dominated the program. Mrs. Milward Adams gave two lectures, which focused on aspects of "personal culture," a form of self-improvement involving comportment and elocution, and Lady Henry Somerset spoke on "woman suffrage."[63]

Besides influencing who and what was excluded, Bull very much determined who was included; like her mother, Amelia Thorp, Bull was committed to women's rights and didn't hesitate to promote women, such as Somerset, who shared her politics.

The lecture series was well subscribed by local intelligentsia and far exceeded Bull's expectations. Charles Lanman, editor of the Harvard Oriental Series and first president of the department of Indo-Aryan Languages, attended, as did William James and Ernest Fenellosa, a professor of philosophy at the University of Tokyo, who had been appointed commissioner of fine arts for the Japanese empire.[64]

The roster of speakers and participants did one thing not even the Parliament of Religions could do for Vivekananda—it legitimized him and his message.

Bull had her hands full over the three weeks of the Annex. Her father was dying, and her daughter was ill. This didn't stop her from opening her home—a large clapboard mansion about a mile from Harvard—to Sarah Farmer and Vivekananda, who stayed with her for the duration of the conferences.[65]

In addition to his lectures, Vivekananda taught a series of smaller classes in Bull's home, quite possibly in her teak-paneled music room (which could seat two hundred) where she had had the Sanskrit phrase *Truth is One; the wise call it variously* inscribed over the fireplace.[66]

There, Vivekananda instructed this small group in Raja Yoga, just as he had the group under the pines at Green Acre. Over six classes, the swami gave his students a step-by-step introduction to the eight-limbed yoga presented in Patanjali's *Yoga Sutras*.[67]

Students took detailed notes, and Sara preserved these for posterity.

Seated in Bull's home, Vivekananda now tried to clear aside the obscurations of tradition, language, and indifference. Westerners had known of Patanjali's text as early as the eighteenth century, and Charles Wilkins briefly mentioned it in his translation of the *Bhagavad-Gita*. But neither Thoreau nor Emerson had devoted any time to the *Yoga Sutras*.[68]

The Transcendentalists' indifference notwithstanding, early Orientalists had hardly ignored the sutras. In a revised edition of his treatise on Hindu culture published in 1822, the Reverend William Ward included a translation of a commentary on them, written by the king of Dharŭ.

More significant, it was here that Ward introduced the notion that yoga is one of six darshanas or "Systems of Philosophy," and Patanjali's sutras, written sometime between the third and fourth century C.E., served as its foundational text or shastra.[69]

At a meeting of the Royal Asiatic Society a year later, H. T. Colebrooke also presented a set of Hindu philosophical systems (Sāmkhya, Nyāya, Vaiśeshika, Vedanta, Mīmānsā) and described each in some depth; his analysis was later published in book form and read closely by Emerson and Thoreau.[70]

These men were trying to figure out what yoga was and how it fit into the larger context of Indian philosophy. Unlike Ward, Colebrooke claimed yoga was a subset of the Sāmkhya system—less of a leap than it may seem since the earliest commentary on the sutras, *The Yoga-Bhâshya of Vyâsa*, also links the two systems. Since then, the two schools have been conjoined in Western minds, even though Colebrooke himself pointed out some glaring theological differences, e.g., the *Yoga Sutras* were "more mystic and fanatical" than the main Sāmkhya text, even if Patanjali's aphorisms had the decided advantage of "recognising God."[71]

Colebrooke can't be blamed for perpetuating confusion about the six darshanas; contemporary scholars are far more cautious about defining each system as a self-contained worldview since the list of six has changed over time. According to the earliest sources of this schema (circa 500–800 C.E.), Buddhist and Jain schools of thought numbered among Hindu schools.[72]

Though Vivekananda clearly quotes from the *Yoga Sutras*, if the class notes are complete, he never mentioned them by name. And he would hardly have pointed out this essential fact about the *Yoga Sutras*: these present a markedly different conception of divinity than Vivekananda's own Vedanta.

As Vivekananda and most neo-Hindu leaders preached it, Advaita Vedanta proposes a universe in which "every soul is omnipresent" and indestructible. The *Yoga Sutras* describe a comparatively dualistic theology, in which nature, prakriti, is distinct from spirit or pure consciousness, purusha; once the goal of yoga is realized—disentangling spirit from nature—the sutras suggest many purushas, or liberated spirits, persist.[73]

Despite these theological differences, Vedantists (as well as other schools) have freely exploited the *Yoga Sutras* for centuries for its practical instruction.[74]

Likewise, Vivekananda skirted Patanjali's metaphysics and dove right into the techniques he described for perceiving spiritual truths.

He began his first lesson boldly. "Raja-Yoga," the swami explained, "is as much a science as any in the world." It was a powerful one at that, which, if Vivekananda wasn't exaggerating, "teaches us to make matter our slave." Not even "electricity" promised such mastery.[75]

Vivekananda went on to a more precise explanation: "Yoga is the science by which we stop Chitta from assuming or becoming transformed into, several faculties." Here, Vivekananda translated the second of Patanjali's sutras.

Soon thereafter, Vivekananda instructed the small group in the technique: he told them how to sit and what to focus their minds on (information Thoreau had had to infer from his reading).

The swami explained that, after bathing, cleanliness being of vital importance, his students were to sit down, "as firm as a rock," and "hold the head and shoulders and the hips in a straight line, keeping the spinal column free; all action is along it, and it must not be impaired." Once they were seated this way, he instructed them to think of each part of their bodies as perfect, beginning with their toes, going upward, bit by bit, until they reached their heads.

Next, they needed to "think of the whole as perfect, an instrument given to you by God to enable you to attain Truth, the vessel in which you are to cross the ocean and reach the shores of eternal truth."

The following step was to take a long breath through both nostrils, "throw it out again, and then hold it out as long as you comfortably can." Finally, he told them to pray for illumination and meditate on the "glory of that being who created this universe" for ten or fifteen minutes.[76]

While these exercises seem tame compared to poses and practices familiar to many today, it's hard to imagine Sara or Emma Thursby or any of the other women present inhaling deeply or holding their breath, particularly since by the end of the nineteenth century corsets had become even more effective at conforming a woman's body to an idealized hourglass figure (this because steel boning had replaced whalebone). Under the best of circumstances, fully attired ladies of the era would have had difficulty breathing deeply.[77]

As for Vivekananda's assertion that yoga was a scientific method to quell the fluctuations of the mind and thereby see God, it's clear from his instructions that what he actually offered was a sort of spiritual empiricism. You could test his philosophy by using his techniques, but he made no claims to objectivity, nor were his theories about the mind or God open to alteration based on new evidence, as is the case in scientific inquiry.

If yoga fell short of science, it still had the potential to upset Americans' worldview, since the discipline posited a radically different relationship to one's own body. In the privacy of Sara's home on Brattle Street, Vivekananda's students were forced to regard their toes, hands, feet, shoulders, chest, and even their sex organs as "perfect," rather than as symptoms of some original transgression.

In his second lesson, Vivekananda enumerated the eight limbs (or ashta-anga) of Raja Yoga. The first two limbs emphasize morality and purity; Vivekananda insisted they are "for lifelong practice." These overlap with many of the Ten Commandments: not injuring, in word, thought, or deed; not coveting; perfect truthfulness; as well as bathing daily and performing appropriate rituals. The third limb, asana, is most familiar to Americans today. Vivekananda skipped over it and focused on the fourth limb, pranayama, which involves "restraining the breath."

Vivekananda's third lesson, however, veers off Patanjali's tracks. Rather than moving on to the fifth limb, the swami introduced Kundalini and the subtle body, not of Vedanta, but the one more closely associated with Hatha Yoga.

He elaborated on the nerve centers, and the "sun" and "moon" currents, he had mentioned in his previous class and described a passage in the spinal cord called the Śushumnâ. His discussion was surprisingly forthright:

> The nerve centre at the base of the spine near the sacrum is . . .
> the seat of the generative substance of the sexual energy and is

symbolised by the Yogi as a triangle containing a tiny serpent coiled up in it. This sleeping serpent is called Kundalini, and to raise the Kundalini is the whole object of Raja-Yoga.[78]

As Vivekananda presented it, Raja Yoga transmuted "the great sexual force" or Ojas, into spiritual force. With little in the way of preamble, Vivekananda informed his students they must use their sexual energy to see God.

Vivekananda well knew that such information might have shocked many less intellectually and spiritually adventuresome Americans. Earlier that fall, before the Annex commenced, he had observed in a letter to his Bengali friend, "You cannot so much as mention the normal functions of the body [in America]: nobody knows when anyone goes to the toilet— one has to live so circumspectly."[79]

The swami's next two lessons returned, more or less, to Patanjali; he discussed various levels of meditation, instructing his students on the best ways to "get hold of the mind."

He ended his series of classes on a vivid note, depicting the Śushumnâ as a brilliant thread, strung with six lotuses. The aim, he says, is to "awaken the Kundalini, then slowly raise it from one lotus to another till the brain is reached."

The image achieved two things at once: it gave students a potent and poetic visual metaphor for spiritual awakening. It's not hard to remember the idea of Kundalini when figured as a snake moving along a brilliant thread, piercing lotuses.

The image, and Vivekananda's earlier explanations, also laid out a physics to this process, which reversed the usual movement of the elements through the body. (However, it's never clear whether Kundalini is purely symbolic or something quite real, since Vivekananda shifts back and forth between metaphor—the lotuses—and anatomy—the pineal gland.)

In his "Six Lessons on Raja Yoga," Vivekananda had turned that most tantalizing of Oriental mysteries—samadhi, superconsciousness, union, bliss—into a process akin to digestion. He promised that if you controlled your breath and trained your mind on a certain set of thoughts, your sexual energy would ascend your spine, whereby you'd achieve this vaunted superconsciousness.

Like digestion, this process operated in a logical and predictable way that made it accessible to even the most committed rationalist and anyone willing to practice.

This was a radical departure from mainline Christianity or Judaism at the time. Most of Vivekananda's students would have considered themselves Protestants of one variety or another; they were Unitarians, Episcopalians, or Presbyterians, denominations in which the rewards of one's spiritual labors were realized in the next life, not this one, and in which prayer was a mental petition that had little if anything to do with one's breath, body, or sex energy.

Yet if you were to observe Vivekananda's students practicing Raja Yoga, what you would have seen was a small group of people, dressed formally, sitting either cross-legged on the floor or, more likely, in chairs, eyes closed. Aside from the breathing exercises, which involved pinching one nostril and then the next, most of their efforts would have been invisible to the naked eye. As they meditated on the perfection of their bodies, these aspiring yogis and yoginis would have looked as if they were sleeping upright or maybe quietly praying.

In retrospect, the most striking aspect of Vivekananda's lessons on Raja Yoga is how seamlessly they combined elements of his own guru Sri Ramakrishna's teachings on yoga and the metaphysical jargon then in vogue in America.[80]

First a disclaimer of sorts: Ramakrishna was notoriously hard to pin down on this topic (and many others). In a single day, in June 1883, Ramakrishna told some of his devotees yoga wasn't possible in these times, then went on to say, of the two types of yoga (Hatha and Raja), Raja Yoga was better.[81]

Mostly, when Ramakrishna talked about yoga techniques, he spoke of raising Kundalini through the six lotuses. "Spiritual consciousness," Ramakrishna said, "is not possible without the awakening of the Kundalini." One of the fastest ways to do this was the path of devotion, or Bhakti. "Sing earnestly and secretly in solitude," he urged his devotees, and then he sang them a little ditty: "Waken, O Mother! O Kundalini, whose nature is Bliss Eternal!"[82]

On another occasion Ramakrishna insisted it's the awakening of the Kundalini that elicits devotion to God, presenting a confounding chicken-and-egg dilemma for his disciples.

That Ramakrishna never offered a coherent system for God realization, or even a defensible opinion of yoga, follows from his own experience. From the time he was a boy, Ramakrishna (then called Gadadhar), an unschooled Brahman, tended to spontaneously fall into ecstatic, trancelike states. His mother worried; local village women considered this a sign of his spiritual precocity.[83]

Later, as a priest in Dakshineswar, Ramakrishna would spend days, sometimes weeks, so deep in meditation he'd forget to eat. The ease with which Ramakrishna seemed to achieve samadhi didn't stop him from experimenting with different disciplines and philosophies, including Tantra, which differs from Vedanta in one fundamental way: it "takes into consideration the natural weakness of human beings," as one of Vivekananda's disciples put it.

While Tantra, like Hinduism, is a debatable category, encompassing a wide variety of practices and philosophies, these are linked by a heuristic of reversal, predicated on Vedic notions of purity. What Vedanta rejects, Tantra transforms; what Vedanta negates, Tantra affirms.[84]

During a period his followers have since termed his Tantric "phase," Ramakrishna experienced his Kundalini rising. A female Tantrika had guided him through various rituals and yogic exercises.

These practices mostly took place on the Dakshineswar temple grounds. Ramakrishna is said to have acquired the eight supernatural powers of yoga in record time and then had a vision of Kundalini awakening in his own body and ascending through his Śushumnâ, making each of the six lotuses bloom along the way.[85]

According to one account, this experience, which happened shortly before his disciples arrived, convinced Ramakrishna of the importance of awakening the sleeping serpent.

As far as the record shows, Vivekananda freely discussed the subtle body in his lessons on Raja Yoga but omitted its Tantric implications. (His students were none the wiser; it would be two more years before Max Müller's sketch of Ramakrishna's life came out in the magazine *Nineteenth Century* and nearly a century before a more complete picture of Ramakrishna appeared.)[86]

Vivekananda also inserted pithy affirmations such as this one—"This whole universe is my body; all health, all happiness, is mine, because all is in the universe. Say, 'I am the universe'"—into his lessons. These made direct reference to metaphysical religion (Christian Science, New Thought, and Theosophy), then still very much in vogue and familiar to many of his students.[87]

To listen to Vivekananda's discourses on Raja Yoga was clearly not sufficient though. Vivekananda was instructing his students in its *practice*. He wasn't just their teacher. He saw himself as their guru.

"Tell your experiences to no one but your guru," he instructed his small class, in his very first lesson.

Reflecting on the swami's teachings at the Annex, Bull concluded, "I believe the philosophy of the Vedanta to be *practical*."

But she carefully guarded the class notes from his yoga lessons. According to Pravrajika Prabuddhaprana's hagiography (titled *Saint Sara*), Bull suppressed their publication until after her death. (They were then published and distributed privately.)[88]

Bull had essentially bifurcated Vivekananda's teaching. She advocated Vedanta, that is the philosophy, for the general public, but insisted that yoga should be taught only in private, to qualified students.

To be fair, Sara didn't concoct this division between philosophy and its application herself. The guru/disciple relationship presumed a far greater intimacy than a lecture hall or even a crowded parlor. In India such distinctions had been maintained for centuries.

In America, the division between the casual student and the disciple didn't hold up. Most of the material covered in Vivekananda's semiprivate lessons in Cambridge appeared in his 1896 book, *Râja Yoga*, which was published more than a dozen years before Sara's death and sold out its first edition almost immediately.[89]

Sara's continued reticence about Vivekananda's lessons suggests she had motives other than protecting the unwary or insincere from powerful teachings, and the most likely one is simply that she wanted to keep her own practice of yoga something of a secret.

To admire Indian philosophy was, for a New Englander, relatively uncontroversial. But to devote oneself to it, to enact its rituals, was cause for consternation, and Sara clearly didn't want to compromise her station in Cambridge society or her ability to influence Vivekananda's career as a spiritual leader.[90]

The success of the Cambridge Conferences, which went on uninterrupted for several more seasons in tandem with the Green Acre Conferences, deepened Vivekananda's friendship with Sara Bull as well as his indebtedness to her.

The conferences had had the intended effect, consolidating Vivekananda's reputation as a respected thinker who could converse with America's leading intellectuals.

These also lessened the importance of Sarah Farmer, at least vis-à-vis
Vivekananda's career. Fearing that Farmer was getting too mixed up in
Christian Science and astrology, he had asked Sara Bull to intervene and
take over the 1895 Green Acre program as well, which she did to general
praise.[91]

In between the sessions, Vivekananda began teaching in New York
City. He rented a small flat on West Thirty-third Street, in what was then
the famously seedy Tenderloin District, and invited any who wished to
come to hear him. He planned to support himself through contributions
to his lectures alone.

Bull objected. She and her proxies believed the swami should teach
only "the right sort of people," which is to say wealthy ones of a certain
social rank who could make substantial donations.

In general, though Bull had accepted Vivekananda as her guru, she
treated him more like a naughty son whom she needed to rein in lest he
do irreparable damage to himself.

Vivekananda chafed in this role and particularly at the notion that he
accommodate only the wealthy. "Every one of my friends thought it would
end in nothing, this my getting up quarters all by myself, and that no ladies would ever come here," he wrote Sara in April 1895. ". . . But the
'right kind' came for all that, day and night. . . . Lord! how hard it is for
man to believe in Thee and Thy mercies! Shiva! Shiva! Where is the right
kind and where is the bad, mother? It is all He." He signed the letter, as
he did most to Sara, "Your ever obedient son, *Vivekananda*."[92]

By the second season, the Cambridge Conferences had moved to Bull's
home at 168 Brattle Street, and within three years membership had increased to four hundred; professors, graduate students, and undergraduates from Harvard University and Radcliffe College made up more than a
quarter of the total.[93]

So many Harvard professors from the philosophy department participated over the conferences' several seasons that one, G. H. Palmer, felt compelled to clarify the relationship, or lack thereof, between Bull's recurring
lecture series and his employer. "Confusion on this point would be easy,"
wrote Palmer, "and would certainly do injury to us, possibly to you also."[94]

During the 1897 conferences, Swami Saradananda taught in lieu of Vivekananda, who had returned to India. Saradananda, also a direct disciple of Ramakrishna, offered an advanced and a beginner class, suggesting he continued to teach students the practice of Raja Yoga.[95]

The following season ran from November 1898 to May 1899. Students and professors were welcomed into the conferences as long as there was room; for the unaffiliated, a ten-dollar associate membership bought admission to the entire lecture series.

Asian religion continued to be well represented. Nagarkar, of the Brahmo Samaj, who had also participated in the World Parliament of Religions in Chicago, spoke on the "Evolution of Religious Thought in India," and Swami Abhedananda lectured on "Religious Ideas in Ancient India." (That year the roster also included Jane Addams on "The Taint of Institutionalism," William James on a topic "to be announced," and six classes, taught by conference director Dr. Lewis Janes, on "The Relation of Science to Religious Thought.")[96]

Sara Bull also planned to address the conferences in May 1899. Hers was to be the last lecture of the season, and she was slated to discuss "impressions of her visit to India."

4

SWAMI VIVEKANANDA'S LEGACY

Ever the organizer, Sara Bull had decided she wanted to help Vivekananda build up his organization in India. He had plans to create two maths (or institutes), which would serve as both schools for monks, passing on the teachings of Sri Ramakrishna, and social aid societies dedicated to helping the country's impoverished, much like Christian missions.

Her trip would also afford her more time with her guru without the complications of Cambridge society.

Bull didn't travel alone. Josephine Macleod, a fellow student of Vivekananda's, as well as Swami Saradananda, joined her on the journey over.[1]

When Vivekananda first got wind of their plans, he sent a letter advising against the trip. He told Sara India was "the dirtiest and unhealthiest hole in the world," the climate would be too much for them to bear, and they'd be more of a nuisance than anything. He warned Jo Macleod, "The Europeans and Indians live as oil and water. Even to speak of living with the natives is damning, even in the capitals."[2]

But he knew Sara and Jo well enough to realize he couldn't stop them from coming. "You ought to think you are starting for the interior of Africa," the swami urged, "and if you meet anything better that will be unexpected."[3]

Sara had some new gowns made and packed her trunks in early January 1898.

Before Bull and Macleod, few, if any, other American women had undertaken such a journey, though a number of American men had traveled to the Far East seeking spiritual wisdom or at least becoming enchanted by it once they arrived in Japan or India.

The most famous Western woman to have made a similar pilgrimage, Helena Petrovna Blavatsky, had publicly converted to Buddhism within eighteen months of her arrival on the subcontinent.

A Russian émigré, Blavatsky first surfaced in Spiritualist circles in New York and Vermont in mid-1874.[4]

At the time, journalists were fixated on the Eddy brothers and their farm, where manifestations of Native Americans further confirmed, at least to some people, the existence of the afterlife and the possibility of direct contact with divine realms.[5]

Blavatsky quickly attracted attention by calling up numerous exotic visitants and publishing acerbic attacks on mediums she considered frauds. She claimed she channeled a Hindu master and described herself as an adept of "Brahma Vidya" or "Eastern Spiritualism."

Just as the missionaries had lumped all Asians into a single category, Blavatsky ascribed wisdom to the East in general, blurring the distinctions between Buddhism, Hinduism, and Zoroastrianism, among other "ancient" philosophies.[6]

In 1875 Blavatsky cofounded the Theosophical Society with Henry Steele Olcott, her "Theosophical Twin." The organization was loose and not hugely productive until after she left the United States for good.

In the short term, her tome, *Isis Unveiled*, did much more to extend the reach of Theosophy.[7]

The book identified an invisible government of God-realized masters based in India, Tibet, and the Gobi region and posited a theory of the universe that rationalized magic and her own intercourse with the spirit world. (Blavatsky argued such phenomena are based on an understanding of the relationship between three principles: matter, immortal consciousness, and an invisible energizing spirit.)[8]

Though her own theories mingled numerous Asian traditions, Blavatsky had great respect for the yoga system of Patanjali. "For six years now, we have been publicly asserting that Indian Yoga was and is a true science, endorsed and confirmed by thousands of experimental proofs." She never tired of reminding readers that the Theosophists had promoted yoga despite skeptics, and that the evidence in its favor was quickly mounting.[9]

About a year after the publication of *Isis Unveiled*, Blavatsky decamped to India and Ceylon. There, on May 25, 1880, Blavatsky, along with Olcott, announced their allegiance to Buddhism.[10]

Today it's hard to appreciate how dramatic Blavatsky's conversion was. Aside from her companion Henry Olcott, no other Westerner had publicly sought initiation into Buddhism, and until the close of the nineteenth century, it was considered an even more repugnant spiritual option than Hinduism. (To Gilded Age Americans, Buddhism was "'atheistic,' 'nihilistic,' 'quietistic,' and 'pessimistic,'" and completely at odds with their values.)[11]

Sara Bull's own trip to India to help solidify a neo-Hindu organization and spend more time with her guru clearly bucked convention, which as usual was of no great consequence to Sara herself.

Sara and Jo's voyage to India was luxurious. They had their own rooms, ate oysters on the half shell most days, and traveled through London, Paris, and Rome before boarding the ship that would take them to the subcontinent.

The trio—Sara, Jo, and Swami Saradananda—arrived in Bombay on February 8, 1898, none the worse for wear, and immediately left for Calcutta, since the Ramakrishna Order occupied a monastery, really a modest house, in Belur, a few miles up the Ganges from the Bengali capital. For much of their visit, Jo and Sara stayed in a whitewashed bungalow nearby, close enough to their guru that Vivekananda could take morning tea with them.[12]

Their quarters were comparatively spare (the house had just two bedrooms, a large drawing room, a kitchen, and veranda); however, Sara and Jo had the usual suite of servants to cook and clean and so felt no more importuned by housework than they did in America.

The two women found the help more than adequate and the other monks sweet, hardworking, and pious. Unlike Mark Twain, who had wrung nearly a chapter of humor out of his attempt to find a suitable "man servant" in Bombay in *Following the Equator*, they were well disposed to India and Indians.

They also had a great advantage over most Western travelers to the subcontinent, though Vivekananda didn't see it as an unqualified one: they had come as the guest of a newly minted Indian savior. "Swami Vivekananda has received the ovation of a conquering hero, returning home," reported the *The Amrita Bazar Patrika* in January 1897.

Through Mohini Mohan Chatterjee, Sara and Jo also had introductions to members of the Bengali intelligentsia.[13]

Even Sarada Devi, Sri Ramakrishna's widow, known to thousands as the Holy Mother, welcomed Sara and Jo. They were the first foreigners ever to meet her.

Occasionally, as Vivekananda had predicted, Sara and Jo met resistance. When they traveled with their guru into the Himalayas, crowds cheered for Vivekananda but shouted, "Unclean women! Be off with you!" to his companions.[14]

Vivekananda had been right about another thing: conditions in much of India were abysmal.[15]

A severe drought had struck, the second in less than two decades. Famine quickly followed; and yet the British continued to export huge quantities of grain. Since the uprising forty years earlier, the colonial administration had merely become more efficient at extracting the resources upon which England had come to depend.[16]

Moreover, the colonialists were more convinced than ever of their role as saviors of a primitive people. "There never has been, in the history of the world, such a body of rulers as the Indian Civil Service," remarked William Cunningham in an *Atlantic Monthly* essay published at the height of the latest wave of devastation, "—so earnestly anxious as they are to study the people whom they govern, so free from corruption of any kind, so deeply conscious of their responsibilities, and so careful to make the very most not only of that marvelous country, but of all the various races of men who inhabit it."[17]

In exchange for their grain, cotton, tea, and indigo, Indians got "development"—railroads, telegraphs, and the like—and a government that would "keep the Hindus and the Mahommedans from flying at one another's throats." It's hard to overstate the cost to India of British benevolence. Estimates of deaths caused by the famine of 1896–1902 alone range from 6 to 19 million people.[18]

Newspapers around the world published photographs of emaciated victims, and Christian missionaries brought the crisis to the attention of American readers.[19]

But Bull and Macleod, cocooned by the privilege accorded any Western traveler and the Indian goodwill frequently shown them as friends and supporters of Vivekananda, witnessed little of this privation firsthand. "One cannot think of the people suffering here," Sara wrote her friend Emma Thursby shortly after she arrived in Calcutta, "since those we have seen all look well fed and healthy, quiet-nerved and free from anxiety."

Bull even convinced herself that the people living in the streets did so "willingly" and was particularly impressed by the cleanliness of the poorest, who in "great contrast to the Italian poor" bathed once a day.[20]

By mid-May, finding the heat unbearable, the two American women left Belur for the Himalayas, traveling first to Almora, a hill station, and then on to Kashmir, where they spent weeks on and off in the area of Srinagar, then a fashionable retreat for British civil servants. There, they lived in houseboats on the Jhelum River.

When Vivekananda's health permitted, Jo, Sara, and Nivedita, an Englishwoman whom Vivekananda had initiated into the Ramakrishna Order a few months before, would spend hours in his presence, absorbing his thoughts on all manner of topics; he spoke more freely with them, sharing details of his life and stories about his guru.

They also practiced Raja Yoga, which entailed meditating twice a day, at dawn and again at dusk. Vivekananda would begin their morning sessions with a reading. He'd then chant, "Hari Om," and the three would silently meditate for twenty minutes, after which Vivekananda would chant in Sanskrit, closing with "Hari Om! Hari Om! Hari Om! Shanti! [peace] Shanti! Shanti!"[21]

Because Bengal and the Himalayas were among the regions least affected by the famine, geography insulated Sara and Jo too. As they moved from hill station to river valley, India's natural beauty, not its poverty or subjugation, impressed Bull most. "We are now making an excursion to see a famous garden and spring," she wrote from Srinagar, "[the Jhelum] is a lovely winding river and we are facing the mountains as our boats are being poled through the sedges."[22]

For their part, the monks wanted to show the Western women a proud India, replete with spiritual riches. As hosts, they also felt responsible for their well-being and understandably wanted to protect Bull and Macleod from the harsh Indian climate and exotic diseases (which claimed one of Vivekananda's British disciples that same year).

Throughout their travels, Saradananda had kept Bull and Macleod abreast of the Ramakrishna Mission work and how the association had disposed of its modest funding.[23]

While failing in its ultimate goal to raise large sums of money for the uplift of India's poorest, Vivekananda's trip to America had transformed the Ramakrishna Order. People such as Sara Bull and Henrietta Muller, an accomplished British woman who had spent much of her time fighting for women's rights, now donated thousands of dollars between them. These women were committed to yoga and Vedanta. In India, more and more young Hindus were taking the vows of sannyasis, committing themselves to the order's ideals of service and devotion. And here's part of the paradox of Vivekananda's success: the Western women cleaved to the Indian aspects of the organization, particularly yoga, while the monks acted much like Christian missionaries, aiding India's needy.[24]

By the fall of 1899, the order had moved into the Belur Math, a permanent site near the Dakshineswar temple, and temporarily absorbed the Ramakrishna Mission.[25]

Predictably, success brought rivalries and dissent, both inside and outside the organization. Other monks of the Ramakrishna Order sharply criticized Vivekananda's approach and suggested he was leading them "astray from Shri Ramakrishna's teachings."

In a sense he was. The Master (as his disciples called him) considered reform movements a waste of time since they focused so much energy on impermanent and, to him, unimportant concerns, when only God mattered.[26]

This was only one of many points of difference between Ramakrishna and his most famous disciple.

The two had nearly opposite temperaments. Ramakrishna worshipped Kali, a fierce goddess who embodies feminine energy (shakti) and is often depicted in a necklace of skulls and a skirt of severed arms standing astride a prone Shiva. Passionate as he was about her, his spiritual ardor was not reserved only for "Mother." Sometimes he would wear women's clothes and imagine himself as Radha, swooning for Krishna.[27]

Of Vedanta, Ramakrishna had little good to say. He found it "dry" and "boring." Ramakrishna preferred a God with form, be it Krishna or Kali, over the formless Absolute, revered by Vedantins. Once, absorbed in contemplation, he cried, "Mother, don't make me unconscious with knowledge of Brahman. . . . I want to be merry. I want to play," and he then repeated, "Mother, I don't know the Vedanta; and, Mother, I don't even care to know."[28]

Vivekananda was equally disdainful of Ramakrishna's infatuations. He once said he never believed in all that "Krishna-fishna nonsense" and dismissed his guru's brand of devotion as "sentimental nonsense, which makes one impotent."[29]

If Vivekananda was to identify with any deity, it was most often Shiva, a name that he rarely uttered when preaching in the West. Shiva is closely associated with yoga and is often depicted with long, matted hair, his body smeared with ash, wearing a necklace of skulls—all signs of his renunciation. A snake coiled around his neck in these images symbolizes Kundalini, the spiritual energy Vivekananda had described in his Cambridge Raja Yoga lessons. Shiva is also figured as the god of destruction and the Lord of the Dance. Vivekananda's affection for this fierce deity apparently dated to childhood.[30]

There was another crucial difference between guru and disciple. Unlike Vivekananda, an urban Bengali, educated in Western institutions and committed to the written word, Ramakrishna never wrote anything down.[31]

It was entirely up to his disciples to transmit his message. With no written teachings, each one could craft the version of Ramakrishna that best served him, and no one, save other direct disciples (a comparatively small group), could dispute this portrait.

Not surprisingly, Vivekananda presented Ramakrishna as a Vedantin, who taught "the essence of existence in each man" is spirituality, "and the more a man develops it, the more power he has for good," rather than a mystic who danced and sang, drunk on his love for Kali. His Ramakrishna, like his mission project and his Western tours, would help restore India's virility.[32]

When a fellow monk challenged Vivekananda's image of their Master, the swami retorted, "Who cares for *your* Ramakrishna? Who cares for your Bhakti and Mukti? . . . I am not a slave of Ramakrishna, but of him only who serves and helps others."[33]

The politics of the nascent Vedanta movement were made even more complicated, beyond its having a contentious figurehead, by its international character. The Belur Math served as official headquarters, dispatching swamis (at first only direct disciples of Ramakrishna) to the United States to preach and teach yoga. Meanwhile, Americans and Europeans contributed most of the operating funds.[34]

Vivekananda depended on Sara Bull and her prodigious management skills to keep the Belur monastery's finances in order. By the time Sara left India, Vivekananda had relinquished control of his own life and, for all practical purposes, handed it to Sara. "Ere this I had only love for you, but recent developments prove that you are appointed by the Mother to watch over my life," he wrote on the eve of Sara's departure. "As regards me and my work, I hold henceforth that you are inspired and I will gladly abide by what Mother ordains through you."

Having departed for India with the intention of staying a month, Sara returned eighteen months later, "in good health and very much refreshed," according to a report in the *Cambridge Tribune*.[35]

Once home, she met unexpected difficulties; the Vedanta movement in America was gathering strength, but she was losing power.

Ever the devoted son, Vivekananda had overestimated Sara's merits as a leader and underestimated her faults. She was decisive, extremely intelligent, devoted to her guru, and well connected.

Sara was also controlling, elitist, and aloof, and she would not or could not recognize her own waning influence in the movement she had nurtured.

Vivekananda claimed students in Chicago, Los Angeles, San Francisco, New York, and Boston. He had initiated two disciples, both New Yorkers, in 1895, and the movement's center, such as it was, lay in New York.[36]

Vivekananda had left it up to followers in each city to organize and institutionalize however they wished. While Sara Bull had been preoccupied with her Cambridge Conferences and traveling in India, and Sarah Farmer consumed by Green Acre, the New Yorkers had spent their time building the Vedanta Society, which had been established there in 1894.

Compared to the Boston students, the New Yorkers had been slow to take up Vivekananda and his ideas. "But when they get hold of anything," the swami observed, "they do it with a mortal grip."[37]

Miscommunications had plagued relations between Sara and the New York society from the start, and shortly after Sara returned from India, Swami Abhedananda upset this tense but until then workable situation.

As the swami in residence at the New York society, Abhedananda was sought after; according to some reports, several hundred students attended his classes.

But he had substantially departed from Vivekananda's teaching of yoga. Swami Abhedananda had begun to instruct students in Hatha Yoga.

He taught them poses, or asanas, that would be familiar to many yoga students today. He taught lotus position ("Sit cross-legged on the floor, placing the left foot on the right thigh and the right foot on the left thigh, and keeping the body, neck, and head in a straight line"); Paścimatānāsana ("Sitting on the floor, stretch the legs straight in front, hold the great toes with the hands without bending the knees . . . [then] touch the knees with the forehead"); and for the more advanced, Mayūr-āsana ("Plant hands firmly on the ground, support the weight of the body upon the elbows, pressing them against the sides of the loins. Then raise the feet above the ground, keeping them stiff and straight on a level with the head").

He also guided them in pranayama, the breathing exercises Vivek-ananda recommended, including breath retention for more advanced students: "The student should then breathe in through one nostril for four seconds, hold the breath counting sixteen seconds, and breathe out through the other nostril counting eight seconds. This exercise, if prac-ticed regularly for three months, will generate new nerve-currents and develop the healing power that is latent in the system."[38]

Some of his students would practice these exercises in loose, pajama-like clothing or gowns, others in suits and ordinary dresses.

He also recommended several methods for internal cleansing such as "swallowing a long piece of fine muslin three inches wide" and an enema, which the advanced yogi could perform "with the help of breathing exer-cises without using any instrument," both of which would rid the alimen-tary canal of impurities. However, it's not at all clear whether his American students abided this advice.

The purpose of all of these exercises was threefold. First, through the poses, the student would "gain control over the involuntary muscles of the body." Second, the various practices together, along with a strict vegetar-ian diet, would rid the body of disease. And in Abhedananda's formula-tion, physical maladies were "obstacles to spiritual progress." Finally, Hatha Yoga would prepare the spiritual aspirant for Raja Yoga.

But there was an even more basic reason to bother with these unusual practices. The swami believed Hatha Yoga was particularly useful for "unawakened souls," who had had no contact with yoga in any previous lifetime. Since Americans didn't generally subscribe to the theory of me-tempsychosis (the transmigration of the soul after death into another body), in Abhedananda's terms we were a nation of unawakened souls, and Hatha Yoga was a necessary first step toward spiritual realization.[39]

Bull was irate. "The address on Sri Ramakrishna that I heard you deliver emphasized his yoga-training and you conveyed by your statement that His disciples had powers, the impression that occult teaching could be given by them," she wrote in April 1900. "In my judgment, if it is proved best that money should be asked for Vedanta teaching it should not be for Raja Yoga in its Hatha Yoga form."

(Sara's critique is interesting partly because she describes Hatha Yoga as a form of Raja Yoga, rather than its own system. According to Hatha Yoga texts, this form of yoga is a preliminary and complementary practice, preparing the aspirant for Raja Yoga.)

Bull urged Abhedananda "to venture devotional teaching only." Anything else was too dangerous for Americans.[40]

She had good reason to be concerned.

While she had been in India, the *New York Herald* ran a provocative piece about yoga: "There are scores of men and women, perhaps hundreds, well known in New York's fashionable circles, who have taken up Yoga in their ceaseless efforts to do something—well, something different. . . . You might see my lady, clad in the loosest of flowing robes, sitting on the floor for hours at a time in some ridiculous posture, gazing intently at the tip of her nose."

The article also introduced Swami Vivekananda to readers ("a most fascinating Hindoo"), described numerous Hatha Yoga postures, and was accompanied by several illustrations. While some of the illustrations were accurate enough, capturing a man supporting himself on his hands with his legs crossed in lotus position (Kukkutasana) or a seated woman meditating, the piece had clearly conflated Vivekananda's teachings and Abhedananda's. Sara Bull was the only yoga student mentioned by name.[41]

Swami Kripananda, a renegade American disciple, one of only two Vivekananda had initiated, had been the source for this article and was the author of an accompaniment, "Just What Yoga Is," which is by turns informative and critical of the subject. It too diverges quite a bit from Vivekananda's message; Kripananda refers to "eighty-four million" postures and relied on the *Hatha Yoga Pradīpikā*, one of the most widely used (and the most frequently commented on) treatises on Hatha Yoga.

Leon Landsberg was Kripananda's given name, and he had been an aspiring young journalist and art critic before devoting much of his time to yoga and Vedanta. Bull had supported Kripananda despite his conflicts with other Vedanta Society members and at one point sent him money to purchase a winter coat.

Though Kripananda was devoted to yoga and described it as "a good thing," the articles left the impression that frivolous society folks were searching for amusement hither and nigh, finding in it an activity that, while not especially dangerous and possibly uplifting in some forms, was rather ridiculous. Assuming a difficult yoga pose in a parlor filled with books and fine furniture looked as incongruous as playing a Bach concerto in the middle of a stable.

And yet, these *New York Herald* pieces were among the most compelling depictions of yoga in America to date. Hatha Yoga is far more visually arresting than Raja Yoga, and this gave it power. Raja Yoga might transform you, but it's primarily a mental activity and the changes internal. The second of Patanjali's sutras concisely defines what has come to be known as Raja Yoga; Vivekananda translated it this way in his Cambridge lessons:

> Yoga is the science by which we stop Chitta from assuming, or becoming transformed into, several faculties. As the reflection of the moon on the sea is broken or blurred by the waves, so is the reflection of the Atman, the true Self, broken by the mental waves. Only when the sea is stilled to mirrorlike calmness, can the reflection of the moon be seen, and only when the "mind-stuff," the Chitta, is controlled to absolute calmness, is the Self to be recognised.[42]

A more colloquial way of putting it is that "*yoga* is the stilling of the changing states of the mind."[43]

The effects of Hatha Yoga, by comparison, are impossible for an outsider to deny: ordinary people learn how to move their bodies in extraordinary ways.

Sara herself understood Hatha Yoga's power, and she feared it. Perhaps she was right to since her loyalty lay with Vivekananda and Raja Yoga, whereas Americans had always found Hatha Yoga—though they might not know it by name—immensely appealing. Audience members in almost every city Vivekananda had visited between 1893 and his return to India in 1896 had asked the swami if he could read minds or levitate.[44]

"Thought reading and the foretelling of events are successfully practiced by the Hathayogis," he explained. As for levitation, many had tried; however, no one to his knowledge had succeeded, and some had nearly starved themselves trying. In relating these feats, Vivekananda would emphasize there were no miracles, rather "apparently strange things may be accomplished under the operation of natural laws."

The swami in effect admitted that Hatha Yoga could give you occult powers, then tried to recast these powers; there was nothing magical about them, which meant that nothing need be kept secret.

Still he took pains to distance himself from such activities and denounced the Hatha Yogis who performed them, just as his guru had. "What have those things to do with religion?" he asked a particularly persistent Memphis woman.[45]

His (and Sara's) vehemence on this point seems almost comically misplaced since the crux of his own teaching—raising Kundalini, that is, moving your sexual energy from the bottom chakra at the base of the spine up to the top chakra at the crown of your head—is central to Hatha Yoga and a very late and somewhat contested dimension of Raja Yoga (which is often termed "classical" yoga). There's no mention of the subtle body in Patanjali's sutras outside a single reference to the nabhi (navel) chakra and one to the "subtle tortoise channel." The bulk of commentative literature and recent scholarship agree that Patanjali propounds a system for achieving samadhi, or superconsciousness, which has no use for Kundalini. As yoga scholar Edwin Bryant puts it, "Liberation is attained entirely differently in classical Yoga, and the *cakra/nāḍī/kuṇḍalinī* physiology is completely peripheral to it."[46]

It's the *Hatha Yoga Pradīpikā*, not the *Yoga Sutras*, that explicitly tethers spiritual attainment to the awakening of Kundalini. Moreover, Hatha Yoga is essentially Tantric by nature, having been passed down from realized masters such as Goraksha, who were identified with Tantric sects.[47]

The swami's departures from classical yoga say less about his pedagogy or knowledge of Patanjali's *Yoga Sutras* and far more about yoga, which has always encompassed various distinct but overlapping traditions, each with its own key scriptures and commentative literature. Much of this interpretive and explanatory work has been preserved, but some has been lost in successive waves of colonization, some was transmitted orally and never written down, and other key texts have fallen prey to the elements.

Then too, much like cooking, regional differences have inflected the discipline and its metaphysics. And, just as the best recipes are often closely guarded secrets passed down through a single family, yoga is by and large transmitted from guru to disciple.

Lineage, far more than scriptures or even locale, is the biggest determinate of what yoga is.

Vivekananda explicitly propounded Vedanta and Raja Yoga, but his guru held that awakening Kundalini was essential to spiritual realization, a belief more characteristic of Tantra. Rather than choose one system over the other, Vivekananda blended elements from classical yoga together with elements from the Tantric tradition.

Still, Vivekananda had a number of reasons to distance himself from Hatha Yoga per se. Most important, his guru disliked this form of yoga. Ramakrishna told his disciples Hatha Yogis were interested only in "longevity and the eight psychic powers" and dismissed their methods. Vivekananda often echoed such sentiments.[48]

There was another problem. Vivekananda wasn't good at Hatha Yoga. He was out of shape and hadn't exercised since his college days (against his doctor's advice). When he had tried to learn some Hatha Yoga poses during his 1890 tour of India, he found them too difficult and quickly gave up.[49]

The swami's attempt to cloak practices drawn from the Tantric tradition and Hatha Yoga in the rubric of Raja Yoga didn't completely succeed.

Years before Abhedananda crossed the line, critics had challenged Vivekananda's version of Raja Yoga, insisting that he lay far too much emphasis on the breathing exercises (pranayama), which purified the nerves and roused "the coiled-up power . . . called *Kundalinî*."[50]

By the time the Weed-Parsons Printing Company published an edition of his lectures on Raja Yoga in 1897, Vivekananda was on the defensive. Purifying the nerves, he contended in his chapter on First Steps, "has been rejected by some as not belonging to Râja Yoga, but as so great an authority as the commentator Śankara advises it, I think it fit that it should be mentioned."

Vivekananda admitted elsewhere Patanjali didn't make much of this method; it was later Yogis who "made of it a great science." And this was true, the reconciliation of Patanjali's system and elements of Hatha Yoga was a late development, put forth in the fifteenth century. Some scholars even go so far to say that the subtle body and its spiritual pneumatics, in which energy rising through the central channel makes the lotuses bloom, is peripheral to mainstream Hinduism.[51]

As it stood, Abhedananda refused to stop teaching Hatha Yoga in New York.

In a countermaneuver, Bull urged Vivekananda to draft a will granting the Belur Math, and Sara, as one of its trustees, control of his estate, including his published works, a profitable and now contentious part of his legacy. Vivekananda complied.[52]

"Did you reveal to Abhedananda that I have given over to you the charge of the entire work?" Vivekananda wrote Sara in 1900. "Well you know how best to do things."[53]

The schism between Bull and the New York center was irreparable.[54]

Sara Bull's death at the age of sixty in January 1911 set off a maelstrom of bad press.

Through her final illness, Sara had leaned on her faith in Vedanta and Vivekananda, and her extended family of Vedantins. (Vivekananda had died in India nine years earlier; on hearing the news, Sara had fallen ill for several weeks.)[55]

And just as she supported the movement in life, she did so in death. Sometime during these final months, Sara bequeathed sums to Nivedita, Swami Saradananda, Mohini Mohan Chatterjee, the Indian scientist Jagadish Chandra Bose, and some others connected to the Vedanta movement, at her daughter Olea's expense.

Olea distrusted Nivedita, who cared for Sara up to the end, and feared that her mother, previously unbalanced, had gone completely mad.

Less than a month after Bull died, the *Cambridge Chronicle* reported the details of her will and suggested the "possibility of a contest over the estate," valued at five hundred thousand dollars (about $10 million in today's dollars).

Sure enough, Olea challenged the will, and a long court battle ensued.

Olea's case against her mother's will rested on highly circumstantial and even farcical information: Sara had traveled to India from England *after* hearing Olea was sick with peritonitis; Sara had spoken to Vivekananda's spirit; several other prominent women "influenced by the Yogi cult" became "insane as a result of the practices." Olea's lawyers had also argued that Sara had been under "the dominion of a 'band of psychic conspirators.'"[56]

(In the end Olea's version of events carried the day. On July 18, 1911, the court decided in her favor.)[57]

The case attracted attention far beyond the Cambridge dailies. "Hindu Love Lore in Bull Will Case," "Crazed by the Cult," "Mrs. Bull's Visions," blared *The New York Times* and *Washington Post*.[58]

Worse was yet to come, in no small part because yoga was now far more available to Americans, and a surprising number had taken to the discipline.

By 1907, *Pearson's Magazine* reported that there were six outposts of the Vedanta Society in the United States—in New York, Brooklyn, Washington, D.C., San Francisco, and Los Angeles, and at a peace retreat in Santa Clara County, California, as well as any number of freelance swamis, such as the Mahatma Sri Agumya Guru Paramhamsa, who visited America but didn't stay for long or leave much in the way of an organization in their wake.[59]

In October 1911, *Hampton* magazine merged with the *Columbian*. Theodore Dreiser had briefly edited an earlier incarnation of *Hampton*, which had developed a reputation for muckraking, a concern for (and conservative take on) women's issues, and an interest in psychic research.[60]

The new *Hampton-Columbian* boasted a circulation of 550,000 and a readership of more than 3 million. Asking readers to "believe in it," the revamped magazine's first salvo was a long, sensational feature titled "The Heathen Invasion" by Mabel Potter Daggett.

Besides an untimely death, insanity, reported Daggett, "is another disaster that threatens as a coincidence in the practice of yoga." May Wright Sewall, "the club woman of national repute," was just one of its many victims.[61]

Yoga also posed a direct threat to the American family, which ranked as much more of an offense than the loss of an idle socialite or two to posh New England sanitariums. Daggett recited a chilling list of domestic abdication. On her deathbed Bull refused to see her daughter; Laura Glenn, daughter of a wealthy man and Vassar graduate, became a nun of the Ramakrishna Order; and the wife of the president of Purdue College disavowed her family, explaining, "My religion teaches that they have no claim on me and I am free to seek the perfect life alone."

When speaking about specific practices, Daggett contradicted herself: "Only those who reach the inner circles become acquainted with the mysteries revealed to the adepts." There was a grain of truth to this. If you attended the bigger public lectures given by Swami Abhedananda in New York or Swami Paramananda in Washington, D.C., you wouldn't learn the techniques involved, the breathing exercises and meditations that constituted the Vedanta Society's version of Raja Yoga or the poses and other elements of Hatha Yoga that Abhedananda recommended. The swamis held smaller classes for teaching "practical instructions of Yoga."[62]

But no one was explicitly barred from these classes, and most of their instruction was available to the public by now. Vivekananda's *Raja Yoga*, which provided detailed descriptions of pranayama, had been out for fifteen years, and the Vedanta Society had published Abhedananda's book, *How to Be a Yogi*, which included a chapter on Hatha Yoga and instructions for assuming eight poses, in 1902.

Daggett knew this. She had availed herself of these same sources to provide her readers with details about the subtle body and Kundalini: "It is taught that the spinal column contains a hollow canal called the Susumna, at the lower end of which is the 'Lotus of the Kundalini,' the source of all power. The practice for its development consists in meditation and concentration and exercises in breathing and posture."

Moreover, Daggett had gotten a taste of yoga at a retreat run by Abhedananda in West Cornwall, Connecticut, and she had liked it. "Then with closed eyes and clasped hands we passed with him to meditate on the Oneness of God," Dagget reported. "A summer breeze swayed through the apple trees. A thrush called," she continued reverently. "Then all the world receded in the twilight. We were folded with God in the soft falling dusk. The waves of eternity beat gently against the soul."

Given her own positive experience and what she could gather from books—that the aspiring Yogi seeks communion with God—Daggett's most effective weapons against the discipline were insinuation and conjecture. She insisted that the yoga you would casually encounter, the prayerful contemplation, simple breathing exercises, and postures, was bait, luring women, like so many unsuspecting fish, to partake in ever more lurid, secret rituals.

The Washington Post, picking up where Daggett left off, ran a long story on the front page of its Sunday-magazine section early the next year.

A drawing of a woman kneeling at the feet of a swami loomed over the copy, and an ad for Berberich's High-Grade Footwear filled the rest of the page.

Headlined "American Women Victims of Hindu Mysticism," the *Post* story opened with some startling news. The lead paragraph read:

> Governmental inquiry has been set on foot in an effort to discover how many American women converted by the various swamis and Hindu priests have left this country for India, in the hope of elucidating the Oriental mysteries. Governmental agents are now quietly at work investigating the strange spread of these Oriental religions throughout this country.

The *Post* article also summed up Sarah Farmer's life in a single grim sentence: "Miss Sarah Farnum [*sic*], a New England spinster, gave her entire fortune to found Green Acre, a summer school of Hindu philosophy, and ended her little journey into mysticism by being incarcerated by her friends in a lunatic asylum."

Here in these clippings was a good part of Vivekananda's legacy in America—women seeking eternal youth through yoga and finding instead mental instability and even complete derangement.

These pieces objected to Vedanta. But yoga was figured as the gateway to infamy.

In Daggett's view, yoga classes had made Eastern teachings more popular among a "wider clientèle than . . . the society set," and in promising mastery over natural laws, health, and "the power to stay the ravages of time," the discipline was an irresistible temptation for "the feminine mind." Yoga was dangerous, in her syllogistic logic, because it was popular and appealing.

Of course, Vivekananda and yoga lived on elsewhere in America and its imagination. His legacy was in a sense as bifurcated as Sara had wished his teachings had been.

In sensational magazines he was a charlatan and yoga was a dreadful weapon.

In more hallowed publications, he was an "eloquent writer and preacher, whose thought is one of the most important influences in the awakening of Indian life."

And when William James turned to the subject of yoga in *The Varieties of Religious Experience*, published in 1902, he turned to Vivekananda.

Though James didn't have much use for Vedanta, he saw yoga as a valid form of moral, physical, and mental training that led to "experimental union of the individual with the divine." Yoga, in his view, was a sort of applied mysticism, and it worked.[63]

"All the different steps in yoga," he wrote, quoting from the 1896 edition of Vivkenanda's *Raja Yoga*, "are intended to bring us scientifically to the superconscious state or Samadhi."[64]

5

THE MAKING OF AN AMERICAN GURU

In the summer of 1919, Pierre Bernard, a vigorous man in his mid-forties, and his younger wife and partner, Blanche De Vries, expanded their Manhattan yoga school, adding a center in Nyack, New York.

This swath of Rockland County runs from the edge of the Hudson River into the wooded hills, punctuated by the Hook and Thor mountains.

Sanford Gifford and other Hudson River School painters had depicted the area as an earthly paradise, and this had been its main selling point. An 1890 catalog for Rockland College described Nyack as "a place of rare attractions and very properly called the 'Naples of America,' proverbial alike for the healthfulness of its atmosphere and the beauty of its scenery."[1]

In addition to being a resort area, it had been a manufacturing hub for a few decades at the end of the nineteenth century. By the time De Vries and Bernard opened their center, Nyack had already boomed and resolved itself into a semisenescence.[2]

Hotels and docks lined the river, but these had long since been abandoned.

In 1919 the drive from midtown Manhattan to Nyack took about two hours, and hundreds of residents commuted by train. However, Nyack retained its rural complexion—the area still supported hundreds of working farms as well as newer suburban homes—and the promise of uplift that city folks associate with the country. In this, Nyack was quite a bit like Eliot, Maine.[3]

Bernard and De Vries leased a sprawling estate running from Nyack's Midland Avenue down to North Broadway. (The couple had convinced Mrs. William K. Vanderbilt, second wife of the railroad magnate, formerly Anne Harriman Sands Rutherfurd, and an avid student of yoga, to finance their expansion.)

Along with several small buildings, two large structures were on the property: Rossiter House, an eighteen-room Tudor, surrounded by exquisitely landscaped grounds, and Braeburn House, a stately brick mansion built in 1835. Most of these structures were in disrepair.[4]

Bernard and De Vries had already turned a five-floor town house on East Fifty-third Street just off Fifth Avenue into a flourishing Hatha Yoga school. There, De Vries oversaw a dozen young female instructors who taught the poses and breathing exercises (of the sort Abhedananda had described in his book *How to Be a Yogi*). The school had attracted a steady flow of wealthy socialites, both young and old, and artists, who practiced these still unusual and demanding exercises in pristine studios on the upper floors.

In Nyack, Bernard and De Vries enlisted ten of their most committed students from the Manhattan school to get the estate into working order. Most of these students, who made up their "Inner Circle," were young women; a number had been dancers with the Ziegfeld Follies and similar troupes. One by one, during weekend trips from New York City, the women restored the buildings, scrubbing and scraping walls, floors, and windows, cleaning out disused stoves, repainting rooms, and trimming back gardens, while a small crew of repairmen did the heavier and more technical work. Inner Circle members worked for free, though Bernard made some vague assurances that they'd eventually get equity in the estate.

"Our tasks started after breakfast, and the work seemed so endless with not a moment to dream," recalls Llellwyn (Smith) Jackson, a teenage member of the Inner Circle who went by the nickname Cheerie, who, along with her friend Clara, had defied their families' wishes to stay under Bernard and De Vries's tutelage. "Miss De Vries checked our work every week and she was an expert in seeing everything was done to perfection, seldom with a word of praise and prompt to find any failures in any of us."[5]

Despite the grueling schedule, these young women were content. "Self-discipline keyed our lives in every way, every day," Cheerie recalled in a deeply nostalgic memoir written many decades later. "This did not mean unhappiness, for most of us were very happy."[6]

Bernard named the Nyack center the Braeburn Country Club and began holding classes in June. It marked the realization of his long-standing vision, which was to get "together a number of pupils" and establish "a school, where the pupils could live and do their work in the proper manner."[7]

De Vries's role was similar to the one she had at the Manhattan school: she oversaw the staff and physical instruction, which meant teaching students yoga postures. She taught simple ones, such as lotus position, more advanced ones, such as back bends, and the positively acrobatic ones, such as Vṛścikāsana—in which you balance on your forearms and pull your feet down to your head, in a deep back bend.

Bernard lectured on yoga and counseled students on all aspects of their lives, from medical to marital.

The one drawback to locating a yoga school in Nyack was the villagers, who were, in Cheerie's words, "clannish and resentful of strangers." They openly spied on the club, and this was no easy task since stands of oak, elm, and boxwood grew dense and insulating during the summer. No matter, the villagers used field glasses to get a better view.

By November the opening of the Braeburn Country Club in a sleepy town on the Hudson had become of national interest. An item in the *Los Angeles Times*, reprinted from the *Kansas City Star* and headlined "Was the Club Yogi Colony?" reported that Nyack residents had discovered "men and women, all garbed alike in black bloomers and white stockings, romping on the broad lawns or practicing strange exercises—exercises which appeared to be some weird fantastic form of calisthenics."

What's more, Bernard refused to admit the few locals who applied for membership. Most offensive, according to the *Times*, were the "mystic religious rites" Bernard performed and residents observed before they sounded the alarm.

When interviewed by a reporter for the *New York American*, one of William Randolph Hearst's papers, Bernard denied that he was running a cult: "The only cult we know about is that of health and the great outdoors. If there be religion in that, we embrace it. Health! Exercise! Life! Those are the things we want here."[8]

The police raided his club anyway.[9]

Pierre Bernard had always been ambitious, just not in the way his family had hoped. When he was an adolescent, his mother sent him to live with his uncle and cousins in Lincoln, Nebraska. (She had remarried and had four more sons to take care of.) There, Pierre, who was still going by his original name, Perry Baker, was supposed to apprentice with a millwright.

Instead he apprenticed with a Tantric Yogi named Sylvais Hamati, who lived across the street from his uncle.[10]

The details of Hamati's life are sketchy. He was of mixed descent and spent some part of his life in India, most likely in Calcutta, the hub of Bengali Tantrism and the Hindu reform movement. No one, including Pierre Bernard's biographer, knows how or why Hamati ended up in Lincoln.

Fewer than a thousand East Indians had settled in the entire United States by this time, and most were on the coasts, working as sailors or laborers. Missionaries had also brought a number of Indian yogis to the United States for exhibition, and these contortionists became a popular feature of nineteenth-century circuses and fairs. However, Hamati was highly educated and fluent in English and probably came to America of his own volition.[11]

When he first met Perry Baker sometime in 1887 or 1888, Hamati was teaching yoga privately to a few students. Then in his twenties, Hamati made an immediate and powerful impression on his adolescent neighbor. "Hamati made it very clear to me that his knowledge of human nature and life was so far superior to mine," recounted Bernard more than three decades later, "that he gained my confidence in his statements to me thereafter."[12]

Over roughly a dozen years, teaching five hours a day, Hamati gave Perry a thorough education in "Vedic Studies," which consisted of "ethics, psychology, philosophy, religion, natural science, or natural philosophy with a view to solving[?] the development in general of the human system." Perry learned rudimentary Sanskrit but mostly read Sanskrit works "translated in English."

From Hamati, he also learned Hatha Yoga, or what Bernard would later describe as a form of "advanced physical culture": numerous postures, from relatively simple ones, such as Padmāsana (lotus position), to more difficult ones, such as headstands held for minutes at a stretch, internal purifications such as vāso dhauti, which involves threading a cloth down your throat and into your stomach to cleanse the digestive tract, and breathing exercises (pranayama). Bernard's biographer contends that Perry was a "physical savant" and quickly mastered this dimension of yoga.[13]

Most significant, through Hamati, Perry had found his calling: he'd bring Tantra and yoga to other like-minded or at least open-minded Americans.

•

Pierre Bernard's first great exploit took place in January 1898 in San Francisco. There, nearly a decade before Harry Houdini became famous for his escapes from straitjackets, bags, and crates, Bernard demonstrated "'Kali-Mudra' (the simulation of death)." A group of nearly forty physicians and surgeons—many from the Medical Department of the University of California in San Francisco—witnessed his demonstration.[14]

In a later photograph of a similar event, Bernard's body is lax and blood dribbles out of his nose, as a physician, in black cutaway coat (as are all the rest), fingers his wrist, looking for but not finding his pulse. Bernard had used pranayama to slow his heartbeat to imperceptibility.

Thus Bernard and Hamati launched their professional careers.

The two had settled in San Francisco nine years earlier. Soon thereafter, Perry Baker had changed his name to the more impressive-sounding Pierre Arnold Bernard (which suggested a connection to Dr. Claude Bernard, a late-nineteenth-century French physiologist, famous for inaugurating experimental medicine).[15]

But rather than advertise themselves as yoga teachers or swamis, Bernard and Hamati opened a clinic specializing in the treatment of nervous disorders; soon after, in 1905, with the added help of two loyal disciples, Florin Jones, the son of a successful real estate developer, and Winfield Nicholls, formerly an illustrator for the San Francisco Chronicle, Bernard established the Tantrik Order (the T.O.). Bernard was the face of these enterprises, but Hamati was the intellectual and spiritual foundation of both.[16]

The demonstration of Kali Mudra attracted a number of medical men to their work, as did Bernard's lessons on the role of "mental suggestion" in medicine. Though he had no training in medicine besides what he had learned from his grandfather and uncle, both doctors, and of course, Hamati's lessons, Bernard referred to himself as a "physician."[17]

Bernard later claimed he taught pranayama and meditation to seventy-two doctors, each of whom paid one hundred dollars (a huge sum, worth more than two thousand in today's dollars). Marketing his techniques as a form of "self-cure," Bernard also opened a free clinic in San Francisco, where he taught breath and mind control, and possibly some simple yoga poses (asanas).[18]

The clinic was what Bernard offered the general public. The T.O. was his exclusive club. The order was coed, and members would attend meetings in private homes, the women wearing floor-length skirts, jackets, high-collared shirts, and hats as wide as platters, not a bit of skin visible besides their faces, the men in three-piece suits and high, starched collars. Membership in the T.O. cost one hundred dollars.

Bernard, who had assumed the title *shastri* (or esteemed teacher), would don a dark velvet cape, pinned just below his neck, with the T.O. insignia—a winged globe framed by a gold Star of David, itself encircled by a snake eating its own tail. In a photograph from this era, Bernard has a handlebar mustache and long sideburns. The cape sets off his pale skin and high forehead, while his famously piercing eyes are trained disconcertingly away from the camera.

Secrecy was the T.O.'s most salient feature, and it operated on many levels. Membership required initiation by Bernard himself, and initiates had to take an oath, which they wrote or typed out and signed, and Bernard countersigned. In so doing, members, who were mostly well-to-do professionals, pledged "unreserved" compliance, obedience, and resignation to the order's teachers, and "promise[d] perpetual silence to the uninitiated."[19]

Newer initiates wouldn't have been able to divulge much even if they had wanted to, since activities were hidden within the organizational layers Bernard and Hamati created. The two had outlined seven degrees. Much like grade levels, graduating from one to the next required mastering a body of knowledge and proving to Bernard, via a written examination, that you had. (One such test asked members to "write seven points peculiar to the nature of Brahma"; "give number of years taken in completing the Vedic hymns"; "expatiate on the birth of the Tantrik Doctrine"; and "give the name of your rite, degree number of attendant, culture chamber, jurisdiction and providence," among other questions.) Only then would Bernard advance you, so a member in the first degree wouldn't be privy to the teachings he gave to second-degree members, and so on.[20]

But the secrecy Bernard insisted on had an even more fundamental purpose than segmenting his membership or protecting his teachings from prying outsiders. It was itself a lure, a kind of theatrics that created an atmosphere of mystery and excitement. Secrecy heightened the experience of his members, who spent much of their time trying to master the proper rhythm of inhalation and exhalation for rudimentary pranayama, or the correct pronunciation of mantras, or memorizing the sacraments appropriate to their degree, or learning the Hatha Yoga postures.

As often as not, the dozen or so men and women assembled would sit in upholstered chairs and sofas and simply listen attentively to Bernard as he discoursed on various topics—the nature of Kundalini and its role in spiritual realization or the philosophy of the *Upanishads*.

Though the T.O. positioned itself as a far more exclusive and esoteric organization than the Vedanta Society, you could find much of what Bernard and Hamati taught, even instructions for some of the practices themselves, in one or another of the books put out by the Vedanta Society or at Swami Abhedananda's Hatha Yoga classes in New York City. One of the main differences between the two organizations was that the T.O. actively promoted Tantra and gave the impression that all of its teachings, regardless of provenance, were Tantric, whereas the Vedanta Society sidestepped the Tantric origins of some of its most fundamental lessons, especially yoga.

Vivekananda and his successors had good reason to steer away from Tantra, particularly when addressing Westerners. If Tantrics had a bad reputation in India, which they generally did, the Western response had been even worse. Early accounts of Indian Tantrism and the Tantras (the texts upon which Tantric practice is based) by missionaries and Indologists had ranged from uncharitable to hysterical.

When the Reverend William Ward introduced the Tantras to the West in his compendium, all he could say was that these detailed "a most shocking mode of worship" involving naked women, usually a prostitute or an outcast, and rites "too abominable to enter the ears of man and impossible to be revealed to a Christian public."[21]

Yet Ward's disgust wasn't purely a symptom of Christian zealotry or Enlightenment disregard. None of the earliest Western observers had been initiated by a Tantric guru, and initiation is essential; without it, you simply can't engage in Tantric practice. So the earliest Western investigators had to rely on the Tantras—highly coded texts compiled during and after the sixth century A.D., which were meant to confound outsiders, and native informants, who weren't always sympathetic to the subject at hand—to make sense of this aspect of Indian religious culture.

Faced with these difficulties, people such as Ward concluded the following: Tantra was secret; it involved worshipping a comely female deity, usually Kali or Shakti, and ceremonial sex; and it conferred great power on the successful practitioner.

Put simply, Tantra involved "lust, mummery, and black magic."[22]

Naturally, these early observers found it offensive. So did the Indian Brahmans, who played up Tantra's bizarre and scandalous aspects.

And so too did turn-of-the-century Hindu reformers, such as Rammohun Roy and Vivekananda, who were trying to forge a national identity. For them, Tantra was a liability (whether or not they revered specific practitioners of it); it drew attention to the polytheist and ritualist aspects of Hinduism, not to mention the sexual imagery that appears throughout Indian sacred texts and temple statuary, and made it harder to position it as a universal religion that had articulated empirically proven techniques for God-realization centuries before Christ.

Vivekananda was so worried Americans would misconstrue Ramakrishna and his propitiations to the goddess Kali that he didn't mention his guru publicly for many years. And he always maintained, despite his critics, that his yogic teachings hewed to Patanjali Yoga, though they more credibly belong to the Tantric tradition.

Despite their hyberbole, nineteenth-century Orientalists had gotten much about Tantra right. Tantra, or to be more precise, the Tantras and Tantric sects, put a great premium on secrecy (as Bernard and Hamati did); worship centered around the female principle and involved ceremonial sex (though not necessarily enacted); and if successful, the Tantric practitioner obtained siddhis (special powers).

Above all, the Tantras stressed a *practice* (or *sādhana*), and in theory this sādhana was open to men of all castes; the Tantras were in part a pointed reaction to Advaita Vedanta, which was notoriously abstract and elitist.

This doesn't make Tantra egalitarian: sects did exclude aspirants based on caste. And Tantra, like most Hindu ritual, concerns itself primarily with the male aspirant's ultimate liberation. Female initiates are trained to assist men in reaching this goal.

Many also consider Hatha Yoga a central feature of Tantric practice: "All tantrism," noted Agehananda Bharati, a Western scholar of Tantra who had been initatied into a Hindu monastic order, "presupposes mastery of the intricate *haṭha-yoga* training."[23]

This being said, many aspects of Tantric practice are nearly indistinguishable from orthodox, Brahmanical ritual, which is to say, Tantra is demanding, complicated, highly formalized, and at times tedious. Like the Catholic priest leading high mass, the Tantric generally doesn't improvise; he follows excruciatingly detailed scripts.

A case in point: Bharati's abbreviated description of a Tantric ceremony fills more than twenty pages, and about half of what he describes is preparatory: you wake up and recite a lengthy invocation honoring your guru while still in bed, you bathe, you meditate on various deities, you chant mantras, you sprinkle drops of water into a sacred diagram (mandala), and you purify the elements by verbally offering them to "hierarchically higher" substances (i.e., "the act of speaking into the fire").[24]

And this emphasis on purification and prepartion is hardly unique to the particular ceremony Bharati elucidated. Tabulating the contents of thirty-five different Tantras (twenty-five Hindu ones and ten Buddhist), with a median length of six hundred verses, Bharati found that on average "mantra notation and instruction" accounted for 60 percent of the content, and that less than 7 percent focused on the "erotic" rituals or imagery for which Tantra is so infamous.[25]

The most important Tantric ceremony, performed only after completing these extensive preparations, is the Five M's (pancamakara)—usually rendered as taking wine (madya), flesh or meat (māmsa), fish (matsya), parched grain (mudrā), and intercourse (maithunā). Orthodox or Brahmanical Hinduism usually forbids these substances, which is what gives the ritual its potency. In effect, the Tantric aspirant tries to liberate himself by willfully breaking taboos.[26]

How you perform the Five M's depends on your individual disposition and accomplishments as well as whether you're initiated into right-handed Tantra or left-handed Tantra. If you're following the "right-handed" path (Dakshina-mārga), this central ceremony takes place entirely in your mind. As you chant ritual invocations, you visualize sacrificing these transgressive substances, and you visualize conjugal union with a female deity (usually Shakti, who is Shiva's consort and personifies the feminine aspect of the divine).

In contrast, the left-handed Tantric partakes of the Five M's in a ceremony led by a senior sadhaka (practitioner). Seated on an antelope- or tiger-skin rug, in a circle of male Tantrics and female initiates (who are called Shaktis), the Tantric drinks the wine (a glassful), eats small pieces of fish and meat and some parched grain. He then propitiates still more deities, blesses a couch, and, after still more ritual invocation, eventually has sex with a female initiate, all the while mentally repeating certain mantras, until he climaxes (in Hindu Tantra, the aspirant typically ejaculates; in Buddhist Tantra, he retains his semen). The result is a euphoric, nondiscursive state, a hallucinatory level of bliss that, "in Indian theological parlance," according to Bharati, ". . . is tantamount to supreme insight or wisdom," and superior to all other types of knowledge, including formal learning. This inwardly ecstatic state, often rendered *samadhi*, is also the telos of all successful yoga practice, of whatever type.[27]

Since it involves ritual sex, even adherents of left-hand Tantra (Vāma-mārga) describe their sadhana as risky. "It is a very difficult path," Ramakrishna explained when Vivekananda (then still Narendra) asked him about it, "and often causes the aspirant's downfall."[28]

And yet, even the left-handed Tantric isn't much of a hedonist. Too much precedes the sex he does have. Though it's intended to produce bliss consciousness, the intercourse is far too structured and plotted for anyone bent entirely on pleasure and self-gratification. And you can't simply decide to become a left-handed Tantric; you must be initiated into these practices, and your guru must believe you're ready for them.[29]

The Tantric, then, abides in a rulebound, hierarchical world, no less than the Brahman, and ritual intercourse lies near the end of a long, difficult path. Mastering Hatha Yoga alone can easily take years. A married American man at the turn of the twentieth century would have been a far more successful hedonist. He would have drunk more and in all likelihood had sex more often than most Tantrics (though you need to be careful about such generalizations given the number and variety of Tantric sects and practices).

Certain degrees of Bernard's T.O. were eligible for these sexual teachings, and initiated members of the seventh degree had the right to be married in the sacred "chakra circle." These select few were dabbling in ceremonial sex.

Bernard advertised what he called "Kaula rites" in a San Francisco newspaper, and he rented private rooms for their express purpose. Being one of the few who had passed into the seventh degree, Bernard would select his own spiritual-sexual consort or pair off disciples of his choosing. After some theatrical ritual invocations (in all likelihood he would have picked among the hours of preparatory rites that traditionally precede such ceremonies), the selected couple would have intercourse on a raised dais.[30]

Then in his twenties, Bernard had enough knowledge of Indian Tantra to be dangerous—or seductive, depending on your inclinations—and was clearly drawing on other sources, including "sex magic," for these secret rites. Like the Tantras, sex magic linked erotic pleasure to spiritual realization. According to Paschal Beverly Randolph, considered the father of sex magic, "at the instant of intense mutual orgasm the souls of the partners are opened to the powers of the cosmos and anything then truly willed is accomplished." By meditating as you and your partner climaxed, you could, according to Randolph, control the forces of the universe. But sex magic had a far less cumbersome ritual apparatus. The sex was the primary focus.[31]

In an era when premarital sex would quite literally ruin a woman's reputation, rendering her unmarriageable, Bernard's Tantra gave him a powerful tool for his own sexual gratification and empowerment.[32]

But for the majority of his members, such practices remained a secret, and their always imminent revelation kept them coming to T.O. meetings and paying his steep membership fees.

There was one other notable difference between the Vedanta Society's offerings and Bernard's: in crafting the T.O., Bernard and Hamati had heavily borrowed from other new religious sects and practical occultists, such as the Theosophists and the Hermetic Brotherhood of Luxor (known then by its initials, the H.B. of L.).[33]

At the turn of the century, millions of Americans were attending weekly meetings of the various secret and semisecret societies. Besides fraternal orders of ancient pedigree, such as the Freemasons, and reform-oriented ones, such as the National American Woman Suffrage Association, there were "strange religions," structured like the fraternal orders and as dedicated to building up membership.[34]

Many of these religious societies claimed they were based on ancient, Eastern teachings, and most promised members magical powers. Vivekananda feared they would cheapen his own message. (Despite his protestations, some scholars argue that these groups were so influential at the turn of the century, and their vocabulary so pervasive, that they necessarily influenced Vivekananda's formulation of yoga.) Abhedananda was even clearer on this point: he considered the Theosophists responsible for most of the misconceptions about yoga and a danger to the discipline.[35]

Outsiders were also quick to dismiss these smaller, religious groups. "The love of novelty, the constant striving after something fresh and un-hackneyed, the end-of-century passion for mysticism in any form, the hungry, gnawing hope of finding comfort for aching hearts and troubled spirits," observed a *Chicago Tribune* reporter in 1899, "—all these reasons impel people to 'follow after strange gods' and to adopt unusual methods of religious exercise and dissipation."

The piece profiled several groups—the Brotherhood of Silence; the Hermetic Brotherhood of Chicago, an offshoot of the Theosophists; and the Brotherhood of St. Martin among them—without clarifying much, since initiates, like members of Bernard's T.O., were forbidden to divulge anything of substance to noninitiates. The Martinist motto was "Learn to know thyself, but keep thyself unknown."[36]

You can see Bernard's debt to practical occultism most clearly in volume 5, no. 1, of *International Journal of the Tantrik Order: Vira Sadhana*, first published in 1906. Running nearly two hundred pages, the journal was no mere prop in Bernard's order. For more than three decades, it was the T.O.'s touchstone and textbook.[37]

The journal was bound in red, with the T.O. symbol stamped in gold on the cover. Over time, there were several covers, including a red silk one. The frontispiece is a photograph of the moon, which according to the caption represented "the abode of the Tantrik God, Siva (Mahadeva), with the Siddhas as the Moon."

Inside, the editors reprinted a mangled verse of Emerson's "Brahma," as well as citations from various encyclopedias and the works of Rudyard Kipling, Sir Monier Monier-Williams, Max Müller, Schopenhauer, and Victor Cousin, who had influenced Emerson. All of these great men concurred—Tantrism was a "divine science," and Tantrics are masters of the Vedas. This consensus was largely a fiction, the product of the editors' selective quotation.[38]

The journal also published selections from a host of different Tantric texts, including one on Hatha Yoga, titled "Tantrik Yoga: Texts Requiring an Initiate to Unravel and Expound," a portion of the *Maha Nirvana Tantra*, and a "Hymn to Siva."[39]

But the bibliography, "Collateral Reading Relative to the Work of the Third or Vamachari Degree of the Tantrika," consists almost entirely of works of Western occultism, such as *Nature Worship, Culte de Venus,* and *Phallicism, Mysteries of Sex Worship.* These titles purported to detail various sexual rites in ancient cultures and the centrality of sex in all of the world's mystical traditions, including those of the Greeks and the Gnostics.[40]

The Tantric's very education combined equal parts Indian Tantrism as filtered through Bernard and Hamati and a host of Western occult and metaphysical practices. According to the journal, the Tantric initiate would be required to learn "Tantrik Ethics," Yoga, and Postures, and also Word Conjuring (magic), Techniques of Operative Hypnology (mind control), and Phallic Principles (sex worship), among other topics.[41]

In the T.O., Bernard had concocted a winning combination of Western occultism and Indian Tantrism. The overtly occult elements distinguished the T.O. from the Vedanta Society, and the Tantric ones, as well as Hamati's presence, lent the T.O. credibility and authencity that not even the Theosophists, with their imaginary mahatmas channeled by a Russian medium, could claim.

A year after opening their first Tantric clinic in San Francisco, the four men—Bernard, Hamati, Jones, and Nicholls—set up Tantric lodges in Portland, Seattle, and Tacoma. Bernard claimed he attracted roughly sixty pupils in Seattle alone, including Judge Webster and his wife; Walter A. Keene, a lawyer; and Mr. and Mrs. C. J. Challer. These students would then introduce him to others, and so he gathered a small following, concentrated on the West Coast.[42]

Bernard had even more grandiose, and precise, visions of the future. He wanted to open lodges in Europe, and according to his biogropher, Robert Love, he "formulated rules and standards to be applied to everything from the governance of the membership to the design of the physical buildings, their furnishings and the curriculum." Each lodge was to have a large library, full of thousands of Sanskrit texts (in the original and in translation) as well as works on "collateral studies," such as science, ethics, and philosophy. While Sanskrit would be available as an "elective," all members would have to take Hatha Yoga. "Our yoga rooms are padded with four-inch hair mats," Bernard advertised in a letter to the T.O., "and an equable temperature [is] maintained there in summer and winter. Our Lecture rooms are large and the walls entirely covered by black boards in constant use. All through the degrees, we carry the practice of Yoga to the highest point."[43]

Four years later, Bernard was locked up in a New York City jail. Two former students, Zella Hopp and Gertrude Leo, had filed a complaint against Bernard, and the police had summarily arrested him at "a richly furnished house" on Seventy-fourth Street in Manhattan. He was wearing a turban and a gown.

The *Evening Telegram* reported, "It is charged that Bernard conducted séances in which he instructed the class of students attired in strange and scanty raiment in the 'mysteries of the Orient' of which he was regarded as high priest."

In the first week of May 1910, paperboys on every street corner in New York City shouted the headlines: "Court Aghast at Her Story of Hindu Den," "Girl Describes Rites and 'Hindoo's' Oriental Séances," "Mystic Held as Abductor." More than fifty headlines about the case ran that week.[44]

While the most vicious circulation wars between Pulitzer and Hearst had died down, in the first decade of the twentieth century, New York City still supported more than forty English-language daily newspapers. These vied aggressively for readership. Bernard was a reporter's dream subject.[45]

But the accusation that landed him in jail with a bail set at fifteen thousand dollars (worth over three hundred thousand dollars today) was that Bernard was a white-slave trafficker. New York was atwitter with accusations, leveled mostly in the "public prints," that the city was "a centre or clearing house for an organized traffic in women, or what has come to be known as the white slave traffic."[46]

In his first act as district attorney of New York, Charles S. Whitman charged a "vice grand jury," headed by a reluctant John D. Rockefeller, to investigate. In April, not two weeks before Bernard's own arrest, agents arrested Harry Levinson and two others for "trafficking in girls." Levinson's bail was set at ten thousand dollars, five thousand *less* than Bernard's.[47]

For his part, Bernard denied any wrongdoing, explaining to a reporter for the *Evening Mail*, "The whole scheme is physical culture; that's all." But the scandal provided the first real insight into his operations.[48]

A sister of one of the plaintiffs, Mrs. Jennie Miller, identified him as "the active head of an organization known as the Tantrik Order, an East

Indian Black Magic Society, which uses the teaching of alleged Oriental-ism to cloak terrible things." Bernard's practice as a physician, according to Miller, was merely a front for his Tantrik Order, and instruction cost one hundred dollars. This much was true.[49]

When Bernard, Hamati, and Hamati's two other closest disciples had moved to New York City a few years earlier, they had collapsed the clinic for the treatment of nervous disorders and the T.O. into a single organization.

Bernard was teaching Hatha Yoga (the postures and some breathing exercises) to initiates, a wealthy set made up mostly of people in "show business," including the silent-screen star Sarah Bernhardt, and medical professionals. The *New York American Journal* reported details of his actual instruction: "a group of young girls and two or three aged men swaying and gyrating . . . and finally standing on their hands." The girls, according to this item, were "dressed in a sort of gymnasium costume," and the men in "knee trousers." The description suggests that Bernard was teaching some of the more difficult and gymnastic Hatha Yoga postures and that he taught men and women together (something rarely done in India).[50]

Notably, the phrase *Hatha Yoga* appears nowhere in the profligate cov-erage of the scandal. The pressmen didn't know it, and Bernard continued to avoid it, referring to his teaching as "physical culture" or "physical in-struction."

But he was also still dabbling in ceremonial sex. Apparently, he had had a ménage à trois with Leo and Hopp and had promised to marry both of them. When they realized he had led them on, Leo contacted her sister (Mrs. Miller), who came to New York from Seattle to rescue them. It's unclear to what extent the young women, who were in their early twen-ties, were being held against their will, but once Mrs. Miller found them, she marched them down to the police station, instigating the raid.[51]

For such a student of human nature, Bernard was exceptionally dim-witted about his lovers' expectations. "You know, if you pay more attention to one than you do to another, she gets jealous," he complained to a re-porter for the *New York Evening Mail*. "This whole white slave business was too much. Wonder they didn't hold me for murder."[52]

At his arraignment, Bernard appeared in a three-piece suit and white shirt, hair slicked back from his high forehead. He looked more the physi-cian than white slaver or Tantric priest. Failing to make bail, he spent nearly four months in jail before being released. He was never tried. The DA disqualified Leo as a witness and complainant (it came out that she had had a prior relationship with Nicholls), and Hopp moved out of state and dropped all charges.[53]

Pierre A. Bernard's story could have ended here, a two-bit occultist and lothario who, like many a charismatic leader, was felled by a combination of his own recklessness and bad timing, a footnote in the history of yoga in America.

But his story doesn't end here for a number of reasons. The first is that Bernard knew an awful lot about Indian Tantra and yoga. He was arguably the most educated American in the subject then alive, and a sincere student of Indian experts. He was also a canny man, with a knack for launching organizations; and most important, he soon met Blanche De Vries.

In Tantra, it's the union of Shiva and Shakti that produces the entire universe and a complex symbology, in which Shiva is figured as the moon, and the moon represents both passive being and semen, while Shakti is associated with the sun and is seen as the active principle of creation.

The practitioner is ever trying to merge these forces whereby he transcends polarities altogether.

Bernard saw himself as Shiva (and signed at least one telegram this way), and in Blanche De Vries, he had found Shakti. She was his disciple, then his wife. Their union produced something less transcendent than the dissolution of polarities but far more profitable—a fully modern yoga.[54]

Blanche De Vries and Pierre Bernard met in Leonia, New Jersey, in 1913. He was teaching at one of a series of yoga schools that he set up between 1911 and 1916, as he played a protracted cat-and-mouse game with the police.

Then only twenty-two, Blanche had been a modestly successful singer, who had married badly and recently divorced.

De Vries, whose real name was Dace Melbourn Shannon, grew up in Adrian, Michigan, and made her musical debut in New York City in 1908.[55]

Dace had a "high soprano voice of remarkable sweetness and purity"; though not a small woman (she was about five feet six inches), she was well proportioned and, when corseted, managed the wasp waist then in fashion; with thick, arching eyebrows, dark eyes, and masses of wavy, dark brown hair, she was beautiful; and she was imaginative and headstrong. Dace seemed poised for success.[56]

When Dace met Bernard—no one knows exactly how since she was secretive and skittish about their relationship for her entire life—she was singing professionally under the name Blanche Reiss.[57]

Blanche immediately took to the charismatic yoga teacher, who was teaching an elaborate and well-organized curriculum of yoga and Indian philosophy.

An advertisement for one of his schools, a Sanskrit College he set up at 251 West Eighty-sixth and 250 West Eighty-seventh Street in 1911, lists a free public lecture, "'The East Indian Samadhi, Mukti, Nirvana—Salvation Bliss' by Pandit P. C. Shastri," as well as daily instruction in "Yoga and Sanskrit language."[58]

Some universities covered Indian philosophy (typically in courses on comparative religion); however, these didn't consider yoga or any other school of Indian thought as having much practical value. Until the late 1920s, the Vedanta Society did relatively little to advance an appreciation of the broader historical and philosophical context of yoga or Vedanta.

Bernard's instruction was both more comprehensive and more pragmatic than other options.

A photograph of one of his classrooms shows just how extensive and detailed his classes were. Light pours into the room from a window on the left; a dozen or more wooden folding chairs stand against the front wall, waiting to be called into service. The room is decorated with photographs of Bernard's gurus and admired teachers; the Tantrik Order symbol is mounted on the front wall in at least two places.

Most impressive is the blackboard, which stretches all the way across the room and displays, in bold white lettering, the week's schedule:

Sundays	Vedic Philosophy Services
Mondays	Ancient Hindu Vina Music
Tuesdays	Indo-Aryan Phil . . . {Nyaya . . . By Gotama; Sankhya . . . By Kapila; Vedanta . . . By Vyasa; Vaiseshika . . . By Kanada; Yoga . . . By Patanjali; Purva Mimamsa . . . By Jamini}
Wednesdays	Indian History. Illus. by lantern slides
Thursdays, Fridays, and Saturdays	Physiological Yoga—Private Classes Only

The curriculum was broad, and Bernard didn't skimp on techniques either. In his private classes, he continued to teach pranayama, mantra recitation, yoga postures, and internal-cleansing techniques.

Though not listed on the chalkboard, he'd also lecture on what he called Tantrik Yoga. "The purpose of human happiness is the purpose of Yoga," explained Bernard vaguely in a lecture delivered in August 1912, "therefore what we are to understand by the Tantrik Order is simply that it is a body of men, Yogis, who for their evolution, for their happiness follow a certain system, a certain science of Life, which being in accordance with nature is best suited to bring about the consummation which everybody desires, happiness."[59]

Prematurely bald and sporting a curled mustache, Bernard lectured in cutaway coats, trousers, and turquoise cuff links. (He saved his cape, turban, and robes for ceremonial occasions.) He devoted most of this particular discussion to the principle underlying Tantra, that even the basest aspects of human existence can be instruments of liberation. This is nothing less than a reordering of Judeo-Christian metaphysics, which abolishes the very idea of sin. Bernard emphasized a milder version though; he advocated "moderate satisfaction of those desires and carefully considering their usefulness and importance in life," in contrast to other "so-called teachers of Hindu philosophies" who, he claimed, espoused "killing desires."[60]

For Bernard, the identity of body and spirit also differentiated Tantrik Yoga from other types. Whereas Raja, Jnana, and Bhakti Yoga bifurcated "matter and soul, physical body and spirit," then showed the practitioner how to reunite them, Tantrik Yoga considered body and spirit coexistent—one was merely the manifestation of the other.[61]

Clearly Tantric philosophy, as Bernard presented it, rationalized his own behavior. The notion that body was a manifestation of spirit made Bernard's preference for comely young women seem less clichéd and more exalted than it really was. And the idea of "moderate satisfaction of desires" made his womanizing seem prudent, rather than amoral or at the least a violation of Victorian-era mores. (Tantric practice, on the other hand, quite clearly reserved sex for controlled, highly ritualized settings.) But besides women, cigars were his only vice.

During these lectures, Bernard also presented Tantrik Yoga as a yoga for this world, which has always been one of Tantra's distinguishing features. "The best place to learn to control this desire," he told his class, "is in human habitation—anybody can control their desires in the jungle."

Once his listeners had absorbed this basic message, that Tantrik Yoga was compatible with sex and worldly life, and that "every sensible man" ought to practice it, he left them suspended there, no less enlightened about what this kind of yoga involved than they had been an hour before. He made no mention of the subtle body or awakening Kundalini. Nor would he in the next lecture. Abiding tradition, he told his class, "The best way to do [Tantrik Yoga] is to go to the experts known as gurus."

He was advertising his own services. Bernard was the only openly Tantrik guru in town.

As was the case with Vivekananda, there was a huge gulf between Bernard's students' view of him and his teachings and the broader public's. To his students, he was a guru. They took refuge in his knowledge and trusted him unreservedly. At least one, an Englishwoman, had willingly paid him one thousand dollars to be admitted into his third degree.

The neighbors saw him as a nuisance. The superintendent of an adjacent building claimed that "wild Oriental music and women's cries, but not those of distress," emanated from his Sanskrit College. It's unclear exactly what was going on behind closed doors. Robert Love believes Bernard had abandoned the "Kaula rites" by this point.

Whatever they heard, the neighbors were convinced it was amoral and possibly illegal. They filed complaints, and the police raided again. This time, District Attorney Whitman was determined to put an end to the "'Hindu school' game."[62]

A decade into his career, Bernard was doing more harm than good to yoga. Now, every time there was some disturbance, the papers put "Omnipotent Oom" in large type, and many rehashed details of the earlier scandal.

Nor had District Attorney Whitman given up on that first case; besides copies of the *International Journal*, or "Red Book," which contained illustrations of a "questionable character," he hoped to find "one of the two women who complained about mistreatment" in his second investigation of Bernard.[63]

And so over the next few years, Bernard continued to move frequently, teaching in New Jersey and renting rooms all over the West Side of Manhattan.[64]

None of this deterred Blanche. She was a quick study of yoga philosophy and Hatha Yoga, including some of the more advanced postures (such as back bends and balancing poses like Mayūrāsana, in which you place your hands on the floor, press your arms together, and lift your entire body on your bent elbows). By 1914, Blanche had mastered Hatha Yoga so well, Bernard put her in charge of his yoga school for women, then located on East Fifty-fourth Street; that same year, Dace Shannon, also known as Blanche Reiss, renamed herself Blanche De Vries, and soon after, De Vries began teaching at Bernard's Yoga Center on Riverside Drive, where she oversaw a growing stable of young women yoga teachers.[65]

Up to this point, Bernard had relied heavily on Florin Jones and Winfield Nicholls to recruit and teach new yoga students. Nicholls was handsome and could be charming, but he seemed untrustworthy. Jones was a bookish man a few years younger than Bernard, "whose features," according to Cheerie, "resembled Abraham Lincoln."[66]

De Vries, on the other hand, was young and artistic and inimitably vital. One of her earliest yoga students recalls "her large expressive eyes" and her style; apparently she wore "outlandish hats which would have looked ridiculous on anyone else."[67]

Five years after bringing De Vries onto his teaching staff, Bernard entrusted one of his most ambitious enterprises yet to her.

In February 1919, backed by several wealthy patrons, De Vries opened an institute teaching Yoga Gymnosophy—and here, in a five-floor town house on East Fifty-third Street, yoga took on its most refined and modern incarnation to date.

There were marble staircases, brass fixtures, fine Oriental carpets, a library full of books on yoga and Indian philosophy, and a kitchen that served, in Cheerie's words, "healthful and delicious foods." The studios on the upper floors were sunny and spotless.

Students dressed in stockings or bloomers for class and practiced on yoga mats. Teachers would verbally instruct small groups and physically assist those students who needed extra help.[68]

Not much is known about which poses were taught or in what sequence. Bernard generally favored inverted postures, such as headstands and their variations, as well as Nauli, which involves churning your abdominal muscles (after first gaining control of each set individually), and Padmasana, or lotus position, for meditation.

More advanced students learned the postures De Vries had mastered, the back bends, handstands, and balancing poses, and front and side splits. Students also learned some breathing exercises (we don't know which ones), and the more courageous ones may have learned techniques, such as vāso dhauti (whereby you cleaned the digestive tract with a thin muslin cloth).[69]

Once introduced to yoga, students often attended multiple classes during a single week; some came every day.

Much like today, at the Fifty-third Street yoga school discipline and luxury, artists and socialites, young and old, coexisted. All involved felt a sense of purpose, a sense of working toward something more meaningful than mere physical beauty and something more sensual than religion as they had previously understood it.[70]

"The Center stood for beauty, cleanliness and efficiency," wrote Cheerie decades after the fact, "—one more proof to show visitors that Yoga succeeded materially as well as spiritually."[71]

De Vries, who was twenty-eight years old, now managed twelve Hatha Yoga instructors, and they all met her exacting standards.

Some of the young women yoga teachers came from prominent families (one, Hannah Prince, was the daughter of a California millionaire), some not. What they shared was physical beauty and a demonstrated aptitude in the yoga postures. Like ballerinas permitted to go *en pointe*, they had achieved a rare level of mastery of Hatha Yoga (and, not incidentally, many were former dancers). As a result, within the institute these teachers were more esteemed than even their wealthiest, most prominent students. Then, as now, yoga upset the usual social hierarchies.[72]

Cheerie herself had danced in a Ziegfeld production before she began practicing yoga seriously. When she met these "young lady teachers," she was struck by their "radiance and healthful glow, without a trace of make up," which she felt "far surpassed the most renouned [*sic*] of Ziegfeld's beauties."[73]

Cheerie was also struck by De Vries's intolerance of physical weakness. Once, when trying to teach herself handstands, Cheerie fell and hurt her shoulder. De Vries told her (and the other young women workers) a "Yogi should avoid accidents, be strong and healthy and therefore never sick." Such lapses were, in De Vries's view, "only the results of human stupidity."[74]

De Vries had always been an excellent student ("compliant" is how one friend put it) of Bernard's; her equation of physical weakness and human stupidity and her conviction that both could be averted came directly from her mentor and his belief in the exact correlation of one's physical being and spiritual status, something he attributed to Tantra.

Seeing bodily dysfunction as an indication of spiritual weakness had also long been a guiding principle of New Thought, a popular homegrown movement, also known as Mind Cure.

William James had summed up New Thought as "an intuitive belief in the all-saving power of healthy-minded attitudes . . . in the conquering efficacy of courage, hope, and trust, and a correlative contempt for doubt, fear, worry, and all nervously precautionary states of mind."[75]

From its beginnings, New Thought had been intertwined with yoga; Sarah Farmer had hosted its representatives at Green Acre in 1894, the same summer Vivekananda began teaching Raja Yoga there, and in his 1919 history of the movement, Horatio Dresser singles out Farmer as a leader whose "conferences set the example for New Thought meetings" elsewhere.[76]

Through its early years, several swamis in the Ramakrishna Order, including Abhedananda, addressed New Thought gatherings.[77]

As a result of this intimacy, many observers believed there was little, if any, difference between New Thought and yoga. In 1902, the *Chicago Daily Tribune* published a series of spoofs of the movement. Lesson VIII of its "Home Course in New Thought" conducted by Panamahatma McGinnis begins, "Having learned to decombobitate and concentrate yourself, the next step is Meditation. Without concentration you can do nothing, but concentration, without meditation is profitless." The piece concludes with the boldfaced question "? ? ? Are you in Cosmic Tune? ? ?"[78]

In the person of William Walker Atkinson yoga and New Thought came together. Atkinson edited *New Thought Magazine* and wrote many books on the subject, including titles such as *Mind-Power: The Secret of Mental Magic*, which stresses "mental suggestion" as a means to influencing others. Atkinson is also the presumed author of the first books on Hatha Yoga published in America, although he wrote these under the pseudonym Yogi Ramacharaka.[79]

Bernard was familiar with Atkinson's work. But if Bernard's Tantra and New Thought shared a premise—the identity of mind and body— they parted ways when it came to solutions when the body failed. The mind curers focused on healing the spirit, which would in turn heal the body.[80]

The Tantric Yogi worked in reverse. "The first duty of every initiate us [sic] to purify his body," advised Bernard in a 1912 lecture, "and through his body improve his spirit, his soul. The finer the body the better will be its manifestations naturally."[81]

This equation of body and spirit also played directly, and even intentionally, into human vanity, and Hatha Yoga, as Bernard and De Vries taught it, gave purpose and spiritual import to the pursuit of beauty and health. In De Vries's yoga school, temple and sanitarium merged.

Besides refining Bernard's operations, De Vries played another critical role: she serviced the wealthy dowagers far better than Bernard, Jones, and Nicholls could. She connected with them, inspired them, and earned their loyalty, and thus increased patronage.

"If I can only put in action all you have both taught me," wrote Mrs. Vanderbilt in a letter to De Vries, "I shall be more than happy."[82]

She also civilized Bernard. The two had secretly married in Richmond, Virginia, in 1918, and for a while their relationship checked his womanizing.[83]

The new yoga institute was so successful, and the Vanderbilt family so committed to the team behind it, that Bernard and De Vries were able to lease the Nyack property.

But even with De Vries in his fold and any number of prominent New Yorkers routinely attending his yoga classes and lectures, Bernard continued to arouse suspicion.

One morning when Cheerie was working at the Fifty-third Street school—De Vries wouldn't let her teach yet; instead she performed more menial tasks, such as polishing doorknobs and scrubbing the marble stairs—the police suddenly appeared. Someone had tipped them off that underage girls were being "held captive and under hypnosis." Barbara and Margaret Rutherfurd, both in their twenties at the time, were in the school's foyer preening; they were just back from Paris, where an adventuresome hairdresser had dyed their hair a silvery pink.

The two policemen questioned Cheerie and another student about their age while De Vries remained out of sight and the Rutherfurd girls melted into the fretwork. The police were eventually shooed out empty-handed.[84]

When Bernard and De Vries opened up the Braeburn Country Club the summer of 1919, it was the combination of the ceremonies resembling "those of a Yogi" and the discovery that the notorious "'Dr.' Pierre A. Bernard was connected to the club" that turned villagers' unease into a "moral panic."[85]

In three separate raids on the club in a single week, the police found nothing illegal. What they did find was becoming a familiar sight to newspaper readers: men and women doing yoga exercises.[86]

Even the optimistic Cheerie began to believe "the Hearst papers" were "seeking to ruin him."[87]

The 1920s (up until that final, fateful year) proved the best of times for the American country club. Numbers tell part of this story: the United States had only one thousand country clubs in 1915. By 1927 that number had increased more than fivefold.

The redistribution of wealth that took place over that same period accounts for much of this growth. The rich got much richer, and they spent lavishly on leisure and entertainment. Automobiles also helped spur this proliferation. In 1920, more than 7.5 million cars and trucks traveled the nation's roads. Seven years later, more than 18 million American families owned a car. No longer did clubs need to locate near railway stations or streetcar lines. With more Americans driving, it was easier for them to get to clubs, whether they were in the suburbs or in even more remote locales.[88]

Bernard and De Vries's Braeburn Club shared many features of the country clubs that dotted the rolling hills of upstate New York and Massachusetts. Members enjoyed plenty of physical activity (though no golf, which had become a staple of many country clubs by this point), holiday parties, dances, and a lecture series, the Open Forum.

In fact, yoga accounted for a relatively small part of the activities in any given day or week at the Braeburn Country Club, which in the early 1920s was renamed the Clarkstown Country Club, or C.C.C.

The list of "Landmarks" for the years 1921 through 1927 found in De Vries's effects includes as many "Teas," performances (weekly vaudeville shows, Chinese opera, circuses), and parties (one New Year's Eve "Poker Party" lasted eighteen hours) as it does Sanskrit, philosophy, "breath work," and physiology classes.[89]

To enter C.C.C. on many a day during the 1920s and early 1930s would have been to stumble into a scene worthy of a prewar, American Fellini. Here was a cast of bored wealthy people (whose boredom was vanquished in preparing for the circus). Here was an assortment of beautiful young women. Over there, a cross-dressing baseball team, the men wearing women's bloomers, skirts, and bathing costumes, the women wearing actual baseball pants and jerseys or men's shirts and trousers.

Under the big top, if it was late August or early September, you might see Cheerie, costumed in rainbow hues, fly giddily above the heads of the audience on the trapeze, or other club members, both men and women, standing on their heads and turning somersaults in designs.[90]

And infusing the atmosphere was the thrill of sexual license: Bernard's theories on sex—his beliefs in women's pleasure and marriage based on love, and his view that yoga and Tantra aided in the pursuit of both—were well-known and widely subscribed to. More than that, extramarital affairs were seen as expressions of "free love" and the "moderate satisfaction of desires" rather than transgressions of a sacred bond.

Yoga was no longer the axis around which the club pivoted; it was a motif woven through all of the activities, the ingredient that distinguished Bernard's club from the others.

De Vries was particularly artful at inserting yoga into the club's entertainment program. With Cheerie and Clara, she adapted yoga to dance and performed intricately choreographed pieces, costumed in shimmering silk with bare feet, plunging bodice, and bare midriff. She gave some of the dances names such as "Buddhamas Festival," "Dance of the Five Senses," and "Birthday of Krishna."[91]

De Vries, however, wasn't breaking new ground so much as picking up where popular culture had left off.

A little more than a decade earlier, the dancer Ruth St. Denis had found a quick route from a seedy vaudeville house on Twenty-third Street into high society and the legitimate theater, performing sequined and barefoot in her first production of "Radha."[92]

On an amber-lit stage, ringed by Brahman priests (played by Indian sailors and clerks) and smoke from burning incense, St. Denis whirled, arched, and writhed. As she twirled and twisted, her skirt sparkled, and her jeweled jacket bared her midriff. The dance centered around the five senses—sight, hearing, smell, taste, touch; by the end of it, St. Denis had collapsed in delirium, symbolically exorcising temptation.[93]

William Hammerstein hired St. Denis as a special feature of his 1911 Victoria Roof Garden season to perform "two Egyptian dances" and "three Hindu numbers"—"The Cobra," "The Spirit of Incense," and "The Nautch Dance." Besides a forty-piece orchestra, St. Denis was to be "supported by a company of Hindus."

By the 1910s, artists of almost every medium had realized the usefulness of India, Japan, and China. As a lead stage designer for the Ziegfeld Follies, Joseph Urban, whom Cheerie knew personally, made his name creating Oriental tableaux such as the "Harem Scene" and the "Temple of Color."[94]

("In all of Mr. Urban's scenes there is a touch of the fantastic," was *The New York Times*' analysis in 1915. "The Oriental note is strong and he makes frequent use of mosaic patterns.")

At C.C.C., the combination of entertainment and edification, layered with a veneer of exoticism, was quite profitable. By the mid-1920s, the club had expanded to include an estate previously owned by the Hilton family and a six-acre, riverfront manor called the Moorings. Three years later, C.C.C. boasted 283 members and a budget of about $110,000. It was also a major contributor to Nyack's finances. The 1927 *Rockland County Redbook* reported, "The Club has, within the last five and one-half years of its existence, actually disbursed in Nyack a total of nearly a million dollars."[95]

With revenues at C.C.C. approaching an all-time high, Bernard was at the height of his career. Almost everyone treated him as a guru, bowing to his unquestioned authority.

Many called him Doc or Dr. Bernard. Some, including the composer Cyril Scott, believed he was a trained medical doctor. Though he was in his fifties, he was still tremendously alluring to women. Cheerie, always a bit of a naïf, saw him as a father figure; Margaret Rutherfurd was obsessively in love with him, though he doesn't seem to have returned her affections; and a young club member, Viola Wertheim, found Bernard and his theories so compelling, she offered to hand over her substantial inheritance (a transaction that never came to pass).[96]

Bernard insisted members take club names, partly to erase distinctions between some of America's wealthiest individuals and the intellectuals and artists who found their way to Nyack. (F. Scott Fitzgerald could easily have modeled Tom and Daisy Buchanan on Mr. and Mrs. Ogden Mills or Mr. and Mrs. Cyril Hatch or nearly any one of the numerous moneyed couples who filled the club's roster.)

In Bernard's cosmology, the philosophy professor Edmund T. Dana became "Coulton"; the actress Beverly Sitgreaves became "Lamont"; Lillian Russell became "Millard"; Mrs. William K. Vanderbilt became "Stanley"; and Countess Mira de Karzybska became "Gregory."[97]

Bernard also actively involved himself in his students' personal lives, urging them to marry each other when he thought it appropriate, or useful, and, in other cases, preventing a couple from spending time together. According to his biographer, Bernard believed in monogamous marriages based on love and tried to steer his members into these sorts of couplings. (There's no small irony here; Bernard's marriage to De Vries was highly secretive and in its latter years troubled. In the 1930s, he tried to replace De Vries with one of his girlfrends and kick her closest allies out of the club. A power struggle ensued, and De Vries eventually left.)[98]

As for his teachings on yoga in these years, they varied widely.[99]

"The simplest way to translate the word yoga is Evolution," he remarked in a lecture in 1924. "It is a process analogous to tending a seed in the ground. The soil has to be watered and fertilized and ideal conditions have to be created to assure rapid development of the plant. That is yoga." He had, at this point in his talk, already rejected seven other definitions of yoga, including "a pecular [sic] combination of stunts," "union of the individual with the universal," and "management, whether of work or play" as being either "about as clear as mud" or too specific. "Yoga," he continues, "is the art of more rapid evolution."

In this lecture, he also outlined the "eight degrees" of yoga "theory and practice": "Yama-niyama, Asanas, Mudras, Pranayama, Pratyahara, Dharana, Dhyana," and finally, "Samadhi" or "Mukhti, Moksha, etc." Here he was reciting the limbs of Hatha Yoga. "Asana," he explained, "means posturing; mudra movements; pranayama breath control; pratyahara sense control; dharana concentration or mind control; dhyana meditation or contemplation; samadhi isolation, and isolation means 'in the world but not of it.'"[100]

But what yoga was at any given moment seems to have depended to a large extent on *whom* Bernard was addressing. Like any good teacher, Bernard tuned his message to his audience.

By the mid-1920s there wasn't much difference between initiated and uninitiated members. Bernard referred to the entire C.C.C. membership as the "American Tantrik Order."

But there was a big difference in how any given student arrived at the club. Some came voluntarily for the country living, educational program, and yoga instruction; others were *sent* there, often by relatives, to dry up or straighten out.

This first group needed to be encouraged and entertained, the second, disciplined. (Though members could and did float between the two modes.)

Barbara Rutherfurd spent much of her time in this latter category. Writing to her mother from C.C.C., she described her tasks: "My day includes cooking lessons, typing . . . keeping books, organization, mantra, dish washing. . . . To be still more specific . . . I am on the mat at 7:30AM every morning."[101]

It seems likely Bernard stressed the ethical dimension of yoga for members such as Barbara, going so far as to threaten a "probation of seven years," during which time he'd "see how much yama-niyama"—the ritual observances and rules of conduct by which the aspirant must abide—"you can practise [*sic*]" before he'd teach lessons "in asanas." The poses would be Barbara's reward, if she reformed, which meant not stealing, lying, harming others, or sleeping around.[102]

However, three pillars of Bernard's yoga philosophy stood fast through his entire career. The first was his adherence to Tantra (testimony to his loyalty to Hamati). His hierarchy of yogas was fixed from his earliest days: Bhakti—good for "sloppy females" who delight in "'God is love' stuff"— was forever at the bottom, and Tantra at the top. "Any 3rd degree Tantric can beat any so-called Paramahansa," he declared, no less adamant in 1928 than he had been in 1912, "in every Yoga test of body, brain, and heart."[103]

Bernard believed Tantrik Yoga was the best kind because it was the most complete and almost vexingly adaptable: "'To all men something'— crumbs in the most cases—'To some men all,'" he explained in a lecture, "You see that is what [Tantriks] do. It is all the elasticity of the text of the doctrine. How does the doctrine come to be elastic? The doctrine is so big, you see, that there is always some of it that you could give even to Wop, the dog, here; it is so big; there are so many sides to it."[104]

Western scholarship on the subject was beginning to catch up to Bernard. Arthur Avalon had recently put out English translations of key Tantras, *Principles of Tantra* (1914) and *The Serpent Power, Being the Ṣaṭ-Cakra-Nirūpaṇa and Pāḍukā-Pañcaka: Two Works on Tantrik Yoga* (1919), among them. Avalon was actually a pseudonym for Sir John Woodroffe, who had been a High Judge in Calcutta, and his collaborator, Atal Behari Ghosh, a Sanskrit pundit. Together they cowrote numerous books and shaped the Western exposition of Tantra for decades to come. You could find much of both Avalon's and Sir John Woodruffe's oeuvre in the C.C.C. library.[105]

However, in practice, Bernard had largely abandoned the most outré aspects of Tantra, and certainly the sex rites, possibly due to pressure from the Vanderbilts.[106]

As a partisan of Tantra, Bernard co-opted many neo-Vedanta swamis to his cause. Bernard told his students, "It is so damnably notoriously known from Ceylon on the south to the foothills of the Himalaya Mountains on the north that Vivekananda was a Tantrik and a notorious one." And, said Bernard, so was Swami Abhedananda. (There was no question about Swami Bodhananda, since he had taken Bernard's Tantrik oath.)

In most cases, Bernard intimates to his students he was letting them in on a big secret and that what was common knowledge in India had to be "covered over in this country."[107]

(Recent studies by Jeffrey Kripal and others have shown that Bernard was more right than not, on this point. Certainly Ramakrishna was far more of a Tantrik than his monastic disciples had made him out to be; and Vivekananda had taught elements of Tantric practice and theory under the rubric of Vedanta or Raja Yoga.)

The second unwavering principle Bernard adhered to was that yoga was scientific.

Yoga, Bernard liked to say, was "all branches of science applied to the individual."[108] Bernard read widely in the sciences, everything from astronomy, biology, and zoology to sexology and even eugenics, and commanded an elaborate scientific vocabulary. His "Medical Books" alone—which included such works as H. Head's *Studies in Neurology* (London: Henry

Frowde, 1920) and A. Keith's *Human Embryology and Morphology* (Edward Arnold Co., 1923)—took up four shelves in his extensive library.[109]

He also acquired most books related to yoga and Tantra then published in the English language.[110]

His collection of books on Indian thought was comprehensive enough that after his death representatives from Yale asked De Vries to bequeath it to their Oriental Library. (She refused and sold it.)[111]

As a result, Bernard was much better equipped to describe in scientific language how yoga worked than any previous teacher of it, and his technical explanations of yoga bolstered his claim that yoga contained within it all the sciences.

His 1924 lecture that covered character is a startling, prescient case in point. "Character, as we see it in Yoga," said Bernard, "is the result, in the first place, of the physical development of brain or memory cells. . . . So by the term character we mean, first, the development of a certain brand of memory cells . . . and secondly, nerve impulses that accord with those memory cells."

Altering character could then be achieved by altering these types of cells, and this is precisely what he claimed the postures and mudras did. "They are designed to effect some change in the building of brain cells, and especially of memory cells."[112]

In Bernard's hands, character development wasn't the product of one's moral choices, or at least not solely that. It was a physiological process that anyone—at least anyone who practiced yoga—might control.

Vivekananda had clearly seen the need for these types of explanations but couldn't quite deliver on them.[113]

Current neuroscience does a good deal to bear out Bernard's explanations. Regardless of their accuracy, Bernard's speculations pleased his students. "Dr. Bernard's lectures are the most illuminative and scientific expositions of Yoga," enthused Jagadish Chandra Chatterji, an expert in Kashmir Shaivism, who had given a lecture on Tantra at C.C.C. in the fall of 1927, "that I have ever listened to in my entire life."[114]

The third principle Bernard held fast to was his belief in yoga as a form of this-worldly self-improvement.

Bernard espoused a sort of antitranscendentalism. "Divinity," he once said, was just a term for "that which to you is unknown and about which you are superstitious."[115]

Yoga was useful for the here and now; it gave you the tools for "attacking all problems of life better than the other fellow," and Moksha, or liberation, was nothing more or less than "the pleasure, peace, happiness you get out of all that composes life."[116]

Bernard's "spiritual man" was "a man who follows nature's laws." Bernard adduced what he saw as natural laws, translated them into a set of rules for living, and convinced a group of wealthy, open-minded Americans to pay for the privilege of submitting to them.

Some of his rules were abstemious. He forbade his students cigarettes and alcohol save a glass of wine on New Year's Eve. (Bernard himself was the exception; he was addicted to cigars and smoked them incessantly.) His policies on this count insulated him from Prohibition. C.C.C. opened in 1919, the same year that liquor was outlawed in the United States, and succeeded anyway.[117]

Other rules for life Bernard derived from yoga, including some related to "intersexual relations," seemed similarly constraining. In one lecture, he advocated sexual continence, counseling students to have sex only every fourteen days.[118]

But all of his rules, even his most abstemious ones, were designed to heighten pleasure.

His injunction to abstain from sex most days of the month would have intensified any erotic encounters his students did have. (As the parable goes, the longer a man waits for a meal, the better it tastes.) And on other occasions he recommended yogic postures to strengthen vaginal tone and techniques to ensure female sexual pleasure.[119]

Bernard believed yoga offered "a bargain with nature." Practice yoga, he advised, and we can "enjoy life and not pay the price that the ignoramus pays for enjoyment."[120]

Despite his success in Nyack, Bernard's influence beyond his membership was limited. He spoke only to those he felt worthy of his teaching; he never wrote any books about yoga, and he lectured on the subject almost exclusively at the club. Consequently, his reputation in the wider world was rightfully mixed—on the increasingly rare occasions that his name came up, so did "the Omnipotent Oom."

Surprisingly, outside the yoga subculture, Bernard wasn't that interested in shoring up his reputation. He was too disdainful of the average man, and in person he was able to win over his critics (as he had in Rock-land County).

Instead, he'd redeem himself by proving to the world that yoga was a valuable philosophy and science of life.

Yoga could still use some help. "The Yogi's teaching was a pleasing mixture of Couéism, Childs dietetics, first aid to the injured, mysticism, and Bernarr Macfadden, combining the best features of each," wrote E. B. White in *The New Yorker* in March 1928. "He passed quite easily from varicose veins to self-mastery."[121]

White had captured the essence of American yoga of the era. Hatha Yoga postures did resemble elements of Macfadden's physical culture. And the vocabulary of New Thought that permeated contemporary presentations of yoga, including Bernard's, undeniably echoed Émile Coué's autosuggestions. (Coué was a French psychologist famous for, among other achievements, his affirmation "Each day, in every way, I am getting better and better.")[122]

It wasn't so much the content of yoga that White got wrong as the efficacy and coherence of the discipline. No one seemed to believe that these techniques taken together amounted to much or could be part of a meaningful philosophy—with its own metaphysics and theology.

Bernard had an ambitious plan for yoga's redemption. In 1928, he launched yet another organization, called the International School of Vedic and Allied Research (ISVAR). Its stated mission was to "promote a better understanding and more lively appreciation of Vedic culture in its relation to the other cultures of the world." On a practical level, ISVAR members would work to establish professorships in Indian and Eastern philosophy at Western universities and to integrate "Vedic and allied subjects" into the general curricula. They'd also institutionalize student-exchange programs with India.[123]

Bernard had developed an informal version of ISVAR early in his career. Since the early 1910s, he had hosted visiting Indian scholars, pandits, swamis, as well as a number of Indian scholars working in the West. (Several Indian institutions awarded him honorary degrees for his work helping these men.) He was also gracious to any American scholars of Indian thought who sought him out, and he made good use of his acquaintances, collecting letters attesting to his erudition from the most famous and lettered among them.[124]

From the beginning, yoga featured prominently in ISVAR's plans and, less obviously to many, in its name. Isvara is the deity Patanjali invokes in the first chapter of his *Sutras*; devotion to him is presented as a quick route to success in yoga.

The 1928 prospectus for ISVAR listed a handful of works "in preparation," including one titled *Yoga: Its Theory and Practice*. Unlike the American Oriental Society, which promoted knowledge of Indic thought from a safe distance, ISVAR accorded yoga the status of an *applied* science; to learn it was to learn how to live better.[125]

In arguing that Indian religious culture had produced a philosophy that could help Westerners live better, ISVAR also pointedly challenged Katherine Mayo's 1927 book, *Mother India*, a bestseller in the United States for two years in a row.[126]

Mayo had already published a sensational book about the Philippines, titled *The Isles of Fear*, when she traveled to India to see that country for herself. What she found was a miserable, squalid place that had been romanticized by other observers. She wanted to set the record straight.

To her credit, she examined some of India's most pressing social problems: poor nutrition, illiteracy, poor hygiene, women's constricted social roles, and early childbearing, among them.

In elucidating the causes of the suffering, however, Mayo went wrong—drawing reckless conclusions from the bits of information about Indian culture that she amassed.

She notes, rightly, that many Hindus worship Shiva in the form of a lingam ("the male generative organ"). From the erotic imagery of India's scriptures and temples ("there are the sculptures and paintings on temple walls and temple chariots, on palace doors and street-wall frescoes, realistically demonstrating every conceivable aspect and humor of sex contact"), Mayo inferred that sex was the Indian's main occupation and preoccupation, starting in childhood. As a result, "the average male Hindu of thirty years . . . is an old man."

(Imagine if Mayo had been an Indian visiting America. She might have concluded that the Bible, and God's injunction to Adam "to go forth and multiply," had produced overcrowded East Village tenements and heaps of garbage on the street.)

Mayo goes one step further. Because so much of India's adult population had been drained by sex, the country wasn't fit to rule itself.

Once more, then, one is driven to the original conclusion: Given men who enter the world physical bankrupts out of bankrupt stock, rear them through childhood in influences and practices that devour their vitality; launch them at the dawn of maturity on an unrestrained outpouring of their whole provision of creative energy in one single direction; find them, at the age when the Anglo-Saxon is just coming into full glory of manhood, broken-nerved, low-spirited, petulant ancients; and need you, while this remains unchanged, seek for other reasons why they are poor and sick and dying and why their hands are too weak, too fluttering, to seize or to hold the reins of Government?[127]

Mother India was dangerous because it gave the impression—over nearly four hundred pages of vivid description—that "the peoples of India" were almost irredeemably backward, confirming long-standing suspicions about their capacity, or lack thereof, for self-governance.

Indian intellectuals immediately challenged Mayo's book. Gandhi and Rabindranath Tagore, the country's leading poet, wrote lengthy responses, which were excerpted in several American periodicals.[128]

"Her case," wrote Gandhi in November 1927, "is to perpetuate white domination in India on the plea of India's unfitness to rule herself."[129]

As Gandhi wrote, the issue of self-governance was becoming, almost daily, even more urgent. "All shades of moderation over the question of British rule are disappearing, it is hinted," reported *The New York Times* in mid-February 1928, "and the country is lining up in two camps," those for complete self-rule, including India's former moderates, and those against.[130]

The First India Conference, held in October 1928 in New York City, aimed to present a more balanced and positive view of the country. The program of events spanned the entire month and included lectures on Hindu art and music, womanhood, and marriage. There was also the lecture "America's Interest in India," and a discussion on Indian self-rule, "India Free—Within or Without the British Empire?" The editor of *The Nation* participated in one of the panels, as did Professor George C. O. Haas, identified as the "sometime editor of the *Journal of the American Oriental Society*" and assistant director of ISVAR. A young radio network, the National Broadcasting Company, aired four sessions.[131]

Besides Haas, who worked in ISVAR's New York City office, Bernard had recruited two other scholars—S. L. Joshi (of Dartmouth) and E. R. Seligman (of Columbia)—who participated in the First India Conference.[132]

Bernard had also hired Jagadish Chandra Chatterji, who had given a lecture on Kashmir Shaivism to club members and now described himself as a peripatetic lecturer on comparative religion, to oversee most of ISVAR's operations and set up the British Committee as well as a center in Benares. Bernard promised to pay Chatterji a salary for the first two years of ISVAR's existence as well as the organization's operating expenses.[133]

Soon some other renowned scholars lent their names to the organization. Charles Rockwell Lanman, a titan in the field from Harvard, who had attended Sara Bull's Cambridge Conferences and was by then retired, came on board as president; Maurice Bloomfield, an esteemed Sanskritist from Johns Hopkins, initially took the post of vice president; professors from Columbia (including Seligman), Yale, and the University of California filled out the Executive Council.

Chatterji quickly garnered the support of several important British scholars; eventually, Lt. Col. Sir Francis Younghusband, and F. W. Thomas, Boden Professor of Sanskrit at Oxford, agreed to sign on to the British Committee. The *London Times Educational Supplement* praised Chatterji's efforts, noting with "satisfaction" that the organization was comfortably funded, "thanks to the generosity of American citizens and institutions" none here named.[134]

Chatterji wrote to Bernard from London around Christmas 1928, flushed with success: "You have referred, in your letters, to my success in London. But, my dear Friend, . . . It is you alone who are making all this possible for me and for the School. . . . And my Christmas presents to you this time are the sincerest homage and devotion of a grateful heart and fresh resolve to make your good name known and recognized among scholars and the learned of the World in a manner that shall be truly fitting."[135]

During ISVAR's second year of operation, Chatterji published two issues of its journal; one included an article by the famed Yale scholar E. Washburn Hopkins, "The Epic View of Earth."

ISVAR seemed to be well on its way to establishing itself as a reputable, scholarly organization and was cited as a promising "Hindu Cultural

Movement" by Wendell Thomas in the first sympathetic study of Hinduism in America ever published (misleadingly titled *Hinduism Invades America*).

Impressed by ISVAR's ambitions, "nothing less than complete Western appreciation of Aryan culture," and its methods, which are "purely academic," Thomas didn't mention Bernard in connection with ISVAR and noted that Charles Lanman had advanced many of its proposals nearly a decade before.[136]

But by the time Thomas's book came out, ISVAR had effectively collapsed due to a particularly lethal combination of academic politics, financial mismanagement, and personal grievances.

Tension had been building between Chatterji, who spent money at a rapid clip to get ISVAR off the ground, and Bernard, who was supplying the funds. In May 1929, Haas reported the school was moving along well enough, but that "we are hampered, of course, by the failure to receive any gifts of money but that is a difficulty which will be remedied in time." A year later, Chatterji threatened to sue Bernard; each insisted the other had failed to fulfill his obligation. By June 1930, Chatterji completely reversed his opinion of his sponsor (or finally made known his honest appraisal): Bernard, Chatterji insisted, was a faker who "pretends to be a master of a language (Sanscrit) [sic] of which he cannot read a single text . . . and who bolsters up his pretensions by claiming a spurious title, *Sashtri*." He dismissed C.C.C. as "the Nyack love-cult," a partial truth that belied much of what went on there.[137]

The demise of ISVAR was of no great consequence for Vedic philosophy, since the American Oriental Society had a similar project under way. It was a loss for yoga, since ISVAR had made it a priority and approached it both as a subject for academic inquiry and of actual practical value.[138]

Bernard remained, perhaps perversely, optimistic. According to the theologian, founder of the humanist movement, and teacher of comparative religion Charles Francis Potter, who became a C.C.C. member in 1929 and served as president for two years, Bernard "was confident the pioneering work he was doing in human-body building and character training would be understood sometime and he was willing to wait for his later vindication."[139]

6

THEOS BERNARD'S SPIRITUAL HEROISM

One winter morning in February 1937, Theos C. Bernard set out from his bungalow in Kalimpong, India, a border town nestled in the foothills of the Himalayas, as was his routine.

He had leaped out of bed at 5:00 a.m. to cram in pranayama (his breathing exercises) and a brief review of his Tibetan lessons, this in a room that by Western standards lacked the most basic amenities—heat and hot water. Without so much as a cup of tea to fuel him, Theos walked the mile or so to his teacher Tharchin's house.[1]

The route was banked with citrus, banana, and eucalyptus trees, and once spring arrived, it would soon be canopied with the pink and red blossoms of poinsettias, orchids, and rhododendrons, the result of the 350 inches of rain that fell on this corner of the Himalayas annually. On some days, great shelves of clouds would hover above town and the sun would play off them, stippling the sky with flares of red, orange, and purple, a Mardi Gras that engulfed the heavens.[2]

The sight alone made Theos's spirits soar. But few other Western travelers made it to Kalimpong, and those who did couldn't make sense of Theos's life there. When a visitor "does arrive," he wrote in a letter to his wife, Viola, "about all they can think of is why on earth come to such a lonesome place and study Tibetan of all things, and then they are off, on their whiskey and sodas or what have you."[3]

On this particular morning, Theos arrived at his teacher's house and was also greeted by a man he'd often see around town. This "chap," an Indian man, had heard that Theos was interested in Tibet and Tantric Yoga and had come specifically to meet him.

Then he was at Tharchin's the next morning too, this time with a special yoga scripture in hand. It was written in Tibetan—a script based on a seventh-century Indic alphabet. Theos was still new to the language and assumed Tharchin would read it. When he went to open the book, its owner immediately grabbed it, insisting he couldn't let Tharchin see it. Theos chastised the poor fellow, telling him he "was just like the rest of the Yogi Racketeers of India." Tharchin told him his teachings were "tommy rot," suggested he go back to his cave and stay there, and threw him out.

This wasn't the end of it though.

Theos followed the man out, and they walked together through the dusty streets. By the end of their interlude, the man had revealed to Theos that he was a Yogi and could do "just about all there is too [sic] be done" in Hatha Yoga. He had mastered the basic asanas and the purificatory practices (Naulī, Netī, and the various Dhautis), as well as the mudras, and no longer bothered with them, focusing all of his energies on pranayama. In addition, he spoke several languages fluently (including English, Hindi, Urdu, and Sanskrit) and had a photographic memory of English literature, reciting it well and at will, including page numbers.[4]

A few days later, Theos reported the encounter in a letter to Viola. "I have myself a Yogi who is a Yogi," he typed jubilantly. The Yogi ate almost nothing, slept only two hours a night, and, like Theos, was continuing his search for knowledge about yoga in Tibet. "It looks as tho. I am going to wind up getting some real dope from this chap. It really is amazing the things that he knows and can do."[5]

It was as though Theos had discovered some rare species of bird, previously thought extinct, which in a sense he had, since he had spent the preceding few months scouring India for teachers.

Theos was Pierre Bernard's half nephew. His father, Glen, was one of Pierre's younger half brothers. He wasn't close to his uncle, and he was a relative newcomer to C.C.C., having attended his first event there in the spring of 1934. But his wife, Viola, had been a member of the club for nearly a decade, had served as assistant secretary of ISVAR, and was close to Blanche De Vries.

Theos had originally planned to practice law; he had earned a bachelor of law degree in 1931 and worked as a court clerk during the summer of 1932 in Los Angeles. Finding law impractical given his interest in yoga, Theos had changed course. Now he was pursuing a doctorate in the anthropology department at Columbia University and had submitted his master's thesis—"An Introduction to Tantrik Ritual"—just before leaving the States.[6]

In the fall of 1936, with Viola, Theos had traveled from Calcutta to Bombay and then south, to Bangalore, Mysore, and Madras. They had many advantages in locating those Indian Yogis who might help them. The first was motive: their trip to India was neither a honeymoon nor even much of a vacation; Theos planned on writing up the results of his investigations in India as his dissertation.

Secondly, Theos and Viola were young and indefatigable tourists. Theos was only twenty-eight and Viola was just a year older. They could pack more into a single day or a single week than seemed reasonable and were none the worse for wear, most of the time. In the first ten days or so of their stay, their breakneck pace took them from Calcutta more than 260 miles southwest to Puri (a coastal city on the Bay of Bengal), back to Calcutta, then nearly 400 miles north to Darjeeling, and back once again to Calcutta. They visited Hindu and Jain temples, the Royal Asiatic Society of Bengal (the seat of Oriental research established by the esteemed philologist William Jones), the University of Calcutta, the ghats along the Ganges to watch morning rituals, Tiger Hill (an eight-thousand-foot peak from which they could see the tip of Mount Everest), and a Tibetan Buddhist monastery, among other attractions, and barely caught their breath before they set out for Benares.[7]

And as members of C.C.C., the two had connections to a number of sympathetic Indian intellectuals and yogis. Pierre had sent his half nephew off with an enthusiastic letter about where to go, whom to talk to, and whom to avoid (namely his new nemesis, Chatterji). Fellow club member S. L. Joshi also supplied numerous letters of introduction to well-connected Indians, including Sir Mirza Ismael, then the dewan, or chief administrator, to the maharaja of Mysore.[8]

Within three days of their landing in India, Dr. Bannerji, Pierre's former colleague, had taken Theos and Viola to Vivekananda's original Ramakrishna Math in Belur. They left with an open letter of introduction to the Ramakrishna monks across India, complete with addresses.[9]

Apart from these introductions, Theos had an even greater advantage: his own father, Glen Bernard, who had gone to India specifically to do preliminary research for his son.

The yoga bug ran in the family. Glen was one of Pierre Bernard's younger half brothers and had also been a committed yoga student since his youth (though the two brothers had little else in common).[10]

Glen had had a number of teachers. In the States, he was a student of Swami Dhirananda, who had come to help Paramahansa Yogananda run the Self-Realization Fellowship (though the two later had a falling out); Hatha Yogi Wassan; and Sukumar Chatterji (a young Indian Brahman who came to America in 1912 and almost immediately got caught up in Indian nationalist Gadar party).

In the early 1920s, Chatterji had taught yoga in San Francisco's Haight-Ashbury district, lecturing on pranayama, Ayurvedic medicine, and Sāmkhya philosophy, among other topics. Glen had studied with him there, before Chatterji returned to India.

Glen had also traveled to India in the mid-1920s, spending much of his time in Calcutta, the locus of the Bengali yoga tradition, where he developed relationships with disciples of Sri Yukteswar (Yogananda's guru) and of Swami Vivekananda and began a close friendship with Atal Behari Ghosh (one-half of "Arthur Avalon," author of the most famous Tantric books in the English language at the time) and Swami Vimalānanda and his family.

For an American, Glen was exceedingly well connected to Indian Tantrics and yogis, and his contacts would be invaluable to Theos.[11]

However, by the time Theos and Viola arrived in Calcutta in September 1936, Glen's patience for travel in India was beginning to flag. He accompanied them on much of their tour anyway, to Viola's endless irritation.

Together, the two and often the three of them, Theos, Viola, and Glen, stopped in on some of the most famous Yogis then alive. In mid-October, they traveled to Lonavla, about sixty miles from Bombay, to see Swami Kuvalayananda and his clinic.

Kuvalayananda was among the first Indians to scientifically investigate the physical effects and possible benefits of yoga, starting in the mid-1920s. In one of his earliest experiments, the swami tried to measure the physiological effects of Uḍḍiyāna (intense abdominal contraction combined with breath retention) and Naulī (abdominal churning) using a device of his own invention.[12]

Theos and Viola caught up with Kuvalayananda for what turned out to be a long and disappointing lecture "on man." They were more impressed by a copy of the *Vira Sadhana*, Pierre Bernard's Red Book, which they spied on a table at the institute.

The couple much preferred Yogendra, who had done some work with American medical doctors and had set up a Hatha Yoga clinic in Harriman, New York (about thirty miles from C.C.C.), in the early 1920s. Yogendra was convinced that scientists could record only external manifestations of yoga and, hence, missed the point. He stressed the spiritual goal of yoga, as opposed to "street 'stunts,'" such as fire walking, discounted celibacy as a prerequisite for practicing, and told the couple women should do yoga "per the old texts."[13]

Theos and Viola were also advised to visit Sri Aurobindo Ghose, but cryptically, they were told they could find him in Calcutta, a place he had not ventured for more than two decades.[14]

In Theos's estimation, the Kalimpong Yogi ranked at least as high as, if not considerably higher than, some of these other Yogis.[15]

Most impressive to Theos was his skill in Kumbhaka, the practice of retaining your breath for extended periods, which the Yogi could do for two hours. After years of practice, Theos could hold his for only six minutes, a feat for most anyone but not long enough for Theos, who had recently discovered that pranayama—the breathing exercises that Vivekananda had taught his Cambridge pupils and that the Red Book detailed— was "the one thing that begins to do things to one's inside."

Lately, Theos's experiments with pranayama had deeply moved him, though he had at first been skeptical of these practices and the extravagant claims made in the scriptures about their effects. "Never have I discovered anything so revealing," he confided in another letter to Viola. "However, today I can only speak as a child would who was wading ankle deep in a pool where others were swimming. He has found out that the water is wet, refreshing and will not bit [sic] him, but more, he cannot say."[16]

These glimpses of something indescribable made him eager to push his Kumbhaka even further.

Unfortunately, his new Yogi friend, adept at the practice himself, couldn't show Theos how to extend his own Kumbhaka; he simply didn't know how he managed to do what he did or the "laws involved."[17]

Such explanations were at the crux of Theos's entire project. Theos didn't just want to master the specific practices, but to learn "the fundamental principles" and to find out the best ways to surmount the various obstacles other students of yoga might face.

While Theos didn't hold much store in his actual program of study at Columbia, he thought a doctorate would be useful precisely because it would legitimate him to a Western audience. Not incidentally to Theos's thinking, a Ph.D. would also give him a leg up on his uncle.[18]

In letters he penned to Viola at odd hours in his cold quarters in Kalimpong, Theos mapped out his future. He imagined studies on yoga's physiological effects as well as more philosophical works that would present yoga as a sort of applied ethical theory.[19]

He'd break Hatha Yoga down for the average man, who now enjoyed automobiles, refrigerators, and radios. With logic and reason—and living proof of yoga's effects—he'd whittle away at American indifference and even disgust.

In so doing, he would, as he put it to Viola with characteristic immodesty, help people the world over "attain to a small degree . . . toward the real purpose of life."[20]

Though he had no great affection for his half uncle, if he succeeded, Theos would also be the one to vindicate Pierre's vision.

Were Americans ready for a presentation of yoga that didn't shy away from the intense, even grueling, Hatha Yoga practices Theos mastered? Would they have the patience to learn Kumbhaka? Perhaps.

In the late 1930s, Americans' interest in yoga still leaned toward the philosophical and spiritual dimensions of the discipline, for the simple reason that Raja Yoga and books on yoga philosophy were widely available, and despite Pierre's success in Nyack, Hatha Yoga remained comparatively obscure. However, this more physical yoga was beginning to attract attention.[21]

A few months after Theos met the Kalimpong Yogi, *Time* magazine published a flattering profile of Dr. Kovoor Thomas Behanan, a graduate student in the psychology department at Yale who had studied the work of Swami Kuvalayananda, the very same guru who had bored Theos and Viola when they had visited his clinic in Lonavla, India, in the early 1930s.

Behanan had concluded that yoga was "hygienically beneficial" and later wrote a book on the subject, *Yoga: A Scientific Evaluation*, which was as clinical as the title sounds. *The New Yorker* called it "an authoritative appraisal and description which seems more sensible than similar guides to infinity."

The various postures and breathing exercises, said Behanan, toned frayed nerves and weak "sex glands" and induced relaxation. He devoted a chapter to each, with photographs of Indian men demonstrating several of the more difficult poses and alternate-nostril breathing.

The odd thing was, for all his praise of the physical dimension of yoga, Behanan never mentioned Hatha Yoga by name, preferring the more generic *yoga*. Nor did he refer to any of Hatha Yoga's main scriptures, relying instead on Patanjali's *Yoga Sutras*, among the most psychological of yoga sources.[22]

Time dubbed Kuvalayananda "the most extraverted yogin to appear in centuries," and the publicity around Behanan's book briefly made him into something of a spokesperson for this more gymnastic yoga.[23]

Behanan had hit on something. He left out the supernatural and translated yoga into the language of modern, scientific psychology.[24]

In May, *Yoga: A Scientific Evaluation* sold record numbers in at least one town—Atlanta, Georgia. There, shoppers at Miller's Book Store and Davison-Paxon's Department Store put Behanan's study, along with Dale Carnegie's *How to Win Friends and Influence People*, on the best-seller list.[25]

When Theos returned to New York in November 1937, American syndicators plied him with offers for the rights to his story and photographs. These were the slow ones. Newsmen had already tracked him down in India, contracts at the ready.[26]

The New York Times ran an early account of his travels on its front page a few days after Thanksgiving. "Buddhist Worship in Tibet Pictured, Young Explorer Is Returning Tomorrow with Results of Five-Month Study." The story ran on to page two and included a photo of Theos looking like a clean-shaven, young professional.[27]

From Kalimpong, Theos had gone on to Gyantze, Tibet, in search of more teachers. Through all his travels in India, he felt he had met "some fine personalities" but no true masters of Tantra and had concluded that he'd find such men only in Tibet. That view was shared by many, even Indians, since centuries of colonization by the Moguls and then the British had driven Tantra underground in India, with many Tantric texts, which were often written on palm leaf, having been lost as well.[28]

Eventually, high government officials granted Theos permission to enter Lhasa and, even more unusually, their temples. His mission to learn all there was to know of yoga had taken an exhilarating and unexpected turn.

Theos the unknown scholar studying what looked to most of America like démodé occult practices quickly became Theos the heroic adventurer. The press made much of the weird feats he described and said little of his purpose for going to Tibet. While Theos would have preferred a more nuanced depiction of the religious rites he witnessed and even partook in, he himself had banked on and fanned the press's interest in his Tibetan material and decided any publicity he received would ultimately serve his larger project.

In fact, he had been courting the press before he left India. In Calcutta, he told a reporter for the *Daily Mail* that he was "the first White Lama—the first Westerner ever to live as a priest in a Tibetan monastery, the first man from the outside world to be initiated into Buddhists' mysteries hidden even from many native lamas themselves." This was quite an exaggeration. Theos had participated in religious rituals at Tibetan monasteries, and he had spoken with numerous Tibetan Buddhist lamas in his continuing research on Tantrik Yoga. But he had fabricated the "White Lama" bit. The *Daily Mail* went along anyway, pronouncing Theos's story "the greatest adventure story of the year."[29]

Once back in the States, Theos signed up with two American syndicators, North American Newspaper Alliance and the Bell Syndicates. They placed stories about Theos in small and large newspapers from coast to coast.[30]

The formula—dashing young hero, exotic lands, forbidding physical challenges—has stood the test of time. But there was an even greater interest in this kind of story upon Theos's return, not the least because the Depression had heightened Americans' appetite for transporting adventures set in distant lands. Publishers and radio stations eagerly invested in (or at least touted their wares as) "escape literature" and "escape music." The whole movie industry was geared to this market.

James Hilton's novel *Lost Horizon*, published in 1933, was *the* crowning example of the genre.

Hilton conjured "Shangri-La," a remote Himalayan valley that sheltered the secret of immortality and became synonymous with paradise. His antihero, Glory Conway, is kidnapped along with a few others and held captive in a lamasery. What Conway discovers, and ultimately risks his life for, is that the lamas have stopped time and attained great spiritual insight through a mix of yoga and other Eastern disciplines.

Near death in 1789, as the story went, Father Perrault "embarked upon a study of certain mystic practices that the Indians call *yoga*, and which are based upon various special methods of breathing." He lived another five years and continued his regimen, which kept him alive until Conway meets him, more than a century later, at his Himalayan lamasery.[31]

Against a backdrop of sheer cliffs, soaring peaks, pristine rivers, and exotic flora, *Lost Horizon* deftly played on Western notions of freedom and success.

A few years later, Frank Capra adapted the book for a motion picture, which was still in theaters when Theos disembarked from the *Queen Mary*. The film differed from the novel in one important regard: it didn't depict yoga or Buddhism, as Hilton's book did at least in passing; instead, the valley air, its peacefulness, and the lamas' devotion to quiet occupations, such as music, art, and philosophy, conferred immortality on anyone who stayed there.[32]

Unlike James Hilton, Theos had lived the story himself and documented it with color moving pictures. The connection was lost on no one. Whether or not the average American was interested in "Tibetan mysteries," more than likely she'd be curious about the discoverer of the "real Shangri-La."[33]

Still, there were some salient differences between the fictional and real Himalayan adventurers. Conway was a rootless and cynical World War I veteran, and Theos, an earnest, fresh-faced student. He also looked like a movie star, not a little like the then popular Tyrone Power.

For weeks, papers across the country ran stories about Theos and his travels in Tibet. Almost as soon as he learned of Theos, Maxwell Perkins, the Charles Scribner's Sons editor who was then one of the most powerful men in publishing, wanted to contract his first book, which would recount his time in Tibet. "I have gone through all your outline very carefully," he wrote Theos in January 1938, ". . . and I am very anxious to have a talk with you about the whole matter of the book. It is extremely interesting to me, and has great possiblities."[34]

Yet, during the months after his return, the public was missing the most remarkable part of the story: that Theos had survived his trek to Lhasa and back at all was a medical miracle.

When he had left for India, Theos had a pronounced cardiac murmur, valve lesions, and an enlarged heart. His condition, which doctors said made vigorous activity prohibitively dangerous, was a vestige of the rheumatic fever he had contracted as a college student.[35]

There was no cure for rheumatic fever when Theos contracted it, and if he lived, his doctors assured him he would be an invalid. Over a long convalescence, he claimed he began reading books on yoga in his mother's library and tentatively began trying out some of the instruction he could make sense of.[36]

In fact, it was probably in the summer of 1931, when Theos met up with his father in Los Angeles, that he first started to learn Hatha Yoga.

At that point, Theos hadn't seen Glen for two decades. He was only two years old when Glen left Theos's mother to raise her son in Tombstone, Arizona, and eventually to remarry there.

Once reunited, Glen taught his son much—from preliminary practices, to simple postures, to Hindu philosophy. From then on, Glen was Theos's guru, and Theos's loyalty to his father and his father's main passion, Tantrik Yoga, never flagged.[37]

The summer after he returned from Tibet and India, Theos visited his cardiologist, Dr. Raisbeck, who reported an interesting finding: Theos's enlarged heart was now nearly of normal size.[38]

Raisbeck was so impressed with the transformation a decade of yoga practice had wrought on Theos that he hooked him up to the electrocardiograph and asked him to slow down his pulse and heart rate, which Theos did using the breathing exercises (pranayama) he had long practiced. Raisbeck also borrowed some books on yoga from his patient. When he returned them, Raisbeck told Theos that he had decided to "attempt to do the exercises and evaluate the effects independently, incidentally making some study of the physiological changes."[39]

Raisbeck, a medical man, a man of science, was one of Theos's early and somewhat incidental converts to yoga. Another was Charles Lindbergh. Theos had met the aviator at a conference in Calcutta in March 1937 and interested him in pranayama.[40]

In the fall of 1938, Theos signed on with Colston & Leigh, Inc., Bureau of Lectures and Entertainments and began the first of several seasons touring the country.

These were not easy tours. Theos had a grueling schedule, traveling mostly from small town to small town and addressing Rotary Clubs and Women's Leagues. In each, he'd give an hour-long talk and, when technology permitted, show his film footage. He was indefatigable, though. Theos crisscrossed the country four times in six months, and he made a point of doing newspaper and radio interviews every place he went.[41]

NBC signed up Theos for a radio series shortly thereafter. According to the brochure sent out to advertisers in January 1939, his show had "tremendous 'escape' rewards" and Theos himself "commands the interest of advanced radio sponsors seeking a powerful approach to the mass-mind."[42]

Three months later, Charles Scribner's Sons published Theos's book on his five months in Tibet, *Penthouse of the Gods*. The book sold less than five thousand copies in the first year, but it enhanced Theos's authenticity. By the next tour season, the White Lama was addressing large venues, such as the Shrine Auditorium in Los Angeles and prestigious organizations such as the National Geographic Society in Washington, D.C.[43]

Publicly, Theos now fully embodied this new persona. He was a daring spiritual adventurer who sought wisdom in the most dangerous locales. He kept the focus on the Tibetan leg of his stay in the East, his initiation into secret Buddhist rituals, and the challenges of traveling in the Himalayas. There was no doubting Theos was physically rugged and knowledgeable about certain branches of Eastern religion. But as his reputation and celebrity grew, his personal life was falling apart.

He and Viola had divorced in the fall of 1938, their visions of the future totally incommensurate. Viola was on track to become a medical doctor; Theos wanted her to play the role De Vries had for Pierre Bernard, handmaiden to and homesteader for a new spiritual community focused around Tibetan Buddhism and Tantric Yoga. Viola also found some of Theos's Tantric Yoga practices offensive. These required that he regulate his sex life and that, when he and Viola did have intercourse, he retain his semen.[44]

Upon their divorce, Viola, who was exceedingly generous and still a little bit in love with Theos, had split the inheritance from her mother in half and set up a fifty-thousand-dollar trust fund in his name. Theos was allowed to draw out up to twenty-five hundred dollars per year, which helped underwrite his continued research into and practice of Tantric Yoga.[45]

His fame growing and his finances at least momentarily stabilized, Theos outed himself.

In August 1939, for the fourth time in a little over a year, *The Family Circle* magazine featured Theos on the cover. There he was, robed, bearded, and cross-legged, addressing the women passing through the checkout aisles in grocery stores in Cleveland, Detroit, and Los Angeles. "Now he tells about Yoga . . . and what he thinks it offers us who live in the nerve racking Western world of today. Would Yoga benefit *you*? See page 14," went the tagline, selling the discipline as if it were the latest diet or hand cream.

Theos was no longer an investigator and occasional participant in Tibetan Buddhist ceremonies. He was a Yogi, bringing Hatha Yoga to a mass audience.

Yoga was still a titillating subject, but *The Family Circle* seemed to think its audience—by and large younger housewives—could handle it, and a fairly detailed discussion of Hatha Yoga at that, illustrated with photos Theos had taken in India of Yogis assuming complex asanas and a drawing of the six main chakras, each represented by a lotus, aligned along the spine of a seated, mustached skeleton.

Flipping to the profile of Norma Shearer, a shopper in Piggly Wiggly or Safeway might innocently stumble on the first image of the subtle body ever printed in a mass-circulation magazine.[46]

The profile was a lead-up to Theos's second book, *Heaven Lies Within Us*. Perkins still believed in Theos and had contracted *Heaven Lies Within Us* as a popular book on yoga.[47]

The book Theos ended up writing recounted his experiences studying yoga in the Bengali jungle with a Tantric and Hatha Yoga master; it was in effect a prequel to *Penthouse of the Gods*.

As the story went, Theos had spent three months in an Indian ashram at some undisclosed location west of Calcutta. His quarters consisted of an adobe room with a thatched roof, which stayed surprisingly cool during the relentless midday heat.

Theos's daily routine at the ashram was even more intense than the one he later had at Kalimpong. He'd rise at 4:00 a.m. to do some of the yogic practices he had already learned in America. He began with Dhauti, swallowing a long piece of cloth to cleanse the stomach; followed by Netī, drawing water through the nose and then spitting it out of his mouth, then reversing the process; then fifteen minutes of stretching his tongue in preparation for Khecari, or "the swallowing of the tongue," an essential exercise in pranayama; then forty-five minutes of abdominal exercises (first Uḍḍiyāna, sucking the abdomen in so that your spine is nearly visible, then Naulī, in which you churn all of the abdominal muscles), then a thirty-minute headstand, and finally pranayama. He'd take lotus pose and do ten rounds of Bhastrika, inhaling slowly until he had fully expanded his stomach, forcefully exhaling through the nostrils, then inhaling and exhaling in rapid cycles, making "a noise which can be felt in the throat, chest, and head." Eventually, he worked up to Kumbhaka, in which he'd inhale through one nostril, then suspend his breath, fixing his gaze on the tip of his nose. The whole routine took him three hours.[48]

His guru had also been up since 4:00 a.m., and by the time he and Theos met up for breakfast, he had already done a half day's work. Discussions of yoga philosophy accompanied their leisurely morning meal. After a noonday rest, student and guru convened again to hammer out the points of philosophy or practice that confounded Theos.[49]

It was an ascetic lifestyle if modern America was your yardstick—there were no radios, moving pictures, or even magazines to read out in the jungle, nor were there cigarettes or liquor to drink. But by another measure, the setting was quite luxurious: Theos could devote every waking moment to his study of yoga; he need not prepare his own meals or even his bath (servants did that) or bother about any of the small details of daily life that so often consume it. And he had an expert in the subject all to himself.

At the end of his stay, he was initiated in a long ceremony, which began near midnight. (Though he noted that relatively speaking it has "probably less ritual to it than any other.") The purpose was to awaken Kundalini and "become aware of it."

He had spent several days preparing for this, fasting a full twenty-four hours beforehand. At the entrance of the temple where it would take place, he drew some shapes on the ground, a triangle inside a circle inside a square, and put a vessel with scented flowers in the center. He recited mantras and made different mudras (symbolic hand gestures). He then stepped inside the shrine and worshipped before the "presiding deity" (unnamed), sprinkled some holy water on the ground where he would be sitting, sat down next to his guru, recited another mantra, and lit incense, filling the place with the scent of sandalwood, saffron, and camphor.

After a few more preliminaries, he took lotus position (Padmāsana). After more purificatory gestures, he offered bhang—a narcotic made with hemp—to the deities before drinking the substance himself, then, after a few more rituals intended to create a protective (if symbolic) barrier around the initiate, Theos began an extended meditation while also performing pranayama.

According to his account, the ceremony had the intended effect and transported Theos to spiritual heights almost beyond description. All he could say was that he was engulfed in a light that grew brighter and brighter, its warm rays penetrating Theos's very being and vanquishing time.

(It's worth noting that throughout *Heaven Lies Within Us*, Theos presents each stage of Hatha Yoga, whether purifications such as Naulī, asanas, or pranayama, as a threshold to be crossed. Once he had perfected a particular technique, he'd abandon it and move on to another, more difficult one. All aimed at a single telos—achieving the kind of meditative state that overwhelmed him during this final initiation.)[50]

On parting, Theos's guru gave him two bits of advice. The first was to go to Tibet to learn more about Tantrik Yoga, and the second was to return to the West and "give an intellectual grasp of your realization for the candidates for humanity."[51]

For all the romance of India, which in Theos's hands is by turns splendid and sclerotic, Hatha Yoga instruction makes up the bulk of his second book. Outside of his half uncle's Red Book, it was the deepest and most accurate discussion of Hatha Yoga yet put out by an American publisher.

The only problem with the book was that Theos had fabricated the entire jungle retreat and many details of his Hatha Yoga training.

Theos had hired the novelist, poet, and critic John Cournos to help him edit *Penthouse of the Gods*. At Perkins's urging and likely with Cournos's help, Theos had penned dramatic opening and closing scenes for his first book. These were completely fictional, but the rest of *Penthouse of the Gods*, all 340 or so pages of it, hewed closely to Theos's journals.

Not so with *Heaven Lies Within Us*. Theos hadn't done any such retreat in the Bengali jungle. His father, Glen, had, however, studied with one Trivikram swami at his ashram in Bhurkunda (about four hundred kilometers west of Calcutta), before meeting up with Theos and Viola in 1936, and Glen had participated in a Tantric initiation in Calcutta.

In all likelihood, Theos appropriated Glen's experiences for his book.

He also altered the details of his own life story, suggesting that even in

America he had been instructed by an Indian guru, who would make sudden dramatic appearances.[52]

Theos had refused to name his Indian Tantric guru or the one who taught him in America. This despite tradition; most disciples are eager to name their gurus as this places them in a specific lineage and legitimates their own practice. So there was no way to check out Theos's story.[53]

No one caught the confabulation until recently (when his biographers were able to scan a cache of documents that had been in private hands for decades and eventually collected at the University of California, Berkeley).[54]

We'll never know why Theos fictionalized so much, but as a narrative device, the initiation had a couple of effects. For one, it turned Theos into a spiritual hero who had conquered his own mind and body. For another, it made the sacrifices Hatha Yoga demanded—after all, on his fictive retreat, Theos gave up almost every accoutrement of modern American life—seem worth it.

Due to the softening market, Scribner's printed only 2,455 copies of *Heaven Lies Within Us* and never printed a second edition.[55]

Still, the book piqued some interest in yoga. By the holiday season of 1939, a good number of readers had expressed interest in instruction from Theos. He'd politely reply to each of them, directing them to his upcoming correspondence course (there's no record that he ever set up such a course).[56]

Given his expertise, Theos also received his share of odd letters. Mrs. Carrie Horne wanted to know if he "took pupils for developing their clairvoyance and if so what are your charges?" She claimed this power came to her "spontaneously" and sought help controlling it. Theos, who was diligent about replying to fan mail, suggested that in the course of a "sincere study of the Truth . . . those things which had seemed unusual become natural." Theos clearly believed that yoga developed psychic powers (or siddhis) and didn't take Ms. Horne for a crackpot as many another author might. As for helping her, he mentioned his upcoming correspondence course and promised to keep her name on file.[57]

He had a similar response to Esther Hankins, who had had some sort of spiritual awakening in part by following Bernarr Macfadden's diet advice. This was proof, after a fashion, of Theos's contention that in transforming matter you can't help but affect the "vital forces." However, since then Esther had married and had children and had abandoned these practices. "It is ever before me," she wrote Theos, "to return to raw foods and milk and fasting" (a diet similar to the one Theos had followed during his fictive yoga studies in India). ". . . I want to return to that glorious state of detachment, but how can I do it with a family?"[58]

It was a good question, one that Theos skirted most of his life. How does one take the time required to follow Theos's yoga program (he claims he'd spend hours in just a headstand) given the daily responsibilities of caring for a family or earning a living?

For the American housewives reading *The Family Circle* or the businessmen attending his lecture at the Commerce Club in Chicago, accepting that yoga could benefit you was only the first and, some might say, lowest hurdle.

Occasionally someone would write Theos who seemed to have read far more in his books than he may have meant to convey, and in one notable case to have pinpointed all of the contradictions inherent in his plan to bring yoga to the ordinary American. Mary Wilkeson described *Penthouse of the Gods* as a polyglot colloquy of the dead, "one voice disagreeing with another, one impatient of religion, another deeply, truly, absorbed in that, and in nothing else."[59]

This was another problem yoga posed to Americans. Born of a culture in which every act is part of a sacred system, in which man embodies and reflects the universe, and creation is variously figured as the lovemaking of Shiva and Shakti or Brahma's fitful dream, yoga was difficult to unhinge from religion.

And Theos only partly wanted to. In both the real and imagined accounts of his travels in India and Tibet, it was Theos's participation in "sacred rites," down to the last detail—twenty-four hours of fasting beforehand, dressing in special robes, chanting specific mantras, imbibing certain substances—that yielded his spiritual ecstasies.

Much as he might suggest substituting "electricity" for various deities as a more appropriate symbol or insist that you need not travel to India to practice it, the yoga Theos offered on the *Hobby Lobby* radio program seemed a paler version than the one he purported to have learned in the Bengali jungle and the one he had in fact tasted on the Tibetan plateau.[60]

In his own home, he built an elaborate shrine and his meditations retained as many of the particulars as he could muster nine thousand miles from his Tibetan teachers, which suggests that the rituals he downplayed publicly were not mere theater. They might even be necessary for yoga to work.

The Hotel Pierre, set along the southernmost tip of Central Park on Manhattan's Fifth Avenue, was a paradox in brick and steel. Schultze & Weaver had designed the hotel, and like its siblings—the Los Angeles Biltmore and the Breakers in Palm Beach—the Pierre embodied Jazz Age luxury. Its neo-Georgian structure soared forty-two stories into the air. The seven hundred suites ranged in size from a single room to ten rooms. There was a dining room, a basement grillroom, and three ballrooms, and guests could dance over more than four thousand square feet of polished maple in the largest of them.[61]

Luxurious as it was, two years after its opening in 1930, the Hotel Pierre went bankrupt. Oil magnate J. P. Getty purchased it in 1938.[62]

Designed as an entertainment complex, the Hotel Pierre was also a hive of social activity for the wealthy and "devastatingly chic," as an advertisement for Macy's put it. On any given week you might be able to attend lecture series, luncheons, fashion shows, benefits, club meetings, or a wedding. Some of these functions, such as the series "New Perspectives on Opera," produced by the Metropolitan Opera Guild, were broadcast directly from its lavish rooms.[63]

In the heart of this grandeur, Theos launched the American Institute of Yoga and the Pierre Health Studios. Classes began in the fall of 1939 and took place in suites 402–7.

Course offerings were extensive, covering the applied philosophy of yoga, seminars on Hatha Yoga, weekly lectures by Theos himself, guest lectures, a library, reading courses, and an Open Forum (presumably modeled on Pierre Bernard's successful program of the same name). Those wanting more personalized attention could make an appointment for a private consultation or a psychophysical analysis. And this didn't encompass the Pierre Health Studios offerings, billed as nothing short of complete "physical re-education, adapting the Science of Breath and the corrective postures of Yoga to modern needs."

To pull this off, Theos had teamed up with Claire Lea Stuart. Claire had been a member of Pierre Bernard's "inner circle" two decades before and was teaching at De Vries's yoga studio on Fifty-seventh Street when Theos set up the American Institute of Yoga. Claire, officially the "assistant director of Pierre Health Studios," did most of the physical instruction.

Glen helped out too, manning the front desk and assisting with research, which turned out to be a particular boon.[64]

Before he set up his own yoga school, Theos had already developed a small but lucrative business in private yoga lessons. He had conceived of the American Institute of Yoga and Pierre Health Studios as a profit center.[65]

Not surprisingly, classes there were pricey.

For steady students, eight one-hour lessons a month cost twenty dollars, a slight discount off the regular price (about three dollars per class). Twelve one-hour private lessons would set you back one hundred dollars (more than fifteen hundred in today's dollars). And those interested in Hatha Yoga instruction by Theos himself would have to part with double that rate.[66]

This wasn't much of a deterrent.

Theos had a full teaching schedule, and his students included professionals and housewives, the young and middle-aged, men and women. Mrs. Wilfred J. Donovan, wife of the vice president of Abercrombie & Fitch, and Ganna Walska, a middle-class Polish émigré who had amassed fame and great fortune by marrying a succession of extremely wealthy men, were just two of the socially prominent women who took classes at the Pierre Health Studios.[67]

As his course offerings suggest, Theos didn't take many shortcuts in explaining yoga. Like his uncle, his father, and many others, he believed yoga was nothing short of a science of life and refused to reduce the discipline to one of its constituent parts.

Instead, he'd circle around his subject, explaining it from every possible vantage point in the hopes of capturing a little of its richness.

All types of yoga, he'd say, allow the individual to gain control of her own energies and tap into the universal storehouse of this power, as if the average person were a malfunctioning engine, overheated and underpowered.

Such a tantalizing idea—that yoga provided an inexhaustible well of energy—might also pique interest in his detailed and technical discussion of the subtle body. After all, to delve into the ideas behind yoga is to delve into a highly detailed, densely coded world, and Americans had to have good reason to bother.[68]

Theos was introducing his students to some of the most up-to-date research by Western Indologists on this very topic.

Glen had got hold of an unpublished copy of the Jung-Hauer lectures on Kundalini yoga, given in 1932 but not widely published in English for more than forty years. From these, and Woodroffe's translation of the Ṣaṭ-cakra-nirūpaṇa (included in *The Serpent Power*), Glen and Theos produced a series of lectures on the subtle body and Kundalini—the energy the Hatha Yoga practitioner must "awaken" and raise through the central channel to gain real spiritual insight and, ultimately, liberation—as well as a poster-size version of Woodroffe's illustration of the six chakras and their locations.[69]

Among Theos's lecture notes from this period is perhaps the clearest explanation of the subtle body and its relation to human anatomy. Vivekananda was so eager to translate yoga into Western terminology, he overstated the correspondence between the chakras and "nerve centers" or plexuses in the body and referred to the sixth chakra as the "pineal gland" as if these were interchangeable.[70]

Theos on the other hand was skeptical of Western science and felt Americans had become too reliant on this mode of inquiry. As a result, he was far more cautious about applying scientific terminology to yoga. "To-date [*sic*] it has been impossible for science to physiologically locate these chakras," he wrote in his lecture notes for his series "The Psychological Basis of Yoga." "They are known only through the instrumentality of the sixth sense, the mind, and this [is] accomplished only by means of Yoga."[71]

Yoga, according to Theos, was also the way to make "man a more perfect instrument through which consciousness can flow." Notice how he makes no mention of divinity or God. Notice too how the word *consciousness* skirts those pesky dichotomies between mind and body, vital forces and matter.

This wasn't all. If mastered, Theos told his listeners, Hatha Yoga allowed you to "extract the spiritual essence out of every circumstance in life" the way the lotus flower extracts nutrients from the muck "without being touched or tainted by it."[72]

The Yogi, Theos elaborated in another lecture, "can hear without using ears and see without using eyes." He enters the "inner world, leaving behind the mind" and "the world of name and form." Once he does that, "the Yogi is no longer concerned with what happens to him; he will never again experience confusion and frustration."[73]

Whichever way he formulated the effects of yoga, Theos staunchly advocated Hatha Yoga for modern Americans. In the age of the Kali Yuga, which began after Krishna's death five thousand years ago and continues for billions more years, he argued, humans needed something more powerful than meditation, mantras, or devotion alone. They needed the force, intensity, and physicality of Hatha Yoga to arouse Kundalini. The Tantras insisted on this, and Theos, despite his avowals of skepticism, took the scriptures quite seriously.[74]

This way of looking at Hatha Yoga had an appealing logic. As Theos put it, matter is inseparable from energy, and if you transform your body, you can't help but transform your "vital forces."[75]

Yoga healed the dualism that plagues us, the dread and, in many, deeply held conviction that our bodies doom us to sin. Not only did Hatha Yoga, and Theos, see the body as a decent vehicle for transcendence, it's the only one we in Kali Yuga have.

"Control of the body leads to control of the mind," he wrote in lecture notes dated May 1, 1940. "If the timid man imitates the gestures of a brave man, he will actually begin to feel courage."[76]

Theos made this point most concretely through his demonstrations. In some lectures he'd take up to seven or eight poses. To see him fold his body into the more complicated among them—Matsyāsana (fish pose) or Dhanurāsana (bow pose, a back bend)—was to witness a sublime level of mastery. You need not believe that one's own Kundalini must be awakened to imagine how much better you might feel if you could do that!

But Theos never suggested that even the grossest levels of Hatha Yoga came easily. He advised students that to be effective, headstands should be held for twenty-four minutes and felt that one should "develop asanas to the point they can be held for three hours." He also offered a "Full Course in Yogic Physical Culture for an Average Man of Health," a two-hour routine that entailed various postures and breathing exercises.[77]

Yet Theos firmly discouraged Claire from making too much of the postures in front of certain audiences. He felt this dimension of Hatha Yoga would deter otherwise interested students.[78]

Teaching yoga was much like teaching someone to play the violin. The result is seductive enough: Who wouldn't want to be able to play a Bach concerto with ease? The trouble was keeping your students interested despite the daunting effort required to learn enough to play well.

Sometimes it was better to rein in ambitions and simply direct his students to those aspects of the practice that suited their abilities. Better to play a recorder well than a violin badly.

Or, as Theos liked to say, "If a man is a jackass, let him be a good jackass, and not pretend to be a thorough-bred racer, excusing his failings on the grounds of a lame foot."[79]

Despite a strong start, the Pierre Health Studios operated for less than two years. A suit against yoga teachers Theos Bernard and Claire Stuart brought by Wilfred J. Donovan, vice president of Abercrombie & Fitch, in the spring of 1940 marked the beginning of the end.

Donovan's tale of woe, gleefully reported in the *Daily News* and elsewhere, echoed the dreadful stories Mabel Daggett had related in 1911. His wife, Nina, had been in a psychopathic condition when she was first introduced to Theos and Claire in 1938. Theos had told the ill woman that he had "spiritual powers" that could help her but instead drove her to complete mental derangement and institutionalization. Donovan also accused Theos and Claire of defrauding him and his wife of "large sums of money and personal property." He sought twenty-five thousand dollars in damages.[80]

Theos and Claire eventually settled out of court for a much smaller, though still princely, sum—five thousand dollars (more than seventy thousand in today's dollars).[81]

Not long after, Theos shuttered the Pierre Health Studios. Claire went out to Los Angeles to join her mother and brother, and Theos accompanied his student Ganna Walska, a striking woman with porcelain skin, thick, dark hair, and fantastic wealth, more than twenty years his senior, to Santa Barbara. Walska had made a protracted attempt to sing professionally, for which she had mercilessly been derided by the press, and during her stay in Southern California, she consulted with yet another voice teacher. Theos had promised yoga could help.[82]

In July 1942, the two married. When the tabloids eventually got wind of Theos and Ganna's relationship, Hearst's *American Weekly* (a Sunday newspaper supplement with a circulation of 50 million) reported that "Ganna Walska, the would-be-grand opera star whose vain, 25-year assault on the citadel of musical fame forms one of the most bizarre dramas of modern times has at long last found consolation for her blighted career. . . . She has found it in Yoga as preached by a fabulous and very handsome young American named Theos Bernard." The full-page story was headlined "Disappointed Diva Yodeling Now with a Yogi."[83]

For Theos, this was clearly a marriage of convenience; almost as soon as they were involved, Walska began to subsidize his life's work, which included completing his dissertation for Columbia, lecturing on Tantra, and, with the help of his father, Glen, building an academy of Tibetan literature based in Santa Barbara.[84]

After more than a year in California, Theos returned to New York City. There, in his second wife's town house, he held a series of evening talks on yoga.

The first night of his lecture series, the parlor was crammed to standing room only, and people happily sat on the stairs. The next day, he received numerous calls from students who wanted to bring their friends. He encouraged anyone sincerely interested to come.

Theos had also deduced, through polite inquiries, that many were concerned he would be spirited away any moment to serve overseas. He laid this worry to rest; his heart condition made him 4F despite his obvious physical vitality.

Since he didn't have much choice about it, he rationalized that teaching yoga was his contribution to the war effort. "It doesn't rob you of anything, it doesn't require you to give up anything . . . ," he offered. "It gives you a certain strength and understanding, and the ability to adjust and adapt to any condition that might come to pass."

That fall evening and for the rest of the series, he ended his classes early, at 10:30 p.m., because of gasoline rationing and the frequent blackouts.[85]

The war affected every aspect of American life, and despite his being spared the horrors of combat, it necessarily checked many of Theos's ambitions, at least temporarily.

He had to abandon his plans to create an academy of Tibetan literature in Santa Barbara. The lamas he had invited to help translate key scriptures in the Tibetan Buddhist cannon and teach yoga philosophy got stuck waiting for visas in Darjeeling, India, when hostilities broke out in Asia.

And wartime paper rationing cut into the distribution of his work.[86]

Theos completed his dissertation by the spring of 1943. (That June, he was the first to receive a Ph.D. in religion from Columbia University.)

Titled *Haṭha Yoga: The Report of a Personal Experience*, this work was in fact a much more technical and *less* personal presentation of his fabricated Hatha Yoga studies in India. Although the preface referenced the fictional retreat Theos had detailed in *Heaven Lies Within Us*, the bulk of his dissertation was a "practical commentary" on the *Hatha Yoga Pradīpikā* with generous citations of the two other main Hatha Yoga scriptures, the *Gheranda Samhitā*, and *Shiva Samhitā*, as well as the work of John Woodroffe/Arthur Avalon.[87]

The most personal elements of his dissertation were the photographs of a slim Theos, dressed in white swimming trunks, performing various asanas. These were among the first published photographs of an American in yoga postures. It was almost startling to see Theos's white limbs folded up over each other, his ruggedly handsome face expressing intense detachment.

As part of the requirements for his doctorate, Theos had to publish one hundred copies of his dissertation and file them with the philosophy department at Columbia. Ganna Walska covered the costs, and in 1944 Columbia University printed five hundred copies of *Hatha Yoga* and, surprisingly, sold out all four hundred of the extra copies.

The book was such a success, Columbia University Press decided to reprint *Hatha Yoga* and recommended turning it into a trade publication, which meant printing one thousand copies and distributing these to bookstores. Paper was so scarce though, they could muster only another 390 copies, and this after months of waiting for supplies.

By the mid-1940s, Theos's campaign to popularize Hatha Yoga—to bring it to the average man—was only a partial success.

His most authoritative book on the subject could reach only the tiniest audience.

And he had only just begun to make this knowledge accessible to novices. Even *Heaven Lies Within Us*, which was geared toward a general audience, lists seventeen possible definitions for yoga and insists that any yoga student must be able to retain his breath in Kumbhaka for at least six minutes before he can begin to learn meditation.[88]

When Theos did simplify Hatha Yoga further, he didn't really make learning it easier. If pressed, he'd say only three practices were absolutely necessary for spiritual advancement: Padmasana (lotus position), Uḍḍiyāna, and pranayama. However, Uḍḍiyāna itself is a demanding technique. To master it, Theos stood, knees bent, hands on thighs, and exhaled so completely that his abdominal muscles vigorously contracted along with the back muscles along his spine. When he ran out of oxygen, he'd relax his muscles. At first, he repeated Uddiyana ten or fifteen times. He claims that he then built up to ten rounds of ten a day. Eventually, he was able to reach his goal of fifteen hundred per day![89]

Distilling Hatha Yoga down to these three practices was a bit like telling someone she can become a doctor merely by studying organic chemistry, molecular biology, and brain surgery. You may have reduced the number of tasks to master, but not their difficulty.

Yoga took hard work, and Theos usually was too devoted a practitioner and too guileless a speaker to say otherwise. At times he seemed to relish this aspect of the discipline, his audience be damned, reminding his listeners at the end of an inspiring talk they had to be willing to "pay the price" for yoga knowledge.[90]

Temperament partly explains Theos's insistence on the completeness and complexity of yoga. He was earnest, ambitious, and proud. He wanted to render this body of knowledge, which encompassed Hatha Yoga and huge swaths of Tibetan Buddhism, in English with as much exactitude as possible.

Again and again, he'd sacrifice clarity and brevity for veracity.

Sometimes this impulse to convey the truest version of yoga he could muster left him, quite literally, at a loss for words: "Hat means sun, Ta means moon. Then they will tell you it is a joining of the sun and the moon. Then they tell you something to make it more mysterious, and they don't make sense, I know. They left me dizzy," he confessed in one of his lectures. "I couldn't figure it out, but when you come down to it, it does make sense and when you understand it completely there is no way of expressin [sic] it in our language because we have no terms for it."[91]

Theos didn't teach in a vacuum, though. His half uncle's career was an object lesson in the hazards of yoga in America. He disdained Pierre Bernard's "bread and circuses," and he wanted to steer well clear of the ceaseless gawking and outright derision, the multiple legal entanglements and questionable business dealings, that had plagued Pierre and his club. Yet Theos shared many aspects of his uncle's vision: to create a center for the in-depth study of Tantrik Yoga and now Tibetan Buddhism, and to have enough personal wealth to pursue his own study and practice unimpeded.

(When Theos first met Viola, he even imagined himself the rightful heir to C.C.C.; however, by 1937, the couple had resigned, partly to protest Pierre's ill-treatment of De Vries.)

Scholarship (or at least real credentials) was Theos's best defense against his uncle's fate as well as the legions of misconceptions about yoga and yoga teachers.

"Lots of people call me up on the telephone and tell me they have got Kundalini up this high and if I'll just tell them a mantra they will be alright," Theos reported to a rapt audience during one of his New York lectures. "But it doesn't work that way."[92]

Perhaps the most damning view of yoga during wartime was the belief that the discipline demanded a complete abdication of responsibilities. This was not at all the case, according to Theos; learning yoga was no more selfish than learning any other new skill.[93]

Theos also challenged the notion that to practice yoga was to sign up for a life of austerity and self-denial, something Americans had had more than enough of by the early 1940s.

The Yogi, Theos averred, sounding almost exactly like Pierre Bernard, can eat and drink and have "sex relations" to his heart's content. The difference, Theos pointed out, between him and the average man is that the Yogi has a sense of his limits and won't exceed them, whereas most of us wear ourselves down in pursuit of pleasure.[94]

(Theos also admitted that "sex was the closest thing in the physical world to spiritual realization.")

Another stereotype, lately personified by Kuda Bux, was that Yogis possessed magical powers. Bux certainly did. He could read blindfolded and could walk through fire in his bare feet, feats tested by scientists in the 1930s and 1940s. Bux, who came from northwest India, what's now Pakistan, claimed that anyone could learn to read blindfolded. All it took was a highly developed power of concentration.[95]

One particularly persistent misconception, which dated at least to Vivekananda's first visit, was that Hatha Yoga amounted to little more than acrobatics.

Lately, the headstand had displaced levitation as the favored shorthand for the discipline. In one particularly representative cartoon published in *The New Yorker*, a plump woman is simultaneously doing a headstand—with legs crossed in lotus position no less!—and reading a book titled *Yoga Explained*.[96]

From one vantage point, this was progress. Here was a fully secular view of yoga. There was nothing supernatural about it now, and little sign of Shiva and Krishna, who never failed to put someone out. The discipline could be and was classed alongside Macfadden's physical culture and other health fads.

People such as Dr. Josephine L. Rathbone saw great potential in this new understanding of the discipline. In the spring of 1940, she taught a class, Art of Relaxation, at Columbia's Teachers College, in which she combined yoga techniques "with American standbys for taking it easy." (She also had a small clinic to help the nonstudent with the same task.)[97]

Rathbone, an instructor in physical education, had traveled in India and sponsored demonstrations of yoga asanas at Columbia University. Bishnu Chandra Ghosh, Paramahansa Yogananda's younger brother, with whom Theos was acquainted, executed the poses to amazed audiences. In her course, Rathbone subordinated yoga to her broader goal of alleviating a variety of disorders, such as heart disease, neuritis, indigestions, and insomnia, which were caused, in her view, by the era's pathological level of tension.[98]

Take away Krishna and Shiva, take away chanting and mantras, take away its cosmology, take away its philosophical underpinnings—from Sāmkhya to neo-Vedanta—and you'd have a yoga, as Rathbone found, that garnered university support and sage nods from busy and likely tense reporters.

But it's a view of yoga so devoid of transcendence that Theos and countless other teachers have had to labor to restore its spiritual import.[99]

Worse than such misconceptions about the discipline, which after all were concrete enough for Theos to at least address, was the stink of impropriety that still clung to every type of yoga.

Katherine Mayo and her *Mother India* haunted Theos's lectures. ("Many of you have probably read this book by a woman called Mayo," he offered in a lecture in the fall of 1942. ". . . There was another superficial presentation of a culture.")[100]

A few years later, when his marriage to Ganna Walska fell apart, Theos faced even more direct censure. Sensing that Ganna wouldn't tolerate him much longer, Theos had sued for divorce first. Ganna countersued. The papers quickly picked up the story.

The coverage of Ganna had long been derisive. Theos fared no better, and in many ways worse, as details of their relationship came to light. One particularly pointed headline read "He Can't Work but He Stands on His Head for 3 Hours." Theos came off as a duplicitous and callous fellow who was incapable of supporting himself despite his obvious physical vigor.[101]

Would Americans ever be able to distinguish between a teacher and a charlatan, between receptive student and hapless victim, between spiritual discipline and self-delusion?

Much as he might have wished to, Theos couldn't blame the tabloids for his predicament. Nor was he a casualty of self-appointed moral guardians, such as Mabel Daggett earlier in the century, who had yet to accept yoga as a legitimate American pastime.

He had exploited Ganna and her wealth to realize his original dream to create an institute for the study and practice of Tibetan Buddhism and Hatha Yoga; he had lied to her about any number of things, including the identity of his father; and he had cheated on her (an affair that led to his third marriage). In the short term, Theos had done no more good for yoga than his uncle had.

7

MARGARET WOODROW WILSON
"TURNS HINDU"

Shortly after the Donovan suit against Theos had made news, a Japanese-American architect and woodworker by the name of George Nakashima told the AP newswire that Margaret Woodrow Wilson, eldest daughter of the twenty-eighth president, had "found peace" at a religious colony in Pondicherry, a seaside town on the southeastern coast of India. Nakashima was a credible witness. He had spent two years building dormitories for the ashram and had arrived there about the same time as Margaret.[1]

Much like Chelsea Clinton half a century later, Margaret retained an air of royalty, and even some of its trappings, long after her father had left office. She had had a brief career as a vocalist, spent endless energy on various causes (the Community School Movement was one of her favorites), and had tried her hand at bond trading and advertising before slipping from public view in the mid-1920s.

Recently, according to Nakashima, Margaret had joined Sri Aurobindo's colony and planned "never to return to the outside world."[2]

Early reports didn't go into much detail about ashram life or Aurobindo (though *The New York Times* noted he was a graduate of Cambridge University). All Nakashima managed to convey was that Aurobindo's disciples kept themselves busy. They "wear white robes and let their hair and beards grow," said Nakashima, but contrary to what you might think, these devout folks "live full lives," mostly studying various unspecified arts.

The Washington Post, which had avidly tracked Margaret's every move during her father's two terms, printed the story under the headline "Daughter of Wilson Turns Hindu."[3]

The most striking feature of the story, if true, was the suggestion that Margaret, who was then fifty-four, had chucked it all for a foreign faith.

This is almost exactly what she had done. Yoga had become as much a vocation for Margaret as it was for Theos Bernard, and she had gone to India to pursue it under the guidance of the one man she felt qualified to supervise her spiritual awakening.[4]

Beyond their commitment to yoga, the two could hardly have been more different. Theos was young, handsome, and brashly confident. Margaret bore a striking resemblance to her father (and had his lantern jaw, close-set eyes, and prominent nose), was in middle age by the time she traveled to India, and was forever denigrating her own abilities.

Theos had married twice and was always getting mixed up with women. Margaret had few romances and never married.

Theos courted celebrity, and Margaret had fame thrust upon her.[5]

Theos mastered Hatha Yoga's most challenging postures and breathing exercises; his route to transcendence was through his own body. Margaret vanquished only inner demons, was in slowly failing health, and favored meditation over any other yoga technique.

Theos profited from yoga (though his spending always outpaced his income); Margaret ultimately consigned what little wealth she had to Aurobindo and his ashram.

Perhaps most important, Theos will be remembered for what he did for yoga, particularly Hatha Yoga, while Margaret, if she's remembered at all, will be remembered for what yoga did to *her*.

Margaret had first picked up Aurobindo's *Essays on the Gita* in the New York Public Library in 1932. She had come across an intriguing reference to Aurobindo in Romain Rolland's *Prophets of the New India*. Reading Aurobindo's *Essays* under the vaulted wood ceiling, she so completely lost track of the time, at closing the guards nearly had to throw her out.[6]

The *Essays* are voluminous and dense and pointedly challenge modern interpretations of the *Gita*. But Aurobindo didn't limit himself to Krishna's message. He reworked the very fundamentals of Indic philosophy, specifically the notion of life as samsara—that cosmic merry-go-round Yogis strive to get off of. Life, according to Aurobindo, represents "a progressive evolution of the soul" through successive phases until "it reaches the complete revelation of Sachidananda [bliss]."[7]

In this schema, developed through essays, books, and an epic poem,

Savitri, man was the penultimate life-form in an evolutionary process that would end when Supramental beings (a race of "gnostic" supermen) roamed the earth. Except, unlike the blind chance of natural selection, men and women could aid in this process, transforming themselves into channels for the divine by practicing his brand of yoga.[8]

As for his method, Aurobindo rejected most techniques, including those practices Theos found essential, as incomplete or superfluous.

He acknowledged the need for intermediaries with the Divine. Krishna or Buddha or Shiva—and the guru—were all fine and even necessary tools for awakening. Concentrating one's mental energy via meditation was also useful.[9]

But by the 1930s, Aurobindo laid the most stress on a sort of passive opening to God's pull.[10]

This antimethodology worked well for Margaret. Born in 1886, she came from a long line of believers. Both grandfathers were Presbyterian ministers, and both parents were religious. (She believed her father "approached seership" and was guided by spiritual intuition.)[11]

Like them, Margaret abided in the nearness and reality of God. However, she couldn't countenance church. As a young girl, she walked out during the middle of Communion and never went back.[12]

According to one friend, Margaret was a sort of spiritual rebel, defying God in order to "make of the shoddy materials of human existence something finer than he seems to intend."[13]

She was also prone to rapturous experiences of nature such as being swallowed up by a beautiful sunset.[14]

But not until Margaret was well into adulthood, around the time of her father's death in 1924, did she encounter yoga. First, a lover, who was an avowed Theosophist, took it upon himself to supervise Margaret's "awakening into bliss."[15]

Not long after, Josephine Macleod, Sara Bull's traveling companion in India, introduced Margaret to the neo-Vedanta swamis then in New York.[16]

Over time, Margaret was drawn toward yoga.

By 1929, she craved only "the Realization of God consciousness" and did "not really care about anything else."[17]

In the early thirties, she began studying with Swami Nikhilananda, a direct disciple of Ramakrishna's wife, Sarada Devi.

The Vedanta Society and its offshoots still dominated the field in yoga instruction, particularly on the East Coast. Nikhilananda had opened the Ramakrishna-Vivekananda Center in New York on Manhattan's West Fifty-seventh Street in 1933, and Swami Bodhananda was still teaching at the Vedanta Society on West Seventy-first Street.

These swamis had relatively little competition, in part because of a particularly painful moment in American immigration history. At the turn of the century, union leaders on the West Coast had formed the Japanese and Korean Exclusion League to, in their heated rhetoric, "help drive out cheap labor" by curtailing Asian immigration. By 1907 the organization had renamed itself the more inclusive Asiatic Exclusion League (AEL) and had begun to target Indian immigrants. Fewer than twenty-five hundred Indians had settled in the United States at the time.[18]

Eventually, the AEL's persistent lobbying—combined with wartime geopolitics—swayed Congress. In its immigration bill of 1917, lawmakers included India in a barred zone designed to keep Asians out. The bill passed over President Wilson's veto. For the next half century, few Indian yoga teachers would visit the United States, and even fewer would stay.[19]

Despite her work with Swami Nikhilananda, Margaret was still leery of committing to any American school or teacher. By nature, she was fiercely independent. ("Margaret had her own ideas," as her sister Eleanor put it, "and seldom asked for advice.") She didn't submit to authority easily or lightly.[20]

Somehow Aurobindo and his Integral Yoga swept aside her earlier hesitations and resistance.

After enlisting Swami Nikhilananda to help her make sense of Aurobindo's work, she began a correspondence with the "Master," as Aurobindo was then known. "The longing for liberation and union with the Highest is obsessing me," she confided in her first letter to him, "and I want it to deepen until there is no other desire left."[21]

In another letter sent sometime in 1936, she requested permission to visit Aurobindo's ashram.

He refused her initial request, coming up with a number of reasons— she was ill, the South Indian heat was unbearable, she'd benefit more from a visit after she had "gone some way in the path." (Margaret did suffer from arthritis, among other maladies.)

Still, he encouraged her in other ways. He outlined the first steps in turning her desire for realization into "spiritual experience," which was to meditate on the heart—the "cardiac centre in the middle of the chest"—or the head, in the "mental centre," or to offer "all activities to the Divine."[22]

In the winter of 1937 representatives of Aurobindo's ashram contacted Margaret. They didn't proffer the invitation to visit she'd had her heart set on. The ashram needed to raise money to pay for construction of additional dormitories, the ones Nakashima eventually helped build, to house Aurobindo's swelling ranks of sadhaks. Nolini Gupta, on behalf of the ashram, solicited Margaret; he hoped her connections (and possibly capital) could aid their cause.[23]

Margaret, however, wasn't a wealthy woman. She had a modest income—a twenty-five-hundred-dollar annuity left by her father (about thirty-four thousand dollars in today's dollars)—and relatively few expenses. She had also inherited another two thousand dollars from an uncle.

Sometime in 1937 she used half of this legacy to purchase a small parcel of land in western Connecticut. She described her eight acres as a "lovesome spot," where two meadow hills met in a hollow, surrounded by woods.

Margaret planned to build a yoga retreat for herself there.[24]

She felt New York City was not conducive to the practice of yoga. Her preference was to travel to Pondicherry and study with Aurobindo, but Margaret wasn't content to wait for that day, whenever it arrived, to make the outer reality of her life match the inner one.

By 1937, after a dozen years spent "mulling" over the discipline and a few studying Integral Yoga intently, Margaret felt her entire life now flowed from the practice. "Indeed, if I were told that I had no call to Yoga I should be without any mainspring in my life now," she had written her friend Lois Roth Kellog. "Don't you feel that way too. Once given a glimpse of this Goal how can one have any other afterwards?"[25]

Such dedication was bolstered by powerful new experiences; through her meditations, Margaret was having regular brushes with a different sort of consciousness. She felt truly alive only during the two or three hours a day that she meditated.[26]

Yet she lacked even a rudimentary vocabulary to talk about what she saw and felt.

Putting the experience into words was all the more difficult because thoughts seemed to get in the way. Theos once described these deeper, inner experiences as "beyond the mind."[27]

In an attempt to capture even a fraction of what she felt, Margaret would jot her impressions down right after meditations. It was a bit like watching "a moving picture very clear while I witness and understand," or "a spring uncovered that bubbles up in a fountain of joy which at the same time seems to be a play of light in my understanding making clear many things that have been dark."

For her, as for Theos, this seeing in a new way was blissful, energizing—and addictive.

She became impatient to remove the veils she believed covered her consciousness and even more determined to go to India, her "Mecca," as she put it.[28]

Fortunately, in the spring of 1938, Margaret received an invitation to visit Aurobindo's ashram before she had spent the last one thousand dollars of her inheritance. That amount covered the price of a round-trip ticket to India by ship almost to the penny.

Margaret was advised to bring simple cotton dresses, light underwear, a sun umbrella, and light canvas shoes and was promised that many American products, such as tinned fruits and vegetables, would be available in the market near the ashram.[29]

When Margaret finally did set sail for the subcontinent on September 6, 1938, not a single reporter was on the docks to record her departure. Her plan, which she confided to only a few sympathetic friends, was to "be gone as long as the Spirit keeps me in India."[30]

To most of her peers, Margaret had made an inconceivable bargain: she had traded a reasonably comfortable life for an alien faith and an impoverished country.

More recently, at least one historian has read in Margaret's departure failure and disappointment.

This telling of her life begins with her spinsterhood.

Though she had several suitors, Margaret never married (this being figured as the first disappointment). Instead, she sought a career. She trained as a vocalist with high hopes for singing professionally. During the

Great War, she gave concerts on behalf of the YMCA and Red Cross and was anointed America's "First Daughter." In Europe, she sang for the troops on the Western Front. (Fortunately for the president, she arrived just a few days before the armistice.)[31]

But the cold and damp and ceaseless performances damaged her vocal cords, and no amount of rest and rehabilitation would heal them.

This was the second disappointment.

She had also dedicated herself to reform work, throwing most of her energies into the community-center movement, which tried to knit together social bonds that industrialization had begun to unravel.

During her father's two terms in the White House, Margaret had dedicated herself to social reform with such ferocity that congressmen frequently objected to her "stirring up unrest among the lower classes." In response she'd scold *them*.[32]

But by the mid-1920s, her reform work had also petered out. She briefly tried advertising and trading bonds. Neither proved satisfying. Within a few more years, all members of her immediate family save her youngest sister, Eleanor, had passed away. In this account of her life, Margaret's departure for Pondicherry looks more like an escape from a life whittled down to inconsequence.[33]

But in another reading of Margaret's life, Margaret isn't running away from something but rather running toward something else.

In setting off for Pondicherry, Margaret was, in my estimation, sailing toward her ideal life. What she might trade for it—a temperate climate, a free and democratic homeland, friends, dresses, and cigarettes—seemed trivial when compared to the benefits of being near her guru.

Anyway, many had already made this trade and benefited from it. Not only that, the body of literature documenting the awakening of spirit that a visit to India reliably produced had exploded. Theos Bernard had plied this literary trope. So did Paul Brunton, an English journalist who found a deep solace in India and devoted most of his life to translating his discoveries into a Western vernacular. Brunton is also often credited with introducing Ramana Maharshi to the world. (Maharshi, a silent Yogi, was based in Tiruvannamalai, a town not far from Pondicherry.)

Margaret admired Brunton's books and recommended them to friends.[34]

L. Adams Beck, aka Lily (Moresby) Adams Beck, was an even earlier purveyor of this seductive tale. Beck began her career writing romantic short stories set in the Orient and historical fiction for *The Atlantic Monthly* and *Asia* magazine. In the mid-1920s, her historical novels appeared under the name E. Barrington. Their success and her simultaneous publication of works on Asian philosophy and religion, these authored by the somewhat mysterious L. Adams Beck, caused something of a stir in the literary world.[35]

As the wife of a diplomat, Beck spent years living abroad in India, Ceylon, China, and Japan and during that time studied yoga at its source.

In 1937, six years after her death, Farrar and Rinehart, publishers of popular romances, released *Yoga for Beginners*, a compilation of excerpts from Beck's stories and other writings about yoga.

The same year, one of Pierre Bernard's longtime students, Francis Yeats-Brown, published his second book on India, this one a frenetically penned travelogue. In it, Yeats-Brown profiles a number of Yogis, including a man he calls the Chidambaram Swami, who became his guru.[36]

By the time Margaret left for India, in the fall of 1938, the notion that the world's riches were dispersed along geographic lines had been repeated often enough to pose as fact. The West was materialistic, industrious, and progressive. The East was spiritual and traditionbound.

The formulation contained within it a reverse chauvinism, one that many who became deeply involved in yoga subscribed to and perpetuated. The West was spiritually inferior to the East, and even worse, the West didn't understand this about itself. As Margaret put it, less poetically than Thoreau but with no less feeling, "The West does not realise the difference . . . between talking about the spiritual life, speculating about it and holding certain intellectual beliefs and emotional convictions about God, and entering into spiritual life by means of spiritual realisations."[37]

When Margaret disembarked in Bombay, one of the Ramakrishna monks from Belur Math greeted her. Vivekananda's organization, now more than thirty years old, had become the de facto jumping-off point for Westerners in India and its monks were friendly guides to seekers such as Theos, Viola, and Margaret.

From Bombay, Margaret took a train down to Pondicherry alone. Swami Nikhilananda, who was back in India, fretted like a mother hen over Margaret, cautioning her to latch her compartment door from the inside, to be "discriminating" about the food she ate on the train, and, by all means, not to drink anything but mineral water. (Unlike Theos and Viola, Margaret had to content herself with seeing most of India through a train window.)[38]

Margaret arrived in Pondicherry without incident. By November, she was settled in at the ashram, delighted by nearly everything she found there. The heat was not nearly so bad as she (and others) had feared; with the sea breezes it felt to her more like a summer day in Connecticut than the heart of the tropics.

More than fifty French-colonial buildings formed the main ashram, surrounding a central courtyard, lush with tropical vegetation. Margaret lived in a house just outside its walls with high ceilings, a garden, and two servants, which made her accommodations more luxurious than her apartment in New York. She was given other special privileges at the ashram, including a seat shaded with a sun umbrella for her meditation.[39]

And though she had plenty of solitude, she was hardly alone. Nearly two hundred disciples were living at the ashram, and their devotion immediately impressed Margaret.

"One has to be here to realize how very practical and actual is the effect of Yoga," she wrote to friends in New York, "particularly this Yoga on the lives of those who practise it—I have never seen such a wonderful group of people in my life."[40]

Margaret also received the occasional visit from old friends. Jo Macleod, who had traveled with Sara Bull, was in India once again. Tantine, as she was known to Margaret, was now eighty years of age. Completely undeterred by her age or the rigors of travel in India, she made a point of visiting her friend in Pondicherry.[41]

But Margaret's was no tropical idyll. She worked hard at yoga, waking at 6:30 a.m. to meditate, then meditating again after lunch, when most in the town were taking their midday "siesta," and again in the evening, after supper. Her evenings ended with chores—she and the other disciples washed Aurobindo's dinner dishes since they wouldn't let the servants touch them—and a short meditation before bed.[42]

Nor were conditions always conducive to yoga. The noise was often unbearable. Margaret had a litany of aural offenses: farmers berating their oxen to make them walk faster, sellers shouting the names of their wares, truck drivers honking at the least provocation, "barn yard" sounds, and this all capped "with the sounds of the forth [*sic*] of July let off all day and literally all night for every Hindu, Mohammedan, and Christian festival."

There wasn't much she could do about it either. When another sadhaka had complained about the noise, Aurobindo suggested that if he couldn't stand mere noise, "he certainly would not be able to stand the far greater difficulties on the path of Yoga."[43]

Margaret, ever the model pupil, took these words to heart. Cacophony became an exercise in patience and self-discipline. The gardening she did in the ashram served a related purpose. "The physical work here seems to be very beneficial to Yoga," she wrote to her sister Nell. "Perhaps one reason is that it keeps the mind sufficiently concentrated without tiring it and so rests it."[44]

Her one complaint? After several months at his ashram, Margaret still hadn't met Aurobindo.

This was the paradox of her entire pilgrimage. She plundered her savings to travel thousands of miles around the world, only to arrive at an ashram whose spiritual head spent most of the year in seclusion. And she knew this about him long before she left the States.

Aurobindo was known in some quarters as the Silent Yogi. Though he didn't have much of a reputation in the United States yet, he was quite famous in India, in no small part because he had been a revolutionary. At the turn of the century, before his spiritual awakening, he had articulated the idea of swaraj or "complete independence" from British rule decades before this seemed plausible.[45]

This didn't sit well with the British, who arrested him twice.

Not long after being released from prison for the second time, he decisively (and perhaps conveniently since the British hadn't given up on him) renounced the world of politics and went to live in Pondicherry, a French territory.

There, in his monthly journal *Arya*, he began articulating Integral Yoga. He quickly attracted a small group of disciples, including a few European students.[46]

What made Aurobindo special as an interpreter and transmitter of yoga is that he tried, and some believe succeeded, in mending the dualism that plagued neo-Vedanta and Sāmkhya. Though the systems differ in their particulars, they both consider the reality we can see, hear, feel, and smell as an impediment to divine consciousness (figured in the two disciplines as

Brahma and purusha, respectively). According to Vedanta, the aspirant mistakes ephemeral phenomena for the unchanging absolute; only when she sees through this illusion or maya will she be able to attain liberation. Sāmkhya holds that there are two categories of being, nature (prakriti) and the transcendental Self (purusha), and that the purpose of spiritual practice is to completely disentangle Self from nature.[47]

Aurobindo's vision was much more in keeping with the basic principles of Tantra—all matter, everything you can perceive, is part of one's own awakening into bliss.

Tantra provides an ontological substratum for much of Aurobindo's thinking, but it by no means explains it; Margaret's guru had been influenced by many different thinkers and was nearly as eclectic in his tastes as Emerson and Thoreau.[48]

Part of a new generation of Western-educated Bengali intellectuals and professionals, Aurobindo had been schooled entirely in England, eventually studying at King's College, Cambridge University. Aurobindo learned Sanskrit and a local Bengali dialect only after returning to India in 1893—the year Vivekananda made his first visit to America.

So, in Aurobindo's writings, karma, reincarnation, and divine immanence mingle with Hegelian notions of historical progress and a suspiciously Nietzschean Superbeing who would rule the world.[49]

Margaret had fallen for a mystic who was as much a product of British Liberalism and German Romanticism as of neo-Hinduism.

She was in good company. French novelist and seeker Romain Rolland had hailed Aurobindo as "the completest synthesis that has been realized to this day of the genius of Asia and the genius of Europe."[50]

Aurobindo was also mentioned as the coauthor of a study on yoga in theory and practice in the 1928 ISVAR prospectus funded by Pierre Bernard.[51]

By the time Margaret discovered his work, Aurobindo had completely retreated. The Mother, a Frenchwoman by the name of Mirra Richards whom he considered an embodiment of Divine consciousness, ran the ashram, and Aurobindo communicated with his growing group of sadhaks entirely via correspondence. His instruction was tailored to each and meted out through thousands of letters.[52]

He did however offer darshan (literally, a "sighting") three times a year. Sitting in a canopied seat that looked like a throne, he'd greet his sadhaks and offer a silent blessing. This was less of a compromise than it might seem. In India, to be near holy people or objects, to merely "see" them, is to partake in their divinity.

Margaret was by turns giddy with anticipation and impatient for this moment. When Aurobindo did emerge, later than usual that year, she was bowled over. Aurobindo was, in her estimation, one of the "fully persuaded world-saviours, like Christ or Buddha." Not even her own father, who helped broker the end of the world's bloodiest war to date, could claim such powers of peace-giving. Unlike her father, Aurobindo had "rent the veil of matter" and existed somehow "beyond mind and speech."[53]

By the summer of 1939, as was ashram policy, Margaret had turned most of her financial assets over to the Mother.[54]

War had come to India. Shortages and inflation made daily life difficult. British mismanagement of food supplies eventually led to a severe famine in Bengal that killed nearly 4 million Indians. But Margaret continued on, unaffected for the most part by the privations.[55]

"I [w]onder so often about my dear friends in America if they are able now to think of much besides war and the future—if they can catch at moments the sound of the voice in the Silence, in spite of all the sound and fury around," Margaret wrote to her friend Elsie Weil in late spring of 1939. "I am not thinking about war much, but I still find that the sound and fury in my own mind are fearful obstacles to the discovery of the Peace of which they are a dissembling covering."[56]

Despite the U.S. State Department's efforts to evacuate American civilians living in the Far East, Margaret chose to stay in India and would live through Pearl Harbor at the ashram.[57]

She was as near to her guru she could possibly get, and in yoga she had found something akin to a career. Yoga focused her prodigious energies and made her feel useful.

Before she had left the United States, Margaret had begun copyediting Swami Nikhilananda's thousand-plus-page translation of the *Gospel of Sri Ramakrishna*, and she completed this work via correspondence from Pondicherry.[58]

Once she found Aurobindo's Integral Yoga, the trappings of reform—the benefit dinners, the press conferences, the fractious boards, and even the organizations themselves, which parceled human need into causes—

seemed superfluous. In changing herself, she believed that she was also changing the world around her.

"You will see from both [books] that there is an element in his Yoga and it's [sic] purpose that is different from any other," Margaret explained in a note accompanying some of Aurobindo's books she had sent to friends in January 1939, "—that it is a work for the race, for mankind as well as the usual spiritualizing and liberating Yoga of the individual with God. Of course the effect of the liberation of every individual who has realized his divinity and been freed from the ego has had its influence in the world and on it, but the effect of this Yoga . . . will be to radically change the make up of man, gradually of course."[59]

Once she settled in Pondicherry, Margaret quickly became a one-woman publicity machine for her guru, sending out dozens of letters to scholars at top universities, requesting that they review one volume or another of Aurobindo's newly completed book, *The Life Divine.*[60]

She never hesitated to trade on her name for Aurobindo or the connections her status as a former first daughter had bequeathed upon her. She wrote directly to university presidents and scholars with whom she had only a passing acquaintance and donated Aurobindo's books to libraries at numerous universities, including Yale, Columbia, Princeton, Johns Hopkins, and the University of Chicago, as well as public libraries in St. Louis, Boston, and New York. She urged both Nikhilananda and her friend Elsie Weil, an editor at *Asia* magazine, to help her get the word out.

This part of her work yielded little in the way of visible results. Only one small review appeared, in *Asia*. And Aurobindo's books didn't initially sell well in the States.[61]

The success Margaret did have can't be measured in the number of books sold or appearances in major news outlets (or even citations by other scholars). Not long after Margaret arrived at his ashram, Aurobindo gave her the name Nishtha Devi, which means single-minded devotion. All of the things she found in India that she couldn't find at home—a large community of like-minded souls, a setting more conducive to practice than not, and inspiration and reassurance from someone whom she invested with unparalleled spiritual authority—fostered this devotion. Despite that, in the spring of 1940, more than eighteen months after her arrival in Pondicherry, she reported to Swami Nikhilananda that "there seems to be spread over Nishtha and her intuitive respo[n]se to all the inspired Indian literature a thick veil of Margaret and God knows how many other personalities that have to be purified and thinned out by a slow process before Nishtha can be liberated, for I have not as yet had even one moment of illumination, much less realization. . . . The patience of an artist and the scientist combined seems to be required to do Yoga—isn't that so?"[62]

Things changed quickly for Margaret. Nakashima told the world Margaret had embraced "an ancient Brahmin cult," in June 1940, and soon after, she noted in her diary "a month of almost daily progress in meditation." This was less a matter of reaching a certain mental state, though she did achieve this at times, than it was a renewed desire to turn off the thought-producing machinery of her own mind.[63]

Progress began to accelerate further. If she longed for those periods of "cessation" midsummer, by August 1940 she began to experience these, or something approximating them, more frequently. What she describes as brushes with purusha, or transcendental consciousness, were nothing short of exhilarating. She wrote to her friend and fellow Aurobindo admirer Lois during that same year, "There is such a thing as getting near the central psychic being and feeling its influence. And the luminousness of mind that comes afterward makes me feel as if I have never lived or understood anything at all before! I feel like a discoverer every day."[64]

By October, her progress was visible, at least to the Mother, who told Margaret she would "surely find the Divine."[65]

But just as she felt she was beginning to make real spiritual progress, to actually taste these moments of luminousness, Margaret fell seriously ill.

For the better part of a year, Margaret couldn't do much of anything. Her correspondence dropped to a trickle, and she made not a single diary entry between October 5, 1940—the evening the Mother had assured her she'd find the divine—and July 23, 1942. When Margaret did sufficiently recover to take up her correspondence again, she was too weak to use a typewriter (and her handwriting, by her own admission, was atrocious).[66]

Once Margaret's friends learned of her condition, well after the onset of her illness, they began to lobby for her return to the States.

In March 1942, Swami Nikhilananda appealed to Aurobindo directly, pleading with him to persuade Margaret to come home.

Margaret replied directly, through the U.S. consulate, "I am in fine shape again. . . . I am making no arrangements to return to America, as my work is keeping me here."

Typically, Margaret never mentions any details about illness or identifies it by name; instead, she views it less as a physical malady, though it certainly affected her body, than as a spiritual test. She believed that had she been a better, more consistent practitioner, she would never have fallen ill in the first place. She described herself as a "jerker" and even "a shirker" when it came to making a "sustained effort," though from all the evidence, she was far more steadfast than she let on.[67]

Compared to Theos Bernard, who records triumph after triumph along the path of yoga, whether real or imagined, Margaret Woodrow Wilson comes off as a far more genuine spiritual aspirant, who was deeply engaged in the struggle of what it means to advance and how one goes about it given the limitations of one's own circumstances. This partly has to do with the types of yoga each one favored. Hatha Yoga offered Theos concrete milestones, which bolstered his sense of progress: he could stay in headstand for fifteen minutes, then eventually hours at a time. And if he ever doubted himself, he needed only to stand on his head or perform Kumbhaka. Margaret sought a state of consciousness, a sense of the presence of the divine. Whatever she achieved—a few minutes of this peaceful stillness, a few hours of it—became a memory as soon as she returned to normal consciousness. This made it harder for her to believe in her progress, and it made it easier for an outsider to ascribe expertise to someone like Theos.

If Margaret couldn't or wouldn't claim mastery, the effects of her long devotion to yoga were striking. During the earliest phases of seeking, she was impatient, fearful, and skeptical. She needed constant reassurance that she was on the right track, up to the job, and that she'd end up in a place far better than the one she found herself in. "You will also find your liberty and your freedom and you will also rejoice over it," assured Pritchett, Margaret's self-appointed spiritual guide in the mid-1920s, "and the desert you are passing through will only be a memory of the past."[68]

Now, she no longer doubted that liberation was possible; she believed even she could become a channel for or instrument of the "One Eternal Being."

"Am I getting there?" she wrote to Elsie in 1941. "I can only say that I have faith that because I aspire to reach the Highest I shall one day do so and that I have," in Aurobindo and the Mother, "the most powerful help and inspiration that it is possible to have."[69]

Then too she believed her life, and even the evils of war, were the workings of divine purpose.

Yoga hadn't freed her. Aurobindo and the Mother hadn't swept aside the obstacles strewing her path. But Margaret had found faith and so possessed the equanimity faith in one's future bestows.

When *New York Times* reporter Herbert Matthews tracked Margaret down in Pondicherry in January 1943, he was impressed by her demeanor and wrote a sympathetic profile that was picked up by the weekly newsmagazines.

Matthews noted that outwardly Margaret had changed little. She still wore dresses and even smoked the occasional cigarette. However, she displayed not a trace of nostalgia for life in the United States. She said she was happier and more at home in the ashram than she had ever felt anywhere else. As for her spiritual progress, all she would let on was that she considered herself a novice in Integral Yoga and that serenity was still a challenge for her "restless Western mind."

A little more than a year after Matthews's piece ran, in February 1944, the *Times* reverted to form: "Margaret Woodrow Wilson Dies a Recluse at 57 in Religious Colony in India."

Her kidneys had failed. (Because of the war, international travel was still all but impossible, and her family had to wait before her body could be returned to the United States for burial.)[70]

Theos Bernard heard the news of Margaret's death almost immediately. He may have read about it himself. And his second wife, Ganna Walska, sent him a clipping from the *New York Herald Tribune*. "In case if you did not read, Marguerite [sic] Wilson died in India," she wrote. "Somehow I am very sorry."

In that same letter, she enclosed another clipping from the *New York Journal-American* headlined "Yogi Priestess Grips Hubby, Says Actress." Walska scrawled on the corner, "Is she not one of the girls that went when you spoke at Miss Barnes?"[71]

Theos Bernard, and until then Margaret Woodrow Wilson, struggled to communicate yoga's most powerful effects, in Margaret's case the sense of divine presence, "a vast stillness," and peace that somehow eradicated her usual sense of separateness from God and people, and in Theos's case an unsurpassable joy and richness of waking experience.[72]

Neither would say they had completely succeeded. Meanwhile, others were more than happy to fill in the blanks. The discipline turned husbands into adulterers, it turned scholars into swindlers, it turned women into lunatics or shut-ins.

Once the restrictions were lifted after the war, Eleanor Wilson-McAdoo decided to leave Margaret's body in peace in India where she had wanted to be all along, a place where few would question her devotion to yoga.

But in America, yoga still summoned all our fears.

8

UNCOVERING REALITY IN HOLLYWOOD

Tucked low in the Hollywood hills on a quiet block is a squat, white building topped with onion domes. Delicate gold pinnacles stretch upward into the improbably blue Southern California sky. A set of brick steps lead from the street to simple wooden doors. Above them, the word *Om*, the sacred symbol of the Absolute, is sculpted in looping Devanagari script.[1]

Like much of the local architecture, the building looks fake and incongruous, an effect heightened by the house next door, a dark, shadowy place with a sloped roof, small windows, and wooden exterior. One looks like a miniature, plaster Taj Mahal; this is the Hollywood Vedanta Temple. The other, which looks like a Japanese farmhouse, is the original headquarters of the Southern California Vedanta Society.

We owe this bit of architectural surrealism to Carrie Mead Wyckoff.

Wyckoff, also known as Sister Lalita, owned the wooden house, originally no. 1946 Ivar Avenue. Sister Lalita was a veteran student of Vedanta and a widow whose only son had died. For a while she had kept house for Swami Prabhavananda when he was in charge of the Portland Vedanta Center.

In 1929, she donated her house on Ivar Avenue to Prabhavananda, and the two moved together from Portland to Hollywood. Over the next few years, several other women joined them there. All but invisible to the public, Swami Prabhavananda depended on their daily ministrations.[2]

As a religious leader, Prabhavananda was more teacher than proselytizer. His lectures ranged from Freud to the Bible to the *Upanishads*. They were learned without being academic, and they revolved around a single truth: the purpose of life is to unite with the divine. All else can be classified as a restatement of that basic tenet, an elaboration of it, or a method for attaining it.[3]

For Prabhavananda there was no fire, no brimstone. God, Brahma, the divine, the Self, was a fact, more real, more implacable, than the mountains or the oceans, and it need only be described.[4]

In similar fashion, the swami felt it unnecessary to advertise or market himself or his center. In public, he dressed in tailored suits and wore fine leather shoes. Youthful-looking for his years, Prabhavananda kept his hair cropped short and was always clean-shaven. Unlike Vivekananda, he didn't look the part of a spiritual teacher. He looked more like a salesman or lawyer.

For the first half decade he was in Los Angeles, he had few followers, besides the women who lived at 1946 Ivar Avenue, and was hardly distinguishable from the other "crystal ball gazers" that crowded certain quarters of the city.[5]

Over time, however, the swami's reputation in Los Angeles grew. By 1936, people stopped calling him for horoscopes or demonstrations of his psychic powers and started requesting him to address various functions. Prabhavananda had become known around town as a moving speaker.

Soon after, the temple went up in what had been Sister Lalita's garden. The temple itself has changed little in the intervening seven decades.[6]

In the summer of 1940, to celebrate the second anniversary of the temple's dedication, British author Gerald Heard gave a short talk. He had spoken the year before as well.

By now signs of a buildup for war were clear. In 1940 President Roosevelt commissioned fifty thousand new warplanes, to be built mostly in Southern California at Lockheed, Douglas, Northrop, and Consolidated.[7]

Heard saw the mission of the center—to uncover "Reality" and harmonize human life with that Reality—as being no less urgent, and really more so, in wartime than in a time of peace. For to heal others was impossible without first healing oneself.

Heard concluded his talk with a paean to the squat, white temple. "That these truths are taught here and that the way to practice them is indicated is of the greatest value." Its value lay in precisely what Heard felt the West lacked, a "system, when in the West we have had only fragments of true gnosis . . . an empirical science in comparison with those happy insights and uncoordinated hints which are all the guidance our own tradition can now yield."[8]

Heard, born in London in 1889, had arrived in California in 1937. A pacifist, he had come, along with his companion, Chris Wood, and Aldous and Maria Huxley, in part to escape the violence gripping Europe.

Before his westward journey, he had been a lecturer at Oxford, author, and BBC commentator on popular science. Though he was less known in America, E. M. Forster had described Heard as "one of the most penetrating minds in England."[9]

His move to California had effected if not a complete then a noticeable transformation. Clean-shaven and elegantly dressed when he lived in London, Heard now wore a beard, jackets with ragged cuffs, and jeans with either holes or patches on the knees.

In Los Angeles, he was forging his own eclectic philosophy out of pretty much any material he could get his hands on—history, anthropology, physics, parapsychology, mythology; one contemporary likened him to Blavatsky.[10]

Prabhavananda put great stock in Heard, who lectured on alternate Sundays.

One note Heard struck again and again was that Vedanta offered a complete system, based as it was on "a clear realisation of the body-mind relationship, of how man may and only may change the aperture of consciousness by a thorough understanding of that relationship." Vedanta left nothing out. Not mind, not soul, not body.[11]

Heard proved as popular as the swami, if not more so, and his "spellbinding" lectures noticeably increased both attendance at the temple and donations.[12]

Sometime in the late 1930s, Prabhavananda initiated Heard and his friend Huxley as well. (However, neither considered himself a *disciple* of the swami; both were congenital eclectics, who refused to commit themselves to a single spiritual path or philosophy.)[13]

Huxley and his wife had arrived in California with Heard about five years after the publication of *Brave New World*, which, along with his other novels, had already earned him literary stardom in America. Tall, handsome, and well-spoken, the author had seamlessly slipped into the Hollywood elite. He wrote screenplays, and his movements across the Southern California landscape were tracked by Hedda Hopper, Lee Shipley, and Ed Ainsworth.

By this time his spiritual questing, and whatever treasure he had found, had become a defining aspect of his persona. In a 1938 profile for the *Los Angeles Times*, Arthur Miller portrayed Huxley, half-blind since his youth because of an eye disease, as a seer who meted out wisdom in koanlike pronouncements.[14]

Like Heard, Huxley was a pacifist.

At the beginning of the First World War, Huxley had wanted to fight. By the end of it, having been rejected by the British army twice because of poor eyesight, he had become a conscientious objector. But it was Bertrand Russell's work, particularly his prison letters and *Principles of Social Reconstruction*, that shaped Huxley's views. He lost faith in war. Over the ensuing decades, his views on the subject crystallized; he saw war as a symptom of mass psychological and spiritual malaise. "People can get more satisfaction out of hating foreigners they have never seen," he wrote in his 1934 travel book, *Beyond the Mexique Bay*, "than out of vaguely wishing them well." War bound communities together. For most people, peace was a feeble abstraction.[15]

Huxley's book on the subject, *Ends and Means*, came out the year he left Europe, to mixed reviews. The *Times* reviewer noted that the "beliefs and principles he states are unimpeachable. He advocates non-violence, charity, good-will, non-attachment, justice." But he was chagrined by Huxley's tendency to go "cosmic on us."[16]

This cosmic turn to Huxley's thinking—much as it might displease or confound readers—wasn't incidental to his pacifism. By the late 1930s, Huxley's views on war were inextricably bound up in his spirituality. He believed that mystical religion was the last best hope for preventing "these enormous suicides" then transpiring in Europe.[17]

What he found in Vedanta was another powerful articulation of perennial philosophy.

The idea of a philosophy that could be distilled from all ages and cultures dated to at least the seventeenth century. In Huxley's formulation, perennial philosophy pivoted around a God that's both transcendent (Brahma) and immanent (Atman) and it made union with God the purpose of human existence.[18]

However, Huxley found the practice of yoga more trouble than it was worth. "The bore of this Yoga mind control is that it's so frightfully difficult and takes so long—also that it probably demands a pretty careful regulation of diet and sexual habits," he wrote to a friend wrestling with insomnia in 1935. "But . . . I think quite a lot can be done in the way of securing a certain serenity by means of breathing."[19]

The association of Heard and Huxley with the Southern California Vedanta Society had an immediate and lasting effect. So far, yoga and its various philosophical raiments had been the province of the women in the Southland, and hence dismissed as a harmless pastime. As the journalist Louis Adamic observed, by the mid-1920s, the Realtors, lawyers, promoters, salesmen, officeholders, and boomers who made up the city's burgeoning middle class were now affluent enough that their wives could while their days away, listening to "Swamis and yogis, and English lecturers," and joining "love cults."[20]

Vedanta had been the pabulum of yet another Los Angeles swami, no better, no worse, and no more worthy of most Angelenos' attention.

Then in came Huxley and Heard, men, first and foremost, and men whose works had changed people's "angle of vision." Their form of suasion was the simplest kind: they spoke with conviction, and their lives, at least from the outside, seemed richer, better, and more filled with meaning than most. Together they lent authority, relevance, and glamour to Prabhavananda's small organization.

"The main reason I felt the unknown Vedanta must be all right," recalls John Yale, who became a lifelong disciple of Swami Prabhavananda's in 1950, ". . . was that Aldous Huxley was one of its supporters. I reasoned that Vedanta couldn't be quackery or ignorant idolatry if a man as perceptive as he had become an admirer."[21]

Los Angeles had long been a locus for European expatriates. Germans, Czechs, and Russians founded the film industry in the 1910s and 1920s. With Hitler's rise, a new generation of émigré intellectuals and artists poured into the Southland, settled in L.A.'s sunny canyons, and got to work in the studios. As Californian historian Kevin Starr put it, "The argument can be made that Hollywood, from the 1920s through the 1930s, was more Berliner and Viennese than Yankee-American in style and feeling."[22]

In 1939, Huxley and Heard were joined in Los Angeles by another Briton: Christopher Isherwood. W. H. Auden had introduced Isherwood to Heard in the early 1930s in London.[23]

Of the three, Isherwood would become the most devoted to Vedanta and its most single-minded advocate. But when he set down in Los Angeles, he was no more of a yogi than the queen of England.

Youthful-looking, even for his thirty-five years of age, and fair, with blue eyes and a trim physique, Isherwood was known for his semiautobiographical tales of rebels, misfits, and what was then considered sexual deviance, and several plays, cowritten with Auden. (The 1966 musical and 1972 film *Cabaret*, and subsequent revivals, were loosely based on Isherwood's book *The Berlin Stories*.)

His "Berlin Diary, 1931–1932" was a particularly vivid augur of what was to come to Europe:

> There had been a big Nazi meeting at the Sportpalast, and groups of men and boys were just coming away from it. . . . All at once, three S.A. men came face to face with a youth of seventeen or eighteen dressed in civilian clothes, who was hurrying along in the opposite direction. I heard one of the Nazis shout: "That's him!" and immediately all three of them flung themselves upon the young man. He uttered a scream, and tried to dodge, but they were too quick for him.[24]

Once in Los Angeles, Isherwood wanted to find "some regular humble employment," something akin to being an English teacher in Berlin, to subsidize his writing and afford him some measure of anonymity as he adapted to his new surroundings. However, the effects of the Depression were still being felt in the Southland, and "humble" jobs were hard to come by. So Isherwood had two options: penury or screenwriting, with its big but erratic paydays.[25]

That he could and did eventually choose the latter didn't stave off bouts of despair. Not long after he arrived in Los Angeles, he confided to a friend, "I am so utterly sick of being a person—Christopher Isherwood, or Isherwood, or even Chris. . . . Don't you feel, more and more, that all your achievements, all your sexual triumphs, are just like cheques which represent money, but have no real value?"[26]

The mood, coupled with Heard's convincing disquisitions on pacifism—"To become a true pacifist," Heard advised, "you had to find peace within yourself; only then," he said, "could you function pacifistically in the outside world"—the nature of God, faith, and reality, slowly pushed him toward a philosophy he resisted. (Rebellious by nature and a leftist in his youth, Isherwood had disdained all religion, and this included yoga too.)[27]

By 1940, Isherwood was pulled into Prabhavananda's orbit.

His first impression of "Heard's Swami," which is how he thought of Swami Prabhavananda at the time, was of a charming, boyish man who looked vaguely Mongolian and chain-smoked. The swami was then in his mid-forties.

"He talks gently and persuasively. His smile is extraordinary. It is somehow so touching, so open, so brilliant with joy that it makes me want to cry," Isherwood recorded in his diary on August 4, 1939.[28]

It was a pivotal encounter. During their first private meeting, Prabhavananda reassured the author that just the act of trying to meditate was a "positive advance" on the path to God. In other words, failure or incompetence at meditation was no reason to give it up, as some part of Isherwood had surely hoped.

Most crucially, Prabhavananda didn't see Isherwood's homosexuality as a particular obstacle to the spiritual life. (This at a time when sodomy laws were still on the books throughout the United States and in some places enforced.) He simply advised Isherwood to try to see his lover "as the young Lord Krishna" and sent him home with a mantra and some basic instructions for meditation.[29]

The effects of the swami's advice slowly took hold. Isherwood recorded one of his meditations not long after seeing Prabhavananda: "This evening, on bedroom floor, in the dark. Unsatisfactory. Stuck at number one," the first step in the swami's instructions, which was to try to feel the presence of an all-pervading Existence. "I couldn't get over the feeling that everyone was asleep and therefore no longer part of 'Consciousness.' Posture is difficult. My back hurts. But I feel somehow refreshed."[30]

Isherwood got past "number one" as he went on. In November 1940 he had two visions while meditating. The first one was of a dirty-white bird that walked stiffly and darted under the bed, like a mouse going into its hole. He had found it unusually easy to concentrate that evening and during his meditation was also aware of an intense silence.

The second vision was of his own face, but handsomer, "rather like a Red Indian, with light blue eyes." According to Swami Prabhavananda, Isherwood had got a glimpse of his own subtle body. (Here Prabhavananda may have been referring to the subtle body of Vedanta, which is composed of five sheaths, or koshas, the least refined being essentially your physical body and the most being the ânanda-maya-kosha, or "sheath composed of bliss.")[31]

During this time Isherwood became curious about Hatha Yoga and sought out some instruction.

In this, Isherwood was openly defying his guru's wishes.

On more than one occasion, Prabhavananda castigated Hatha Yogis as the Olympic athletes of spiritual attainment. They might be healthy, they might live to a hundred, but they are complete idiots as a result, he liked to say. Plus, Prabhavananda insisted that pranayama can cause hallucinations. Though Vedanta swamis Abhedananda and Bodhananda had taken a more liberal view of the discipline, Prabhavananda, like most of his fellow Vedanta swamis, was unyielding.[32]

Fortunately, the Huxleys introduced Isherwood to Claire Stuart. (Isherwood once lovingly described Maria Huxley as "that connoisseur of doctors, clairvoyants, and cranks.")[33]

Stuart had recently fled New York and the bad publicity surrounding the Donovan suit. De Vries had paid off her portion of the settlement, and she had left no forwarding address for the lawyers handling the case.[34]

Despite her somewhat sudden arrival, Stuart already boasted a thriving clientele in Hollywood, thanks in part to her brother, Dr. Franklyn Thorpe, a renowned physician who was often on location to care for the high-priced (and heavily insured) stars.

At forty-one, Stuart was a seasoned instructor who had been teaching and practicing Hatha Yoga for nearly twenty-five years. She was adept at explaining the discipline and equally able to assume complex asanas by way of demonstration.

Isherwood found his teacher exceptionally young-looking for her age and extraordinarily limber.

(Although he knew all about her legal troubles, he blamed them entirely on the "somewhat dubious" Theos Bernard.)[35]

Nearly every day for three weeks, Stuart put Isherwood and his roommate, Denny Fouts, through a demanding ninety-minute sequence of asanas and breathing exercises, all the while maintaining her composure in the face of young, half-clad men, who sometimes farted loudly, having not yet perfected Mula Bandha (root lock).

Even over such a short time, her instruction got results. Isherwood felt "wonderful" and described his insides as a "well-packed suitcase."

When he confessed his experiment to Prabhavananda, the swami replied, "What is the matter with you, Mr. Isherwood? Surely you do not want Etarnal [sic] Youth?" Isherwood was stung and stopped the lessons shortly thereafter anyway. But this is exactly what he had wanted.[36]

"Yes, it is true. Los Angeles is not only erratic, not only erotic," wrote Ogden Nash in a sardonic piece of verse published in *The New Yorker* in 1942. "Los Angeles is crotchety, centrifugal, vertiginous, esoteric and / exotic."[37]

Nash's poem "Don't Shoot Los Angeles" distilled three decades' worth of received wisdom about the place, which by 1930 had insouciantly dislodged Cleveland as the fifth largest city in the nation.[38]

In 1925, Julia M. Sloane insisted she hadn't "had a hairdresser who wasn't occult or psychic or something." *Life* chimed in, damning Los Angeles as a "cuckoo land," where "eccentrics flourish" in unrivaled abundance. "Nowhere do spiritual or economic panaceas grow so lushly. Nowhere is undisciplined gullibility so widespread." Harrumph![39]

By the height of the Great Depression, bashing Los Angeles—for its perceived spiritual excesses and frivolity, for its casualness and physicality—had become sport. Columnists competed on depth of feeling and form. The more ostentatious one's antipathy, the more florid one's prose, the better.

Picking up the baton, Bruce Bliven, then editor in chief of *The New Republic*, described Los Angeles this way: "Here is the world's prize collection of cranks, semi-cranks, placid creatures whose bovine expression shows that each of them is studying, without much hope of success, to be a high-grade moron, angry or ecstatic exponents of food fads, sun-bathing, ancient Greek costumes, diaphragm breathing and the imminent second coming of Christ."[40]

Los Angeles journalist Farnsworth Crowder diagnosed a "cult of the body," an extreme "health consciousness," a sports mania, and in general a proclivity for the outdoors, pleasure, and informality. Crowder, like many other observers, blamed Los Angeles' mild climate for this pervasive derangement.[41]

This Los Angeles of body cultists and sunbathers, of "diaphragm breathers" and food faddists, was ready-made for Hatha Yoga. By all rights, Hatha Yoga should have flourished in Los Angeles long before Isherwood's dalliance. Except that the place Sloane, Bliven, Crowder, and many others described was a Los Angeles of their making, crafted in pointed opposition to the city's boosters, who had spun a myth of mild climes and easy living around a desert town that had no significant natural resources, no geographic advantage, and no real industry to support it.[42]

Yoga came to this half-mythical place in fits and starts, and it took root later than it had in other cities.[43]

San Francisco, for example, went through its "cultish" phase at the turn of the century (which is when Pierre Bernard set up his San Francisco Hatha Yoga clinic and Tantrik Order). At that time, a fairly homogenous Los Angeles was dominated by "prominent," God-fearing Eastern families. And even up until the 1920s, Christian fundamentalists held great sway over the city and its politics.[44]

Vivekananda had brought yoga to Los Angeles in 1899, and there may have been others who, like Sylvais Hamati, had small followings and never rose to prominence. But it was Katherine Tingley who rooted it in the Southern California soil.[45]

A headstrong Theosophist, Tingley founded Lomaland on Point Loma near San Diego at the turn of the century.[46]

Set on five hundred lush acres 130 miles south of Los Angeles, Lomaland had the unreality and appeal of Atlantis or Arcadia. The forty buildings borrowed from Egyptian and Moorish architecture; one of the largest was topped by an opalescent green dome. The colony grew its own food and raised silkworms; residents dressed in robes and acted, danced, and sang. Point Loma became well-known for music, and Theosophists from around the world visited, to take in the atmosphere, which was once described as "poppy scented champagne."[47]

Early on, Tingley set up a Raja Yoga school, though its curriculum bore little resemblance to the Raja Yoga of Patanjali or his modern interpreters. For her, Raja Yoga meant evolving "a royal union of the physical, mental and moral powers." It was a program of socialization and education, primarily for children. Raja Yoga, as she conceived it, was also the norm against which Hatha Yoga was measured. And that discipline fell horribly short.[48]

Helena Blavatsky, Theosophy's founder, had discouraged Hatha Yoga. Tingley's attacks, levied in Theosophical periodicals, were every bit as pointed, if not more so.[49]

(Yoga seemed ever to be the thorn in the Theosophists' side. In 1909, the discipline divided the movement's ranks in Chicago. On one side, supported by Theosophy's international leader, Annie Besant, were those who condemned yoga; on the other, those who took private yoga lessons from a "Hindoo," Sakharam G. Pandit.)[50]

Hatha Yoga, in Tingley's view, was a system that liberated "the forces of the *lower* nature." If practiced, its techniques had horrible consequences. "Since the disturbance of the moral balance is a characteristic of insanity," explained Tingley in her *Theosophical Path Magazine* in 1916, "the abnormal trend of these practices, favoring one-sided development, is toward unsoundness." Tingley indicted Hatha Yoga on the same grounds that Prabhavananda would, decades later. It made you crazy.

The critique was one of several tactics Tingley used to distinguish her version of Theosophy from other movements that crowded the American spiritual marketplace.[51]

But no amount of posturing could protect her or Lomaland. The "Purple Mother," as Tingley was known, irked the state's boosters, including Harrison Gray Otis, owner of the *Los Angeles Times*. His paper was relentless and inventive in its attacks. "Tingley Spookery in Justice Court" ran one such headline; "Mrs. Tingley's Abuse; Her Latest Outburst" ran another.[52]

Otis's bid to discredit Tingley largely failed; she ultimately won a libel suit against his paper. Still, she was a ready target. In 1923, the aggrieved wife of one of her students sued her for alienation of affections and won.[53]

Tingley was at best a mixed blessing for yoga in Southern California.

Fortunately, the Theosophists' monopoly on the discipline in the Southland was short-lived. In 1916, a permanent Vedanta Center opened in downtown Los Angeles.[54]

It would be another decade before Los Angeles became a locus for yoga and the headquarters of a swami particularly adept at propagating his message and organization.

In January 1925, civic leaders received Paramahansa Yogananda with pomp and splendor, honoring him at a private party in the Biltmore hotel. The swami, who traced his lineage to a deathless Himalayan Yogi and was also a member of the Imperial Council of India and representative of the maharajah of Kasimbazar, of Bengal, then went on to lecture on "mastering the subconscious by the super conscious, scientific spiritual healing," and other similar subjects, at the prestigious and capacious Philharmonic Auditorium.

Los Angeles "local lights" sponsored his next series of lectures, held in mid-January at the Music Arts Hall to an equally enthusiastic crowd.[55]

Like Prabhavananda, Yogananda came from a middle-class family in Calcutta. The two Bengalis were the same age (they were born in 1893) and had similar ambitions. Both wanted to bridge Christianity and yoga and did so partly by liberally invoking Christian scriptures; both believed in the power of Kundalini, if properly awakened; and both publicly disdained Hatha Yoga.[56]

But here the similarities ended.

With his close-cropped hair and fine shoes, Prabhavananda might have been mistaken for a businessman.

Yogananda had delicate features and long, glossy, black locks. He lectured to huge audiences wearing an orange robe. The whole effect was feminine and exotic. More than Prabhavananda, he looked like an Indian holy man.

Yet Yogananda hailed from a lineage of Kriya Yogis that was far more worldly than the Ramakrishna Mission. These men married and had families. They had, in effect, "found God in the jungle of city life and taught others how to find God there," and they espoused a philosophy that owed much to Tantra.[57]

God apparently included financial success as well as bliss. Yogananda never hesitated to advertise the worldly benefits of transcendence, nor did he dismiss the body as merely a gross, and distracting, manifestation of spirit, which was Prabhavananda's view.[58]

Yogananda saw physical well-being as key to spiritual well-being and so developed his own Yogoda system, which drew heavily from Hatha Yoga (despite his belief that it was an inferior form of yoga on its own).[59]

During his early years, he'd do brief demonstrations—pushing a sofa across the room with his abdominal muscles, taking lotus position in the wink of an eye—to wow his audiences and prove the power of mind over body.

He wrapped all of this in the vernacular of the metaphysical movement and science. Observers noted that Yogananda out-Couéd Coué, the French psychologist and pioneer in autosuggestion.[60]

Americans found this spiritual synthesis immensely appealing. But it wasn't just what Yogananda said or even how he said it that made him so popular.

He had, as Wendell Thomas put it, a "genius for organization." Before arriving in Los Angeles, Yogananda lectured in cities across the country—Philadelphia, New York, Denver, Cincinnati—typically to packed houses. The crowds were a direct result of Yogananda's advance work. He put ads in the papers and on billboards and had a small staff, headed by his secretary, set up meetings at clubs and liberal churches during his stay. The swami would gear his lectures to local concerns, giving the lecture, for example, "How to Recharge Your Business Battery out of the Cosmos" in Rochester, and also hold "free healing meetings." Then, before he left, he'd appoint a local committee to head up his organization in that area.[61]

In Los Angeles, though, Yogananda was more popular than he had been anywhere else, and even his tactics can't fully account for the level of celebrity.

Clubs, colleges, societies, educational centers, and even newspapers warmly embraced the swami, who protested that he could hardly keep up with the invitations to speak or write and the interview requests. According to his count, thousands were turned away each night he lectured. Prominent Angelenos were drubbed in the society pages for their very public displays of support.[62]

Yogananda decided to make Los Angeles his base of operations, and in 1925 he purchased an aged hotel near downtown called the Mount Washington.[63]

Within less than a decade, the swami was running a thriving movement. His Yogoda Sat-sanga Society of America boasted twelve centers across the country and was governed largely by Americans, including an ex-mayor of New York City, a renowned Cleveland architect, and a textile magnate, among others.[64]

The organization also put out a lushly illustrated magazine, an extensive correspondence course, and a variety of cards, calendars, and other ephemera, most of it emblazoned with Yogananda's face.[65]

A swami this visible was bound to run into trouble. For every advance in his organization or expansion of his services, there was a nearly commensurate attack, often from disgruntled followers within his own ranks. Most were publicized.

"Swami Under Investigation" read one such headline, on page A1 of the *Los Angeles Times* in October of 1925.[66]

Soon after, Yogananda had a falling out with Swami Dhirananda, who had run the Mount Washington operation during Yogananda's long absences. (Dhirananda went on to have a local radio show and teach Glen Bernard.)

A decade later, in 1940, the swami was still dodging bullets. Nirad Ranjan Chowdhury, another former associate, sued Yogananda for five hundred thousand dollars. The story in the *Los Angeles Times* ticked off the usual offenses: "Lives in Luxury," "Girls in Abode." It would be another year and many inches of copy before the swami cleared his name.[67]

In 1941, Gerald Heard sent a letter to Prabhavananda severing his ties to the center.

Ascetic by nature, Heard considered renunciation, in its most literal sense, a grounding principle of the spiritual life. Prabhavananda's domestic arrangements, which included a car and doting female disciples, struck Heard as far too worldly. As Isherwood put it, Heard felt Prabhavananda was "too social, too comfortable, and too relaxed," and that this needlessly opened the swami up to criticism.[68]

It was precisely this laxness, the air of "religious Bohemianism, the superficial disorder, the women dressing up in saris, curry, cigarettes, and oriental laissez-faire," that appealed to Isherwood.[69]

In February 1943, he was one of a handful of probationer monks initiated into the new monastery up at the Vedanta Center.

In honor of the occasion Swami Prabhavananda wore his orange robes and lit a homa, or ceremonial fire. There was plenty of food and chatter; photographers snapped away.

Still, for Isherwood, the initiation was anticlimactic. He wore a Sunday suit, not a robe, and felt awkward and "on display." Heard wouldn't come, and Huxley, who was then staying in Llano, California, couldn't make it.[70]

Perhaps this was fitting since Isherwood had become a monk at least in part to avoid a worse fate: more time at a Civilian Public Service (CPS) camp for conscientious objectors. (Even though Isherwood wasn't yet a U.S. citizen, he was still obliged to serve at the CPS camp.)

The previous September, the author had applied to the U.S. draft board for a reclassification from a conscientious objector to a theological student (or 4-D), which would relieve him of any civilian duties as well. By that December, he still hadn't received any word about his request.

As he noted in his diary a few weeks before his initiation, had he not been slated to go to the CPS camp, he "would probably never have actually signed on with the Swami at all," and by the time he was initiated, the draft board had dropped the age limit to thirty-seven, which automatically relieved Isherwood, then thirty-eight, of any obligation to serve at the camp.[71]

But, having taken his vows, Isherwood went through with his commitment and moved up to the center's monastery.

The Southern California Vedanta Society's monastery was like no other; certainly it was nothing like the Ramakrishna missions in India and wasn't even much like those outposts in other American cities.

Rather than buy or build a larger structure to house the monks, Prabhavananda simply bought up the neighboring houses. The monastery was in fact number 1942 Ivar Avenue, dubbed Brahmananda Cottage. The women, or "nuns," a group that had expanded to about five, continued to live at number 1946, with the temple in between. However, traffic was frequent between the two houses, and the genders mingled for all activities, be they chores or meditation, save sleep.[72]

The addition of the probationer monks heightened the contrast between the center's two aspects; one, the most visible to the public, was an amiable but slightly austere salon well attended by the city's literati, the other was more like a family shrine with Prabhavananda in the role of father and guru.

The temple mediated both aspects. Its interior was spare and monochromatic; walls, carpets, chairs, were all covered in a respectable light gray. Photographs of Ramakrishna, the Holy Mother (his wife, Sarada Devi), Vivekananda, Swami Brahmananda, the Buddha, and the Turin shroud lined the walls. The word *Om* carved on the pulpit was the only touch of exoticism.[73]

This is where Prabhavananda (and in earlier years Heard) would give Sunday lectures.

Pull back the curtains behind the pulpit, and you got to see the beating heart of the place: there, glimmering in polished wood and brass and gold, was a small shrine room. The intricately carved shrine stood on a small pedestal and sheltered an assortment of images—of Ramakrishna, Buddha, Krishna, Christ, and Brahmananda—as well as relics from Ramakrishna and the Holy Mother. During Sunday lectures, garlands hung from the photographs and candles flickered in glass candlesticks.[74]

But the shrine room didn't fully come alive unless you attended an all-night vigil, held on various holy days, or meditated there in the wee hours before dawn, as Isherwood did. The incense burned, and devotees felt the small room was like a wood. Despite the quiet, the air itself seemed alert. Other times, "the whole shrine room becomes your brain," as Isherwood put it, "and is filled with thought."[75]

During vigils or japa, the temple could become downright raucous, with devotees taking turns chanting, "Jaya Sri Ramakrishna," singing, or shouting, in some sort of "holy jam session."[76]

The intimacy of the setting encouraged intense devotion amid the monks and nuns, but communal living exacted its price. One had to put up with petty rivalries, minor conspiracies, and physical inconveniences. Isherwood was particularly irked by sound, whether from a radio or a fellow monk who spent half the night typing up Prabhavananda's talks.[77]

Despite these domestic challenges, Isherwood lived at Brahmananda Cottage for two and a half years.

Outsiders saw Isherwood's as a complete renunciation. In his 1945 study, "Transcendentalism in Contemporary Literature," Dr. William York Tindall—then an assistant professor at Columbia University—noted, "Isherwood fell under the power of Heard's Swami, renounced literature and the movies, and the world, and proceeded to meditate in the convenient desert whence he emerges occasionally to assist the Swami in public devotions."[78]

This was hardly the case. Isherwood was no hermit, nor even much of a probationer monk for long, nor did he "renounce literature."

During this time, he and Prabhavananda collaborated on a translation of the *Bhagavad-Gita* (though Isherwood began the work a few months before moving into the center). Prabhavananda rendered the text in English, and Isherwood refined it, drawing on his skills as a novelist and even some tricks he learned from his old friend Wystan Auden.

At first Isherwood had been concerned that his pacifism was incompatible with the *Gita*. After all, Krishna urges Arjuna to fight, and in the end he does. But the author and now translator was reassured to learn that "the Gita doesn't sanction war . . . any more than it sanctions pacifism. It cannot, from its absolute standpoint, do either. It leaves each individual to discover what his or her dharma"—one's duty or one's role in the moral order of things—"is."[79]

Monk or not, Isherwood's dharma also still involved screenwriting. This is how he continued to make a living, and he clung to some of the social habits of his profession. He lunched with the Huxleys and the Viertels (one of Hollywood's émigré couples), took tea with the Beesleys (Dodie Smith Beesley was the author of *101 Dalmations*), dined with the Brechts, and wandered the beach with his friend Greta Garbo. Sometimes, he'd take weekends entirely away from the center. As time wore on, these departures became more frequent, and his sexual restraint loosened.[80]

For all his limitations as a disciple, Isherwood's devotion signaled much to the wider Hollywood community. His was yet another endorsement from an émigré intellectual of Vedanta and yoga. Clearly the philosophy could withstand scrutiny.

More than that, it confirmed that Prabhavananda had near saintly levels of tolerance for human imperfection. After all, Isherwood's homosexuality was no secret in Hollywood, nor were his bouts of drinking and dissipation. If Prabhavananda could accept Isherwood as a probationer monk (not even just as an ordinary student!), it's unlikely that anyone else's indiscretions would ruffle him.

And so, over the 1940s, the number of actors, screenwriters, directors, and Hollywood hangers-on who made pilgrimages to 1946 Ivar Avenue increased markedly. Some came by word of mouth; some came at the express invitation of Isherwood or Huxley or had initially been drawn by Heard's riveting biweekly performances.[81]

Greta Garbo lunched at the center in the summer of 1943. According to Isherwood, she charmed everyone there, "sighing about how wonderful it must be to be a nun."[82]

Somerset "Willie" Maugham paid Prabhavananda a visit in 1941. It was less than successful. The author reportedly struck the swami as a typical British imperialist who opposed Indian independence.[83]

A few years later, in June 1945, Maugham and the swami lunched at Players restaurant on Sunset Boulevard. Isherwood was there, presumably to smooth ruffled feathers, and it worked. Prabhavananda agreed to help the author and director George Cukor with the screenplay of Maugham's novel *The Razor's Edge* and even suggested some additional material to enhance the film's authenticity. (Cukor was later replaced by a different director, who ignored the swami's advice.)[84]

Robert Balzer was also a regular visitor to the Vedanta Temple throughout the forties. A fixture in Hollywood's "haut monde" and an epicure, Balzer ran the family business, a fine grocery store. His first real job in Los Angeles was assistant to studio head Jack Warner, and he counted among his friends many of Hollywood's most famous celebrities. (Starting in the late 1940s, he was also Gloria Swanson's lover.)[85]

Yoga turned out to be remarkably plastic when it came to the needs and wants of Southern Californians.

During the war the Vedanta Society under Prabhavananda's steward-ship provided a refuge for people such as Isherwood and Huxley whose pacifism was inextricably bound to their spiritual convictions and prac-tice. Many others who spent time at the center were also insulated from war, to the extent anyone could be: they were by and large past draft age and wealthy.

By 1945, Isherwood and Huxley had moved on. But their association with the Hollywood Vedanta Society had furnished yoga with new stores of energy.[86]

Now, postwar, this energy was released, making yoga far more avail-able to Americans, whether veterans trying to make sense of the horrors they had witnessed or middle-class women enjoying a new prosperity, as well as the next generation of Hollywood starlets and seekers.

Putnam had rejected the Prabhavananda-Isherwood *Bhagavad-Gita* translation, but Marcel Rodd put out an edition, with a forward by Hux-ley. The book was well received. In February 1945, *Time* described the translation as "simpler and freer than other [recent] English translations" and mistakenly noted that Isherwood was "now thinking seriously of be-coming a swami."[87]

Others began to publish widely read yoga books. Paramahansa Yo-gananda had long produced pamphlets and spiritual instruction manuals. During the war years he wrote the bulk of his longest, most sustained, and ultimately most popular work, *Autobiography of a Yogi*. It's a fantasti-cal and enchanted tale, filled with miracles (he passed an exam without ever having studied the material thanks to his guru's grace; while meditat-ing, his consciousness entered the body of a captain fighting a fatal battle) and the near miraculous prosperity he and his organization enjoyed in America. The Philosophical Library published *Autobiography of a Yogi* in 1946. While a number of reviewers didn't take the book seriously, many major news outlets wrote it up.[88]

As churches began to swell with new members in a spurt of post-war religiosity, the *Los Angeles Times* counted "hundreds of students of Vedanta," in addition to numerous students of unspecified swamis and yogis. Sales of the Isherwood-Prabhavananda *Bhagavad-Gita* soon neared a quarter million copies, and by the end of the decade, the Philosophical Library had issued a second edition of Yogananda's *Autobiography of a Yogi*.[89]

9

HATHA YOGA ON SUNSET BOULEVARD

In January 1947, a petite woman with pale skin, brown hair, and blue eyes came to Hollywood. She spoke perfect English with a Russian accent and had, according to friends, a ready wit. She was the same age as Claire Stuart, nearly forty-eight. Her usual attire was a sari. She went by the name Indra Devi.

This was a particularly inauspicious year for Los Angeles. The same month Devi arrived, Elizabeth Short's severed corpse was found in an empty lot in South Central. The Black Dahlia has the distinction of being only the most famous murder of the year. Los Angeles counted at least a hundred in 1947; most didn't merit more than a paragraph in the city's rapacious dailies.[1]

The influx of returning servicemen was partly to blame for the steep rise in crime. The City of Angels had welcomed the country's veterans with open arms. Many came to work in the Southland's aviation industry or at new automotive plants and almost instantly populated new suburbs. On a single day in February 1947, forty vets and their families moved into Panorama City, before the sod for the front lawns had been laid. (Two years later, 30 percent of Angelenos had arrived *after* 1940.) To keep pace, subdivisions spread over the Los Angeles basin like kudzu, swallowing up orchards and farms.[2]

Nineteen forty-seven was also the year that Hollywood turned on itself. To save his own skin, studio head Jack Warner gave the House Un-American Activities Committee (HUAC) a list of alleged communists. By the end of the year, a good number of actors' and screenwriters' careers were ruined, the "Hollywood Ten" had become famous for refusing to testify, assorted others had made uneasy comprises to continue working, and a few, including Bertolt Brecht, had fled the country.[3]

Soon after making her way to Hollywood, Devi opened a small Hatha Yoga studio at 8806 Sunset Boulevard, technically West Hollywood, in an office complex at the corner of Sunset and Holloway. The immediate neighborhood was neither ritzy nor run-down—small shops and apartment buildings filled the blocks south and just north of this strip of Sunset.

Her friends warned her that using the word *yoga*, which summoned thoughts of cults, rope tricks, snake charming, and charlatans, would put off potential students. Devi was undeterred. She put up a wooden sign on Sunset Boulevard. Large, white capital letters announced INDRA DEVI, YOGA CLASSES, and an arrow under the text pointed drivers toward the building that housed her studio.[4]

Her school was minimalist; the spare rooms had whitewashed walls, matted floors, and few pictures, and the overall atmosphere was in stark contrast to that of the Vedanta temple. Isherwood had been enchanted by the casualness of the Vedanta center—the big meals, the domestic bustle, and the cigarettes—and had described the atmosphere as festive and feminine, even slightly erotic. The women, many of whom were on the plump side to begin with, "so often seemed to be calling attention to their presence, especially when decked out in their best saris with tin-kling bracelets, and the saris naturally enlarged the bottoms." Most of Devi's pupils, by contrast, were trim or at least well kempt, and her center projected order and discipline.[5]

As a teacher, Devi was both gracious and exacting. Sharp, opinion-ated, and focused, she hewed to a few core principles: Hatha Yoga con-tained all that you needed to know for perfect health, peace of mind, and spiritual realization; it was the only yoga suited to busy modern lives; and it would be dangerous for her to convey anything of a spiritual matter. (You needed a guru for that.)[6]

Her classes typically began with some simple breathing exercises. There was an art to proper breathing. You had to breathe through your nostrils with your mouth closed, contract your throat, and slowly inhale, letting your rib cage expand as you did so. If done correctly, you'd hear a "little hissing sound coming from the back of the throat." To exhale, you had to contract your rib cage and pull your abdomen in slightly.[7]

Devi then directed her students to take a sequence of postures (e.g., "cobra," "locust," "bow," and "arch"), all the while reminding them to breathe correctly.

Though Devi spoke precise English, her rolled r's and softened th's made her sound like nothing so much as a ballet instructor, putting her students through tedious routines that yielded unearthly results.

After the postures, Devi usually instructed her students to lie down, close their eyes, and imagine that they were "a cloud passing over the earth."[8]

The experience was gentle and even relaxing. Her students didn't sweat profusely, the way Theos Bernard had when practicing extended headstands or pranayama, or hold poses until their muscles quivered. No, Devi insisted that to strain was to defeat the purpose. Over time, and with regular practice, tight joints and knotted muscles would release themselves.[9]

Within a few years, Devi attracted A-list celebrities including Greta Garbo, Gloria Swanson, Mala Powers, Robert Ryan, Linda Christian, and Jennifer Jones. A number of her students, like Claire Stuart's, were regular visitors up at the Vedanta Temple.

None had been fingered by Warner, but some were more vocal in their opposition to McCarthy's tactics than others. Despite her personal belief that McCarthy's claims were exaggerated, if not paranoid, Swanson acted briefly as a "goodwill ambassador" for the industry, hoping to shore up sympathy in the broader public. Ryan, on the other hand, was a member of the Committee for the First Amendment, formed in the wake of the HUAC hearings.[10]

Devi's near immediate success in Los Angeles reads like some strange fairy tale: a virtually unknown middle-aged foreigner alights in the City of Angels to teach a relatively obscure type of yoga and is almost immediately patronized by the city's biggest stars.

But there wasn't anything particularly unusual about the course of events. Devi had lived most of her life in the company of royalty of some sort and had the assuredness of wealth, though she had long since dispensed with its outward manifestations.

Born Eugenie Peterson in Latvia in 1899, she was the daughter of a Swedish bank director and, on her mother's side, Russian nobility. The young Eugenie grew up in splendor in Russia until the revolution, at which point she and her mother fled to Berlin, where she joined the city's legendary Der Blaue Vogel theater and became a leading actress and dancer.[11]

On her second trip to India in 1929, a renegade film director spotted Eugenie dancing at a Theosophical Society production. He offered her the lead in his film. She took a stage name, and with a stroke Eugenie Peterson became Indra Devi, trumpeted as "the new rising star of Indian screen."[12]

Shortly thereafter, Devi married a Czech diplomat and for a time lived the life of a hostess in Bombay.[13]

When her interest in yoga was piqued, Prince Mussoorie of Nepal gave her a demonstration of several asanas.[14]

Devi decided she would study the discipline.

Having once witnessed Mysore Palace Yogi Sri T. Krishnamacharya stop his heart (a demonstration Theos Bernard was sorry to have missed), she eventually decided to study with him.[15]

When he refused to teach her—she was a Westerner and a woman, which both immediately disqualified her as his pupil—Devi had her friend the raja of Mysore himself intervene on her behalf.

After a year of study, Krishnamacharya asked Devi to teach yoga in China, her husband's next posting. It was less a request than an order.[16]

She opened a Hatha Yoga school in Shanghai, and when the Japanese occupation made it difficult to run it, she moved her five daily classes (of twenty-five students each) to Madame Chiang Kai-shek's bedroom.[17]

Devi traveled in similar circles in America. She knew the Huxleys, which virtually guaranteed access to Hollywood seekers. (Over a weekend spent at their place, Devi discovered the gulf between American diet doctors' advice and the actual diets of most Americans.)

She was also close to J. Krishnamurti. (Annie Besant had recognized Krishnamurti as Theosophy's next messiah when he was a teen, but in 1929 he abdicated this role and for a while he retreated to a farm in Ojai, California, which became a watering hole for celebrity seekers during the war.)[18]

Several seasons teaching at Elizabeth Arden's beauty farms in Maine and Arizona increased Devi's popularity among America's aristocracy, its movie stars and the wives of businessmen and politicians, seeking in most cases to "reduce."[19]

The coup de grâce, according to at least one friend and pupil, was Devi's acquaintance with Paul Bragg, bestselling author, dietitian, and "health adviser to stage and screen stars."[20]

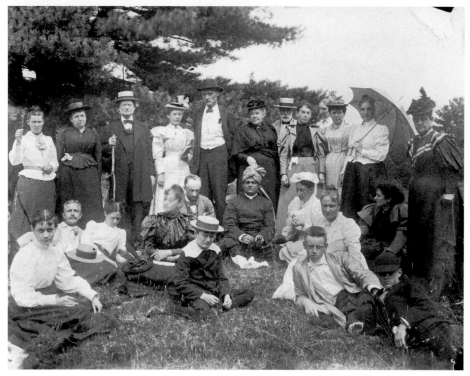

Swami Vivekananda with a class under the pines at Green Acre, 1894. Sarah Farmer is to his immediate left. (Courtesy of Bahá'í Community Archives, Eliot, Maine)

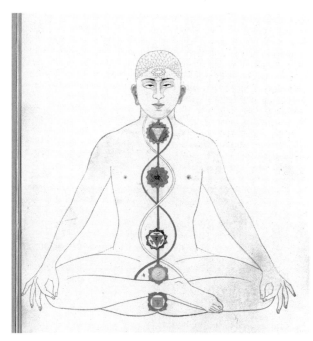

Illustration of the chakras from *The Six Centres and the Serpent Power* by Arthur Avalon, 1919

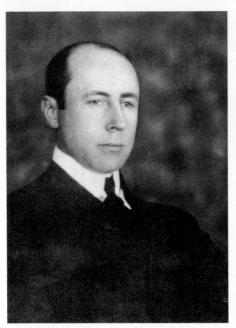

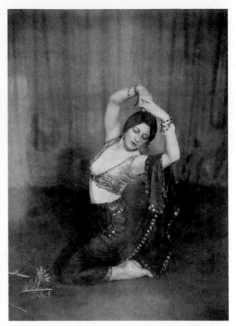

Pierre A. Bernard, circa 1912 (Courtesy of Bernard Collection, Historical Society of Rockland County, New City, N.Y.)

Blanche De Vries, "Summer Follies," 1924, at C.C.C. (Courtesy of Bernard Collection, Historical Society of Rockland County, New City, N.Y.)

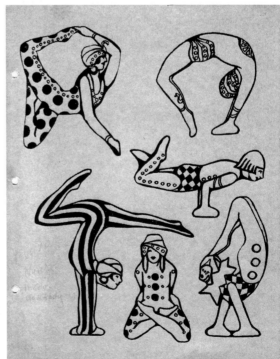

C.C.C. circus program, 1929
(Courtesy of Bernard Collection, Historical Society of Rockland County, New City, N.Y.)

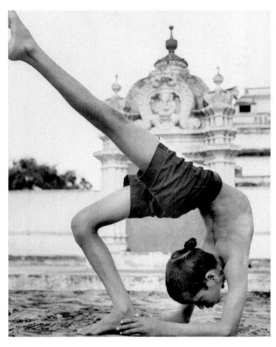

Mysore Palace yoga featured in "Speaking of Pictures . . . This Is Real Yoga" in *Life*, February 24, 1941. This photo shows a boy twisting himself into a yoga position. (© Wallace Kirkland/Getty Images)

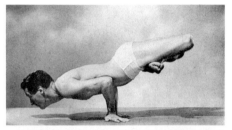

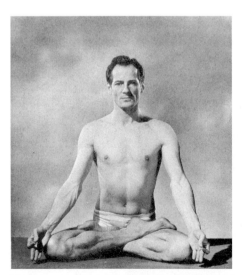

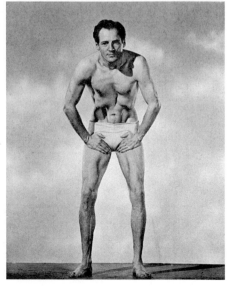

Theos Bernard from *Hatha Yoga: The Report of a Personal Experience* (1944). Clockwise from above: in Padmasana, in Mayurasana variation, and performing Nauli Madhyama

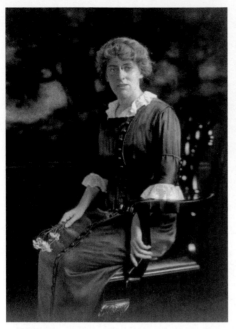

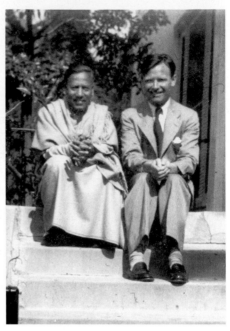

Margaret Woodrow Wilson, circa 1912 (Courtesy of the Library of Congress, Prints and Photographs Division)

Swami Prabhavananda and Christopher Isherwood at the Hollywood Vedanta Temple, circa the late 1940s (Courtesy of the Vedanta Archives, Vedanta Society of Southern California)

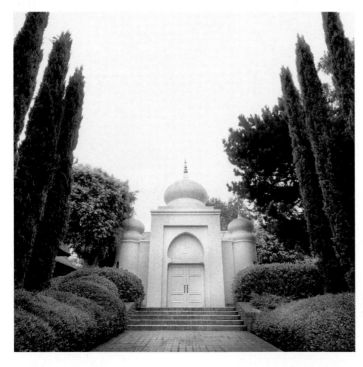

Hollywood Vedanta Temple (© Michael Rauner)

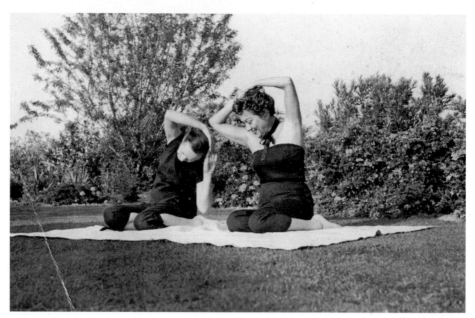

Indra Devi and Gloria Swanson, 1953 (© Mischa Pelz, Jr. Used by permission of Gloria Swanson, Inc., and the Gloria Swanson Collection, Harry Ransom Center, the University of Texas at Austin)

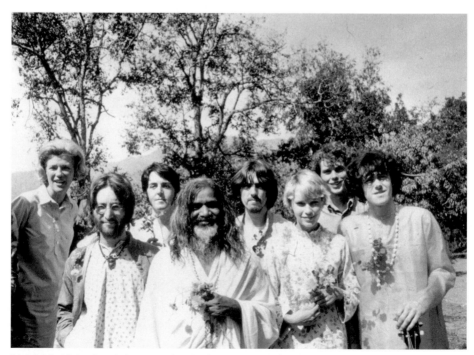

Maharishi Mahesh with (among others) John Lennon, Paul McCartney, George Harrison, Mia Farrow, and Donovan, Rishikesh, 1968 (© Keystone Features/Hulton Archive/Getty Images)

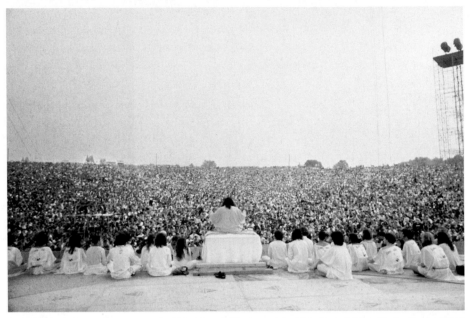

Swami Satchidananda opening the Woodstock Music and Art Fair, Bethel, New York, August 1969
(© Elliott Landy/The Image Works)

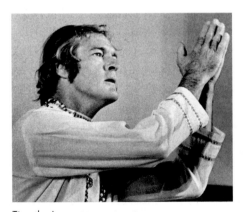

Timothy Leary (© Peter Simon)

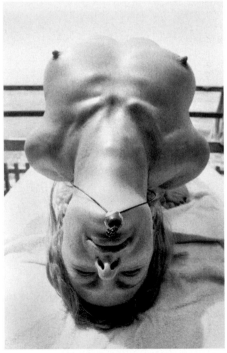

Woman in back bend (Laghuvajrasana) at the Esalen Institute, 1972 (© Peter Simon)

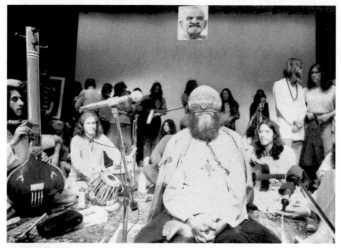

Ram Dass in Berkeley, California, 1973 (© Peter Simon)

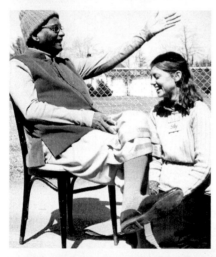

Sally Kempton and Swami Muktananda, from the April 12, 1976, issue of *New York* magazine (© Benno Friedman)

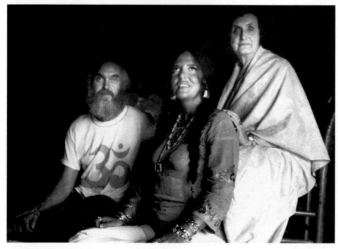

Ram Dass with Joya Santayana and the spiritual teacher Hilda Charlton, 1976

(© Rameshwar Das, 1976)

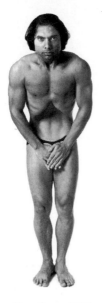

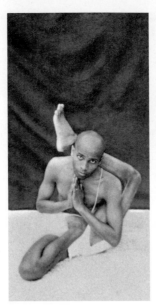

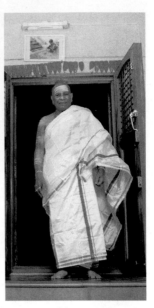

Bikram Choudhury, 1978 (© Guy Webster)

Pattabhi Jois in virañcyāsana (Courtesy of the Sri K. Pattabhi Jois Ashtanga Yoga Institute, Mysore)

Sri K. Pattabhi Jois in Mysore, India, 2006 (© Tom Rosenthal)

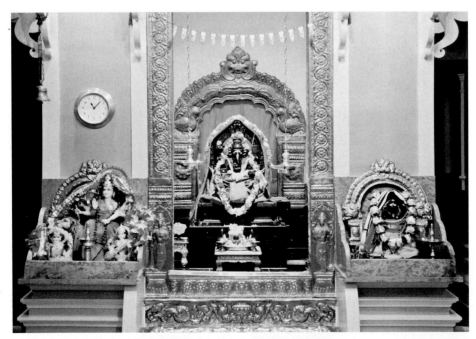

Sri Ganesha Temple at Ashtanga Yoga New York, 2009 (© Alessia Elysee)

In February 1949, Bragg hosted a brief lecture series in Los Angeles at the fifteen-hundred-seat Embassy auditorium.[21]

Bragg's ads tantalized readers with an "Important Health Message from India." In "3 Truth Revealing Lectures," he promised, Indra Devi would show the audience how to "recharge the batteries of your mind and body with Vital Cosmic Energy." Not only that, Devi would give "an amazing exhibition of Yoga Health exercises."[22]

Besides Devi's superlative access to the most influential people in any given place and time, Los Angeles had a huge pent-up demand for Hatha Yoga instruction.

Heard had actually been wrong about Vedanta. It didn't articulate a complete system, based as it was on "a clear realisation of the body-mind relationship," for the simple reason that it didn't adequately address people's bodies.

The only things Prabhavananda had to offer anyone seeking physical, as well as spiritual, transformation were some modest breathing exercises, which were useful mostly for calming the mind.[23]

Prabhavananda promised a system that integrated mind and body and didn't deliver on it. His teaching had always focused first and foremost on philosophy. The techniques he taught his more ardent devotees, the ones Isherwood had practiced daily while he was living at the center, combined Raja Yoga, the meditative yoga detailed in Patanjali's *Sutras*, and Bhakti Yoga, the devotional mode of God realization Krishna outlined in the *Gita*. Prabhavananda's yoga centered on the mind and the heart, not the organ, but the seat of emotions, and the devotee's task was to control the former and turn the latter toward God.

Devi, on the other hand, taught a form of yoga that was intensely physical and made purifying your body the necessary first stage of spiritual training. As a result, Devi's yoga—Hatha Yoga—met far more of the needs of Hollywood seekers, especially female ones, who were under constant pressure to look radiantly youthful, than did the yoga you'd encounter at the Vedanta Society.

Before they discovered Hatha Yoga, many of these actors, actresses, and screenwriters were already being treated by a coterie of physicians and nutritionists, each proclaiming separately that he or she had the key to health and happiness. People such as Gayelord Hauser, who called himself a doctor but had never received an M.D., Paul Bragg, Dr. Kolisch, Dr. Sigfrid Knauer, and Dr. Henry G. Bieler were all regularly consulted.

Much of the advice these men doled out was dismissed as mere quackery at the time, though today it sounds like common sense: eat lots of fruits and vegetables, eat only whole grains, get lots of rest, drink plenty of water, and exercise. Many also advocated fasting as a way to cleanse and detoxify the system. Some focused intently on a few special foods and developed product lines. (Hauser's salt alternative, Spike, is still available, as are Bragg's liquid aminos and apple cider vinegar.)

Garbo was devoted to both Bieler and Hauser, whose recipe for eternal youth included raw-vegetable salads, brewer's yeast, blackstrap molasses, and yogurt.[24]

Isherwood counted the younger, strikingly handsome dietitian Hauser as one of Garbo's prophets. Garbo and Hauser spent hours together, often in public. Gossip columnists delighted in the association, presumed it romantic, and didn't need much of an excuse to cover it. "Greta Garbo and Gayelord Hauser lunched at the Beverly Wilshire on mixed greens, a seafood salad and cold baked potatoes," wrote Hedda Hopper in January 1947, with no further explanation.[25]

There was, after all, some truth to those stereotypes about Los Angeles. However, it was hardly the weather that turned people into health faddists. For many, it was professional exigency. (Gossip columnist Elsa Maxwell claims she once walked in on Garbo studying her reflection in a powder-room mirror and bursting into tears, middle-aged, by Hollywood standards, at just thirty-four.)[26]

Others turned to these men because conventional medicine had failed them.

Isherwood himself as well as Huxley and some of the monks and nuns up at the Vedanta center were patients of Dr. Kolisch's. A Viennese physician and student of Prabhavananda's, Kolisch at one point put Huxley on a "meatless, milkless, saltless diet," which the author believed helped cure a heart spasm.[27]

If you made a Venn diagram of the Angelenos who sought counsel from alternative doctors and those who studied at the Hollywood Vedanta center, you would find a great deal of overlap.

Of course, there *was* a program that united all of these seemingly disparate pursuits—Hatha Yoga.

Its physical practices, internal-cleansing techniques, and dietary strictures are in the service of spiritual realization. Because the Hatha Yogi seeks liberation in this lifetime, the discipline is geared toward creating a divine, or yogic, body, ageless, immune to disease, "adamantine."[28]

What more could Hollywood ask for?

The problem was, until Devi's arrival, Los Angeles had no Hatha Yoga school. One likely reason is that few qualified teachers were in the area, and the institutes that trained them were concentrated in New York State—most notably C.C.C. in Nyack and De Vries's Living Art Center Studios in Manhattan.

Sri Yogendra, whom Theos and Viola had so admired, had set up a Hatha Yoga health clinic in Harriman, New York, not too far from C.C.C.; however, it operated for only a few years in the early 1920s.[29]

Rishi Gherwal, Hatha Yogi Wassan, and Swami Dhirananda had all taught Hatha Yoga in Southern California (Glen Bernard had studied with both Dhirananda and Wassan). They peddled it as a way to build psychic powers, a system of health and healing, and the doorway to "higher consciousness." But these Indian teachers had been most active in the 1920s and 1930s and had not built institutions that could carry on their work or produce the next generation of teachers.[30]

Theos himself might have gone on to train other Hatha Yoga teachers.

After shutting down his yoga institute and Pierre Health Studios, he had settled in Santa Barbara, where Ganna Walska had built him a lavish retreat. However, Theos spent relatively little time teaching yoga. He was focused on trying to get his Academy of Tibetan Literature off the ground. And by 1947, he had left California for Tibet, a contract for another book in hand.[31]

So, until Devi's arrival, most Angelenos had been striving for health and spiritual uplift piecemeal.[32]

Those who knew about yoga often as not didn't make the connection to health. And those seeking health and fitness didn't know to turn to yoga.

Lecturing to a Los Angeles Eaters Anonymous meeting not too long after her arrival in Hollywood, Devi vividly recalls being asked, "How often do you take yogurt?" It took the Hatha Yoga instructor a few minutes, and several more questions about her yogurt intake, to realize that the woman asking the question had misheard her entire lecture.[33]

Hollywood also hadn't woken up to Hatha Yoga for another reason: many of the poses looked almost identical to standard calisthenics and gymnastics warm-ups.

In 1941, President Roosevelt had made physical fitness a national priority, and that August Jack "Strong Man" Kelly was appointed director of physical training for the nation. Kelly recommended that Americans form calisthenics, soccer, swimming, and hiking clubs. His efforts were aimed, in part, at reversing a trend. In 1939, *Life* noted that the "setting-up-exercise fad" was already declining. Whether or not they were exercising more, throughout the war, Americans were treated to descriptions and photographs of service men and women doing long sets of calisthenics.[34]

Postwar, many actresses still favored these sorts of "setting-up" exercises to keep their figures trim.

Susan Hayward, Bette Davis, and Joan Bennett, to name just a few, all included calisthenics in their fitness regimens. As gossip columnist Ida Jean Kain put it, "Another reason the girls are not above calisthenics—nothing short of perfect measurements can pass the camera test."[35]

Once the war had ended, and with it food rationing, "exercise pictures" became one of the best ways to break a new talent. The young, lithe women would often pose in swimsuits; they'd bend and stretch, demonstrating "waist whittlers," "spine stretchers," and tummy "flatners." Many didn't exercise routinely; they were young enough not to need to. The photographs served their purpose nonetheless, getting these women noticed.

In 1948, Marilyn Monroe posed for just this sort of series for Columbia Pictures. Monroe was twenty-one at the time, still nearly unknown, and something of a fitness fanatic. The copy fixed to the back of the prints read, in part: "LOOK PRETTY, FEEL GOOD. Marilyn Monroe, who plays the ingenue lead in Columbia's *Ladies of the Chorus*, exercises her way to beauty and health."

The photos garnered her a bit of publicity, appearing in a number of smaller papers such as the *Portsmouth Herald* (based in New Hampshire) and Ohio's *Coshocton Tribune* in August 1948, just ahead of the release of the film. The following spring, *Movie Stars Parade* ran six poses from the series with an accompanying article titled "Best Shape Ever." None of these publications mentioned yoga.[36]

But several of the poses Monroe struck look identical to basic yoga postures. One of these was a variation of a "stretcher" that Joan Bennett recommended: "Lie flat on the floor, arms and legs straight. Raise legs and arms, and lift torso until hands touch legs, keeping stomach tucked in; then drop legs hard, lower arms, and start again." Monroe had lifted her torso, grabbed her ankles, and held on rather than just touching her legs, as if she had taken boat pose (Paripūrṇa Nāvāsana). Cronenweth also shot a picture of Monroe lying on her belly, clasping her ankles with her hands, which raised her chest off the ground. This is Dhanur-āsana, and Monroe demonstrated it in two different outfits, the white swimsuit and a pair of shorts and a short-sleeved turtleneck, holding a baton.[37]

Whether Monroe had modeled several Hatha Yoga poses or had just improvised on popular calisthenics is impossible to say. As Devi put it, "If you go into any beauty parlor, body culture school, or gymnasium you will be surprised to see how many of the Yoga exercises are performed there." She believed that Westerners had imported these postures and, to an extent, denatured them. But the reverse was just as likely, if not more so.

Modern Hatha Yoga has always been something of a mongrel. Recent research suggests that when Devi's guru Sri Krishnamacharya set about developing a Hatha Yoga program at the Mysore Palace in the early 1930s, he relied on numerous disparate sources, from a twelfth-century text to native gymnastics. Scholars believe the system he ended up creating, which helped spur a revival of Hatha Yoga across India, blended yogic asanas, elements of Indian wrestling and Western gymnastics, and possibly moves found in British military-training exercises.[38]

Keenly aware of the similarities, Devi would always maintain that "deep rhythmic breathing" distinguished Hatha Yoga from mere calisthenics.

Los Angeles, wrote Frank Fenton in his novel *A Place in the Sun*, "was a lovely makeshift city. Even the trees and plants did not belong here. They came, like the people, from far places, some familiar, some exotic, all wanderers of one sort or another."[39]

Entering the 1950s, due to the work of Prabhavananda, Yogananda, Devi, and others, yoga had spread so efficiently through the Southland that, like the eucalyptus and bougainvillea, people mistook it for a native species. Los Angeles could now make another claim: its yoga teachers were among the most prolific, producing more books that sold more copies than any other locale so far.

Following up their successful collaboration on the *Bhagavad-Gita*, Isherwood and Prabhavananda collaborated on a translation of the *Yoga Sutras*. Harper & Brothers released *How to Know God: The Yoga Aphorisms of Patanjali* in 1953. In retrospect, Isherwood was mortified by the title. It made him think of "all those books which tell you *how* to fix the plumbing, plant a vegetable garden, cook on a barbecue, etc."[40]

Of course this was exactly what had appealed to Heard and others about yoga: it offered concrete instructions to ordinary folks—and hope that you might succeed at following them—for a seemingly supernatural feat.

The following year, New American Library issued a paperback edition of the Prabhavananda-Isherwood translation of the *Gita*. Novelist Gerald Sykes, writing in *The New York Times*, called this new edition a "publishing event of major importance."[41]

When Devi had the opportunity to write a book for a big trade publisher, Prentice-Hall, she took it and trained her prodigious energy on the task. (Mala Powers once described her as a butterfly, giving each thing, be it a pose, a beggar child in India, or a conversation, her complete and undivided attention before flitting to the next.)[42]

Devi came up with a winning formula. She yoked Hatha Yoga to the health movement and its most popular advocates, including Gaylord Hauser, whose 1950 book, *Look Younger, Live Longer*, stayed on *The New York Times'* bestseller list for more than a year.[43]

She secured endorsements by celebrity students including Gloria Swanson, Linda Christian, and Ruth St. Denis. She enlisted Mala Powers, who had recently wowed audiences in *Cyrano de Bergerac*, and Swanson to demonstrate a number of asanas.

Swanson was a particularly enthusiastic model. Her photo shoot took place behind a sprawling neo-Georgian mansion on Mulholland Drive, which had been the home of several famed screenwriters and actresses, including Joan Fontaine.

Here is Gloria looking gamely into the camera as she stands on one foot, knee bent in half lotus, one hand clasping her foot, the other brushing her thigh. Her cropped hair is curled off her face. Lipstick gives her smile a ruby sheen. A cummerbund and a bow hanging jauntily around her neck accent her otherwise stark ensemble. She poses on a small Persian rug on a wide lawn bordered by young bushes. A bleached sky and gray hills silhouette her head and shoulders.

In another photograph, Swanson and Devi, who had become close friends, each sit with one leg extended and the other bent in half lotus. They're dressed almost identically in slim black pants and dark tops. Gloria reaches for her outstretched foot; the sun sculpts her arms and bare shoulders. Her eyes are downcast and her brow ever so slightly furrowed in concentration. Meanwhile Indra looks on, spine erect, a look of disapproval (or is it merely the glare?) creasing her forehead.

The irony of Swanson's stint as a yoga model is hard to miss.

Her best "talking" film role was Norma Desmond in *Sunset Boulevard*, who can't accept her mortality or the loss of beauty that attends it. Many fans believed Swanson *was* Desmond, and to her dismay, most directors seemed similarly convinced of this.[44]

In reality, Gloria Swanson remained a beauty icon into her fifties who seemed to defy all the rules of aging and who handily profited from her youthful looks. (A smooth-skinned Swanson smiles knowingly in a 1951 Jergens ad. The copy reads, "Will you look as young as Gloria Swanson at 51?")[45]

Swanson was also indefatigable. In the early 1950s, she hosted and acted in a television series, starred on Broadway, and designed a successful mass-market clothing line called Forever Young.[46]

The photographs taken with Devi in early 1953 were more proof of Swanson's age-defying physique. A mother and grandmother, Swanson looks limber and fit. Her skin is firm, her waist narrow, her belly flat. You can see the faint outline of her biceps. She smiles in lotus posture, as though it's the most natural thing in the world to sit with your legs crossed and feet pressed on opposite thighs. (Anyone who has ever tried this posture knows that it's impossible to do with arthritic knees or hips.)[47]

Swanson would be the first movie star to admit that yoga was her youth and beauty secret, and in so doing she'd boost yoga's profile and possibly book sales. For Devi had rightly calculated that yoga still needed celebrity to sell.

There was only one hitch.

Swanson was writing a book too, tentatively titled "Beauty After Forty," also to be published by Prentice-Hall. In June, Swanson wrote Devi, "I understand from Prentice-Hall, because I am starting my book very soon, that they are going to use the photos of you and I in my book rather than yours."[48]

Prentice-Hall had pulled the photos of Swanson from Devi's book mere months before it was due to come out.

Instead, Swanson introduced Devi and her book, *Forever Young, Forever Healthy: Simplified Yoga for Modern Living*, at the Waldorf-Astoria in the fall of 1953. It was the one publicity event the actress consented to do.[49]

Forever Young, Forever Healthy isn't a book about yoga per se. Devi doesn't detail each limb of Hatha Yoga or refer to its main texts. She alludes only tangentially to the subtle body and not by name.[50]

There are no deities here.

Instead, Devi wrote a broader treatise on health. In her view, Hatha Yoga just happens to be the best way to get—and stay—healthy.

A problem solver, Devi lays out chapters based on specific health concerns such as constipation, insomnia, and headaches and laces her text with testimonials from real students.

First and foremost, there's Devi's own descent into illness, then recovery through Hatha Yoga.

When her husband was stationed in Bombay, she tried to effect a "Yoga healing" on a friend who was ill and had an important meeting to attend. She did little more than wave her hands over him while concentrating her thoughts on banishing his illness. He felt almost instantly better and was able to attend to his professional duties.

Devi, however, came down with a mysterious, intractable heart ailment. Formerly quite active, she was now taxed by the slightest effort. She put on weight and aged, seemingly overnight. No doctor could help her. Devi had, in mere moments, gone from energetic hostess to invalid.

Several years later and in Europe, she stumbled on a young medical student who promised to cure her in five short sessions. He administered no drugs, needles, or tonics of any sort nor, as far as Devi's account goes, does it appear that he even touched her body directly. Yet, he drove out whatever was afflicting her.[51]

Back in India and newly healed, Devi began her own education in yoga at Kuvalayananda's center in Pune. But it was Krishnamacharya who transformed Devi from a pudgy novice into an expert in Hatha Yoga.

To do this, she had to follow a strict diet (for a relatively brief period), give up coffee (for good), go to bed before 9:30 p.m., rise before dawn, and practice asanas and meditation three times a day—morning, noon, and evening. Krishnamacharya got Devi to do a headstand and began instructing her in pranayama.

The stories from her students about the transforming effects of yoga were only slightly less dramatic and had the advantage of being keyed to somewhat more ordinary lives.

Afflicted with terrible stage fright, an actress began using simple breathing exercises and could now perform effortlessly. A female doctor who had had menstrual trouble for years normalized after a few months of yoga. A Danish official suffered horrible headaches for decades; six weeks of Devi's program put him "on the road to sure recovery."[52]

In the drama Devi scripted of well-being lost and regained, of youth squandered and then almost magically restored, Shiva didn't even have a bit part.

But her stroke of genius in presenting Hatha Yoga was to narrow her scope to just the postures and some simple breathing exercises, which she carefully distinguished from pranayama.[53]

You have to applaud the audacity of her shorthand. By page 80, she has retranslated the word *yoga*. Now when she uses it, she's referring to only the asanas, one small part of eight stages of Hatha Yoga.[54]

Just as Charles Wilkins took it upon himself to render *yoga* as "devotion" through much of the *Bhagavad-Gita*, Devi makes the word *yoga* mean what will least offend her audience.[55]

The result was a Hatha Yoga that was simple, practical, and adaptive.[56]

It bore little resemblance to the Hatha Yoga Americans had been exposed to up until then, in publications such as *Life* and *The Family Circle* or in earlier articles about Pierre Bernard.

Take the *Life* photos of Krishnamacharya's students shot at the Mysore Palace in early 1941: The boys range from ten years old to twenty. Their capacity to fold, twist, lift, and balance in the most unlikely combinations is breathtaking. These boys look as wiry and mischievous as young boys everywhere; however, they seem to have exceptional mastery of their bodies. This yoga was not for the faint of heart or even, possibly, for adults.[57]

The pictures of Theos in various yoga postures accompanying his dissertation left a similar impression.

Theos had assumed Kukkuṭāsana—he hovers above the ground, arms threaded through his legs, which are crossed in lotus position—Ardha Matsyendrāsana (a deep seated twist with one leg in half lotus), and Mayūrāsana (he balances his entire body on his elbows with legs extended), among others. In many photos his mouth is set in a line, and he fixes his gaze at a point somewhere beyond the camera. It's a look of intense concentration.[58]

The Hatha Yoga Theos practiced looked to be serious stuff, and it was.

The photographs Devi includes show just how completely she had refashioned Hatha Yoga. Most of the models, famous or not, are pretty young women. They wear leotards and tights, or high-cut shorts. The women smile; their hair is neatly arranged. Though some take challenging poses, there is no sense of strain or difficulty. The impression is that you too might do this, with a little practice.

Reading *Forever Young, Forever Healthy*, you could imagine taking one of Devi's classes, powdering your nose, then lunching at the Brown Derby. You could pick and chose what advice to follow, which poses, what dietary adjustments, depending on your needs and desires.

Where Theos saw a complete system accessible, in theory, to all, Devi saw a system that offered something for everyone but not everything to everyone.

So she reduced *yoga*, a bloated kitchen-sink of a word, down to something that fit more readily into American ways of thinking. Yoga was in effect a health tonic.

This was the paradox of Devi's success. Hatha Yoga held the promise of spiritual uplift and near physical immortality. But she realized that to reach Americans, it was far more effective to sunder the two endeavors.[59]

Devi was so good at packaging Hatha Yoga as a defense against illness and aging, she made this maddeningly complex discipline so accessible and relevant to postwar Americans, that it was easy to lose sight of its real purpose—spiritual liberation.

There were other risks as well. Her Hatha Yoga was far simpler, far

gentler, than Theos's, certainly, but the path to youth and health she describes bucked a good deal of conventional wisdom of the era.

The hourglass figure was fashionable again, as were plucked eyebrows, curled hair, and high heels.

Joan Bennett offered a relatively concise beauty formula in her book *How to Be Attractive*. Her advice spanned makeup application, flattening "your tummy" and developing your bust, "Choosing Your Accessories," and "Staying Dainty."

Most of her advice amounted to creating an illusion of youth and health. Like most of her contemporaries, she recommended lipstick and blush carefully applied to mimic a teenager's cheeks blooming with circulation; eyeliner and mascara to simulate thick lashes and achieve that "doe-eyed look"; and girdles—she advised owning at least two and washing them after each wearing—to mimic the figure of a woman who had never given birth.[60]

Bennett believed there was no longer any excuse for not making the most of one's looks; so many tools were now so readily at hand. "There are beauty salons on every corner," wrote Bennett, "and counters are stacked high with preparations to improve the appearance of everything from toenails to topknot."

Postwar prosperity had merely multiplied the beauty options; Bennett's job was to help women sift through the plentitude. It was assumed that if one applied such lessons assiduously, one would minimize "wear and tear." Eternal youth was not even suggested. (And on a personal note, Bennett considered Swanson, one of Devi's most dedicated students, excessive when it came to her health regimen.)[61]

Devi on the other hand paid no heed to cosmetics and hairstyles. Her advice for beauty, health, and well-being was to practice Hatha Yoga. To a large extent, this meant giving up things: cigarettes, high heels—they had made her walk "like a Chinese woman tottering on bound feet," and more to the point, they strained muscles and put undo pressure on the "female organs"—even food, for anyone hardy enough to take her advice on fasting. Most of all, Devi rejected the idea that beauty was a function of products wisely purchased and skillfully used. "I have been told that here in America people like to go to lectures on health, youth, longevity and peace of mind but will not do anything about getting it if it involves an effort," she cautioned near the end of *Forever Young, Forever Healthy*. "If

that is the case with you, I am afraid you are wasting your time reading this book."[62]

To promote *Forever Young, Forever Healthy,* Devi did more than her share of publicity events. She spoke at women's clubs, health conferences, Theosophical lodges, and Eaters Anonymous meetings. She went on television, still a nascent medium with a relatively small audience, at least twice. At many of these engagements, she would perform a handful of postures.[63]

When she did book signings at department stores, she put on a real show; Ruth St. Denis and starlet Evan Loew would demonstrate poses, and Indian dancers would add a dash of exoticism to Devi's injunctions to forgo sugar, to sleep on a hard surface, and of course to practice "yoga."[64]

Devi was ready to change minds one by one if need be. After a columnist for the *Hartford Courant* complained that her yoga exercises gave him a sore back, Prentice-Hall got in touch and offered him "a personal, private lesson in standing on your head" with Miss Devi.[65]

Forever Young, Forever Healthy found a wide audience, inspiring readers all over the United States as well as in Japan, India, and Canada.[66]

Hatha Yoga quickly became the beauty "secret" everyone was talking about. Many actresses had at least tried it. Some swore by it.[67]

Swanson allowed herself to be photographed while practicing yoga in Italy. The picture, which appeared in the *Los Angeles Times,* shows Swanson seated in a deep twist; she's wearing fitted paisley shorts and a black tube top and looks as unblemished as ever. The caption read, "Vacationing in Rome, actress Gloria Swanson supplies a touch of the ancient East by engaging in a difficult yoga exercise. She says she does the Hindu exercises to keep herself relaxed and in perfect physical condition."[68]

Carol Ohmart, a former beauty queen, now a hopeful Hollywood starlet, told Arlene Dahl that she found yoga especially helpful for nervous tension. "I do [deep breathing] as it is taught in yoga, to the rhythm of my pulse," she explained, echoing Devi's instruction. "Then I do the yoga relaxing routine everyone knows, in which you lie down and concentrate on relaxing each set of muscles in the body in turn, starting at the toes and working up."[69]

Gary Cooper confided to Lydia Lane that he liked two yoga exercises for relaxation: one in which he lay on a hard surface, tightening all his

muscles, then releasing them, and the other a "feet-in-the-air body stand," also known as a shoulder stand.

Even Marilyn Monroe had added it to her regimen by this point. In March 1956, Walter Winchell reported, "Marilyn Monroe's latest kick is Yogi, not the philosophy, just the exercises. To improve her legs, she says."[70]

Hatha Yoga had succumbed to Devi's shorthand. This abbreviated "yoga" was physical, not spiritual or philosophical (though Winchell knew enough, or Monroe did, to make the distinction); it eased tension and erased years. It didn't demand too much of you either. As Cooper said, "You just have to stay in this position a minute or so to have it do its job."[71]

Claire Stuart did her part to push this view of yoga. In the years since her arrival in Los Angeles, she had married (and now went by the name Clara Spring) and was at work on her own book on Hatha Yoga, titled *Yoga for Today*.

"Yoga deals with the physical body, its care, its well-being, its health, its strength, and all that tends to keep it in a normal state" is how Clara explained Hatha Yoga to a reporter for the *Los Angeles Times*.[72]

Credit goes to Devi, though, not Claire Stuart or the scholarly Theos Bernard, for ridding Hatha Yoga of sordid associations and much of the accumulated ill will.

A foreigner for the entirety of her adulthood, in Germany, India, China, and now America, Devi was attuned to the exigencies of assimilation. She understood which rules one must abide by, which ones might be bent.

In India, she had eaten off banana leaves, bathed out of a bucket, and followed all but one of the unwritten laws then governing colonial society: she maintained friendships with people of all ranks, including some of India's most outspoken nationalists. In Los Angeles, she marketed yoga as a beauty remedy but continued to wear a sari.[73]

Pleased by the response to *Forever Young, Forever Healthy*, Prentice-Hall commissioned two more yoga books from Devi.

"Isn't it funny," wrote Swanson to Devi when she learned the news, "we dream about wanting success and spend hours and hours of hard work getting it and then when we succeed in doing so, we want to go off to the desert and be alone."[74]

Devi's second effort, *Yoga for Americans*, came out in 1959. The famed violinist and longtime yoga practitioner Yehudi Menuhin wrote the foreword, and the book included several of the photographs of Gloria Swanson taken under a cloudless sky high up on Mulholland Drive.

In *Yoga for Americans*, Devi once again struck a friendly, if mildly impatient, tone. By dividing the book into week-by-week lessons, she made it even more useful as an instruction manual than her first.

She also added more of the flavor of yoga back into this book.

The Devanagari Om symbol (identical to the one that hovered over the door of the Hollywood Vedanta Temple) was stamped on the book's cloth cover. And this time, Devi went into some detail about the subtle body.[75]

"The subject of our discussion today is the most secret and sacred of all Yoga practices, the awakening of the mysterious *Kundalini* (pronounced Koun-da-lee-nee), or Serpent power," is how she opens "Lesson Four." She then describes the nadis and chakras (with the help of illustrations), unapologetically references the "ancient yogis' clairvoyant capacities," and notes that Kundalini "is closely connected with fundamental sex energy and may be controlled and transmuted by certain Yoga practices."

She was quite clear about the effects of moving this energy up through the central channel along the spine: "When Kundalini finally enters the last and highest center, the Sahasrara chakra, the yogi reaches his highest goal . . . his individual consciousness unites with Universal Consciousness, and he enters a state of ultimate bliss, called *Samadhi*." Raise Kundalini, and you can know God.

Devi did note that it was difficult to do this, few achieve success, and those who wish to must do so under the guidance of a guru.

Still, this was a significant departure. Devi had gone to great lengths in her first book to simplify yoga, and she had largely succeeded. She had excised most of the Hindu and Tantric elements of Hatha Yoga and almost anything that she couldn't talk about in terms of Western science. In so doing, she had reduced a method of spiritual realization so vast and slippery, so varied and mongrelized, that a single book can't contain it down to a set of health exercises.

Violent as it might have seemed to anyone familiar with the tradition, this contraction of yoga had been of a piece with the broader culture. Some observers have described this same era in American literature as systolic—with writers such as Salinger and Malamud delivering "carefully composed dramas of alienation and despair"—and the New Critics putting a "restrictive emphasis on form."

Cold War paranoia, the ever-present fear of atomic annihilation, women's return to domesticity, rapid technological advances from the mainframe computer to the television, as well as Devi's own foreignness, can all easily explain, or at least plausibly rationalize, her initial reticence about the subtle body and Hatha Yoga's real power.

But by 1959, she was showing the way forward. In *Yoga for Americans*, she made available the materials the counterculture would put to use, and she multiplied the kinds of experiences Americans could conceive of having. Even Devi's personal style, which hadn't changed since the moment she'd arrived in America a dozen years before (she still dressed in a sari and, when she wasn't teaching barefoot, wore flat shoes), pointed in this direction.[76]

The hippies and their representatives—Allen Ginsberg, Timothy Leary, Ram Dass, and all the other psychic explorers that came on the scene in the 1960s—didn't need to go to India or Tibet for their spiritual revolution. They didn't need to plumb ancient or obscure texts. All they needed to do was pull out a book geared toward middle-class housewives and peer inside.

10

PSYCHEDELIC SAGES

The helicopters landed alongside a river that cut through a densely wooded valley. They lowered themselves onto the sand, and two Americans disembarked.

Fred Smithline, a lawyer dressed in tennis sneakers and a blue blazer, and his wife, Susan, in a black dress and white boots, had arrived in Rishikesh, India, in the foothills of the Himalayas.

They were from Scarsdale, New York, and they had come on business. Fred represented Kersi Cambata, the transportation magnate who owned the helicopters, which would shortly ferry an Indian holy man, Maharishi Mahesh Yogi, high above his ashram to inspect possible sites for a runway. By this point Mahesh, inventor of Transcendental Meditation (TM), resident holy man, retreat director, and media darling, already owned a Beechcraft airplane, and he had nowhere to land it.[1]

Susan was thrilled to meet Mahesh. *Life* magazine had recently proclaimed 1968 the "Year of the Guru," Mahesh's own face gazing in uncharacteristic solemnity out of the opening pages of the feature. Before she had left New York, Susan's friends had raved about Mahesh specifically, comparing him favorably to the Taj Mahal. He now ranked as one of India's attractions.[2]

A few hours later, Fred and Susan Smithline joined an unusually large assortment of meditation students as well as the resident langur monkeys for lunch. They sat at a long wooden table under teak and sissoo trees.

Fred had brought his home-movie camera, a Keystone 8 mm, which he had turned on as he and Susan got out of the helicopter, and he kept filming during the meal."[3]

Despite his camera, Fred had yet to realize how deeply implicated in the spectacle he and his wife were. They had become part of the story

because everything was being documented here—recorded, filmed, photographed. Fred and Susan weren't famous nor were they in any way connected to any of the actors or musicians in residence at the ashram, which
included, at this moment, all four Beatles, Mia Farrow, and Beach Boy
Mike Love.

They weren't devotees, each of whom paid five hundred dollars to attend the three-month teacher-training session under way. Nor did they
belong to the press corps camped mostly outside the ashram.[4]

They were interlopers.

During lunch Fred casually observed that back home it was hip, it was
de rigueur, to flirt with Mother India.

Said Fred, "You go to a cocktail party in New York and all you hear is
Indian music."

Susan chimed in, "It's very in to be Indian."

After an awkward silence, Susan added, "No kidding, it really is. A lot
of people are doing yoga."[5]

Lewis Lapham was reporting this scene. A young journalist, Lapham
had been sent over by the *Saturday Evening Post* to cover the Beatles as
they attempted to further transcend mundane existence as if they weren't,
in all senses of the word, high enough already.

The problem was that Lapham, who had been half-expecting to go to
Vietnam when he had got this assignment, couldn't get any closer to these
God-men than most of the viewers of the newsreel footage.[6]

He could smell the jasmine and eucalyptus; he could hear the chatter
of monkeys and the scream of a wild peacock; he could taste the bland
vegetarian food; he could see the Ganges, now jade, now brown, now teal
like the Kool cigarette logo, but he wasn't allowed to ask the Beatles a
single personal question, such as why they were interested in yoga in the
first place or if they thought Mahesh's techniques really worked.[7]

Instead Lapham chatted up the other students at the retreat and the
seekers who hung around at the gates of the ashram at the bottom of
the hill.

There was the American John O'Shea. His straight brown hair fell to
his shoulders. He often wore no more than a loincloth, and he liked to
hold a trident. Hash was his yoga, and he smoked it with great and ritual
punctuality when the sun dropped below the horizon. He found Mahesh
disingenuous and venal, "like a politician, you dig?"[8]

There was also Larry Kurland, who considered himself in all ways further out than O'Shea. He wore beads and sandals and many-hued robes. Back home, Kurland had burnt out on the drug scene. He liked Mahesh, and he liked helicopters. Kurland mused, "Where can you buy nirvana for less?"[9]

O'Shea, Kurland, and the Smithlines. Together, in Lapham's story, they stood in for America, its energetic eccentrics, its hardheaded idealists, and (much to the dismay of Fred and Susan) its petite bourgeoisie.

Meanwhile the drama being played out was hard to fully fathom even if you could get inside the head of a Beatle.

Joseph Lelyveld, a reporter for *The New York Times* who like Lapham was an Ivy man, a real up-and-comer, was here too, and he had the same problem. Mahesh had granted little real access to the press, even though this had only heightened the spectacle. Lelyveld's dispatches were short and sardonic.[10]

Americans would have to wait nearly three months for the full story. Patience was a virtue not rewarded in this case, since by the time Lapham had filled in the details, it was all over. The second part of Lapham's two-part article in the *Saturday Evening Post* appeared several days *after* John, Paul, and George explained to the wide world that they were "finished with" Mahesh.[11]

Like many love affairs, theirs was precipitous and passionate, making betrayal all the more likely.

George had met Mahesh first. He had been studying Indian music with Ravi Shankar and reading about yoga. "Like, in the beginning was the word and I knew *mantras* were the words," Harrison told Lapham with little prompting. He introduced John and Paul to Mahesh at the London Hilton. Then all four tramped to Wales for a weeklong TM seminar. There, in August 1967, Paul told reporters, "We don't need [drugs] anymore. We think we're finding other ways of getting there (attaining complete spiritual fulfillment)." The sudden death of their manager, Brian Epstein, cut short their study. Plans were made to go to the ashram.[12]

The Beatles arrived a few weeks into the three-month teacher-training session. They brought their wives or girlfriends and road manager. Over days and weeks at the ashram, they had shed bits of their mod clothing—the skinny-striped pants, the silk shirts, and the brocade blazers and vests. They donned baggy white pants (churidars) and long, white, pajama-like shirts (kurtas). Their beards grew. They got competitive with the meditation. They wrote prolifically.

During their stay, Mahesh orchestrated one big photo shoot. He had them on bleachers, men in kurtas, the women in their best saris, everyone wearing garlands of red and orange marigolds. They all sat blinking in the hot sun for more than half an hour while photographers snapped away.[13]

On February 25, 1968, Mahesh held a birthday party for George, who turned twenty-five. There was a cake and a special chant. By the end of the celebration, George was garlanded with so many marigolds, Lapham thought he looked as if he were wearing a life jacket. It goes without saying that the Beatles got the best bungalows and private instruction.[14]

Although learning to practice TM was easy enough—all you need to do is close your eyes and silently repeat your mantra—Mahesh had written a tome, *The Science of Being and Art of Living*, and liked to discourse on metaphysics. The Yogi insisted that Vedanta and yoga had been badly misconstrued and misunderstood. To counter such distortions, Mahesh created his own system in high-modernist style. There was no color, no filigree, no story, no symbol, nor much ritual of any sort. Though he described Transcendental Meditation as "psycho-physiological," involving both mind and body, he never mentioned the subtle body by name, nor did he talk much about chakras or nadis or raising Kundalini.

Mahesh said TM wasn't yoga; this was true, TM dispensed with many aspects of yoga. Mahesh also said his technique would achieve the same thing yoga promised, just more efficiently.[15]

Paul admitted to getting lost in the upper reaches of Mahesh's philosophy. John said during meditation he often had "music playing in me head."[16]

None of the Beatles stayed for the duration of the teacher training. Ringo left after ten days or so at the ashram. He and his wife missed their kids and anyway had never planned to stay long. Paul left after five and a half weeks. "I'm going away a new man," Paul is said to have confided to Nancy Cooke de Herrera, whose job was to minister to the foursome's more prosaic needs. George and John stayed on for a while longer.[17]

Then rumors started to circulate: Mahesh, an avowed celibate, had made advances toward at least one female student. The Beatles could tolerate Mahesh's politics (he wouldn't oppose the Vietnam War, despite his professed desire for world peace). They could tolerate his inconsistencies (students could use alcohol, but not acid). They could tolerate his

solicitousness. But they couldn't tolerate sexual hypocrisy or even the appearance of it. They felt Mahesh was abusing his power.

George and John left abruptly. "We believe in meditation, but not the
Maharishi and his scene," said John on the *Tonight* show, in mid-May of
1968. "But that's a personal mistake we made in public."

"Yeah. I mean, he's good. There's nothing wrong with him," explained
Paul. "But we think the system is more important than all the two-bit
personality bit."[18]

So many writers have told the story of the sixties. Yet here's another. My
only advantage in telling the story again is that yoga is like a Rorschach test:
students and teachers see in it the contents of their own minds, their fanta-
sies and desires. Pick up yoga books from the 1960s or look at the rise of a
guru such as Mahesh, and you'll quickly discover the indelible traces of that
moment (and there are many and contradictory ones, but I'll get to that).

In any event, what happened in the 1960s was first a reversal. All
those teachers—American and Indian—who had fought so hard to make
yoga secular and practical had won.

They had in effect yanked yoga from the bosom of religion and its in-
explicable mysteries and delivered it to science. (That science still hadn't
fully accepted this child didn't matter.)

Pierre Bernard had begun the process in earnest, and he was soon
aided and abetted by Behanan's work and then Indra Devi. The most
popular among them and the most invested in broadening the appeal of
yoga, Devi can be credited with the most radical reduction of yoga—
down to a set of "health exercises," which functioned like a doctor's pre-
scription, curing this or that ailment.

Though Devi never submitted yoga to scientific investigation (as Swami
Kuvalayananda had), was suspicious of the medical establishment, and
had already begun to restore some of the more esoteric and explicitly
spiritual aspects of the discipline, in the short term she did more than
anyone else to adapt yoga to an age in the thrall of technology and the
power of scientists.

Yoga might speak of those things beyond the ken of microscopes and
telescopes, but Devi, in this middle phase of her career, would only wave
wanly in that direction. She had measured Americans' appetites fairly well.

(Although Theos had struggled with such a reductive view of yoga before Devi arrived in America, the version of yoga detailed in the pages of *Forever Young, Forever Healthy* was the one that had mass appeal and a bigger postwar market.)

Yoga's phases have a rhythm, one that loosely follows the dialectics of the broader culture. If the 1950s were a time of contraction, at least in American letters, the 1960s were a diastolic period, a time of expansion and experimentation, of giddy abandonment. The next generation of writers, people such as Pynchon, Vonnegut, and Sontag, set about upending formal conventions and abandoned any pretense of realism. This new expansiveness applied to yoga too.[19]

But the mechanics of this enlargement are laden with irony.

For it wasn't the swamis who revived yoga as a spiritual pursuit. It was a couple of social scientists—Timothy Leary and Richard Alpert—armed with a handful of psychoactive chemicals (psilocybin, mescaline, and lysergic acid diethylamide) extracted or synthesized in American and European labs. They stole yoga from the health seekers and weight-conscious, and they put it back in the temple, where they believed it belonged. They sacralized yoga, which ultimately yielded the year of the guru and its disillusionments.

Though Leary and Alpert come on the scene in the early 1960s, the enlargement of yoga had begun almost a decade earlier, in the 1950s, with two Brits, Aldous Huxley and Alan Watts, even though neither particularly recommended yoga. The discipline's expansion wasn't so much a revolution but a culmination, and it was ultimately a conservative move. What Huxley, Watts, and others managed to do was restore yoga's original purpose.

In 1951, Watts drove from upstate New York to California with his second wife, Dorothy. He was in his midthirties and had left behind his first wife and three children, a job as chaplain at Northwestern University, and the high esteem of a community of Episcopalians in Chicago, who had seen in the precocious, articulate, and charismatic Watts some hope for their own sort of spiritual regeneration. Watts's divorce and the unusual family arrangements that had preceded it shattered his reputation as a clergyman. He resigned his post.[20]

Redemption came after only a single winter in a drafty farmhouse, in the form of an invitation to teach at the newly formed American Academy of Asian Studies in San Francisco. Watts saw salvation in Eastern religion. And this, despite his chaplaincy, had long been the case.

He had come to the United States in 1938 from Chislehurst, England, and had brought with him a youthful interest in Buddhism, which had yielded a book, *The Spirit of Zen*, published when he was just twenty-one years old.[21]

For anyone not already convinced, Watts's 1947 book, *Behold the Spirit: A Study in the Necessity of Mystical Religion*, gave him away as a diviner of Reality, a lover of Eastern philosophy, a would-be mystic dressed up as a minister.

"God and union with God are Reality; nothing is more real, more concrete, more actual, and more present," he wrote. The trick is to let "go of all devices and methods for realizing union with God" so you can "live and move in the Now."[22]

However, outwardly, even after his exit from Northwestern, Watts looked more like a midlevel bank manager than a spiritual maverick. His hair was short and neat, setting off a high brow and peaked eyebrows. He wore the requisite suit and tie.

Alan and Dorothy Watts had taken the southern route from New York to San Francisco, and during a stop in Los Angeles, Swami Prabhavananda invited Alan to a tea party up at the Hollywood Vedanta center.

In Watts's telling, the swami had taken it upon himself to try to clear up some potential confusion, defending yoga against the sort of spontaneous enlightenment that Watts cherished and that animated his syncretic mysticism.

Making matters worse, in a talk a few evenings before, Watts had suggested (as Theos Bernard had too) that there was "some analogy between the ecstasy of *samadhi* . . . and sexual orgasm."

The idea was anathema to the swami, a staunch advocate of both abstinence and yoga.[23]

Hence the tea party.

Prabhavananda received Watts in his apartment. Aldous Huxley and Christopher Isherwood joined them, as did a steady stream of women in saris, the swami's disciples, who entered one after another through one of several doors.

To Watts it looked like the making of a French farce.

The conversation quickly turned into a debate of sorts.

"Your *Upanishads* say very plainly, *Tat tvam asi*, 'You *are* That,'" said Watts, "so what is there to attain?"

To which the swami answered, there is a huge difference between knowledge of this fact and *realizing* it, and that "it takes a great deal of work to go from one state to another."

"Well, I wonder," Huxley interjected soon after, "isn't it rather curious that there has always been a school of thought in religion which attributes salvation or realization to an unmerited gift of divine grace rather than personal effort?"

From the vantage point of 1951, the observation, made by such an erudite student of religion, seemed straightforward enough, even if it only further discomfited Prabhavananda. Now though, Huxley's remark seems eerily prescient, except that Huxley was so implicated in creating the future, it's hard to say whether he's merely prescient or, like Vishnu, calling into being the thing he's talking about, which is a world in which you can purchase such unmerited gifts of divine grace for a pittance.[24]

Prabhavananda then says, "You are saying that you yourself, or just any other person, can realize that you are the Brahman just as you are, without any spiritual effort at all!"

"Just so," Watts replied to Prabhavananda's further irritation.

The debate was never resolved. Each went away convinced he was right.[25]

Almost as soon as Watts arrived at the American Academy of Asian Studies, the institute faced financial troubles, and less than a year later, its founding dean, Frederic Spiegelberg, stepped down. Watts took over, running the AAAS out of a rambling manse on Broadway in San Francisco's Pacific Heights.[26]

The project was ostensibly to create a sort of information clearinghouse about Asian culture and religion for businessmen, travelers, and others.

The mission Spiegelberg and Watts had in mind was far more ambitious.

"We were concerned with the practical transformation of human consciousness" is how Watts described it, "with the actual living out of the Hindu, Buddhist, and Taoist ways of life at the level of high mysticism."[27]

This AAAS was very much in the vein of Pierre Bernard's International School of Vedic and Allied Research (ISVAR). Both sought to apply yogic knowledge to life and its problems; both subscribed to a more holistic notion of education, putting equal emphasis on theory and practice.

However, the AAAS was far more eclectic in its sources, drawing much from Zen and its Japanese teachers, such as Sabro Hasegawa, a printmaker and disciple of tea master Soshu Sen.

And unlike ISVAR, the American Academy of Asian Studies had enrolled students—and these would come to include beat poets Gary Snyder, who showed up in a black formal suit, complete with a rolled umbrella, and, more occasionally, Allen Ginsberg.[28]

Although the Korean War and the growing distemper in Vietnam suggested the quite urgent and practical need for some deeper understanding of Asian culture, funding the AAAS was nearly impossible.[29]

Watts was no good at covert operations or catering to appearances for the sake of the greater mission. As a result, the AAAS "roiled everyone," including the people who might support it. To burden an academic program with salvific aims was bad enough; to burden it further with Asian techniques, in the early and middle fifties, was dooming it to almost sure failure.[30]

This in no way seems to have affected the spread of the ideals it stood for.

Once the academy folded in 1956, Haridas Chaudhuri—who had taught Indian philosophy heavily inflected by Sri Aurobindo's Integral Yoga—set up an urban ashram, where residents could live and meditate.[31]

Unmoored from an institution of any sort, Watts had to make his way solely through his books and on the lecture circuit.

At this point in his career, Watts wore his hair like a newly minted Mercury 7 astronaut, shaved on the sides, buzzed flat on the top, part of what he called his "square disguise." He drank more vodka in a day than one man should, smoked like "a paratrooper," fielded invitations from Columbia, Harvard, Yale Medical School, Cornell, and Rochester, and starred in a nationally broadcast public television show, *Eastern Wisdom for Modern Life*, which required only that he show up and speak.

Traversing the country, he was a vagabond, a raconteur, a reluctant proselytizer for a philosophy predicated on the impossibility of saying much about it.[32]

Soon enough, Watts was recognized as one of the country's foremost experts on Zen, and by some as a defender of "Square Zen," or the traditional forms of Japanese Zen. This title he refused. For Watts was forever insisting that there was no path or system, no organization or school that could profitably be adhered to—"the experience of awakening (*satori*) is not to be found by seeking" is how he put it in 1959, "and is not in any case something that can be acquired or cultivated."[33]

By now, Huxley too was even more convinced than ever that liberation could happen in the here and now, with, as Watts would say "no fuss." The reason was simple: Huxley had had the experience, or something mighty close to it, for himself.

About two years after the tea party up at the Hollywood Vedanta center, Huxley had taken four-tenths of a gram of mescaline—the synthetic version of peyote, the psychoactive chemical found in a cactus (*Lophophora williamsii*) native to Mexico and the Southwest—dissolved in a glass of water.

"My eyes traveled from the rose to the carnation, and from that feathery incandescence to the smooth scrolls of sentient amethyst which were the irises" is how Huxley famously described a vase of flowers he observed once the drug took effect. "The Beatific Vision, *Sat Chit Ananda*, Being-Awareness-Bliss—for the first time I understood, not on the verbal level, not by inchoate hints or at the distance but precisely and completely what those prodigious syllables referred to."[34]

His mescaline trip was the occasion of one of his most famous essays, *The Doors of Perception*, which Harper & Brothers put out as a small book in 1954. Huxley received mostly positive, if cautious, reviews of his slim volume. But he hadn't convinced everyone of the merits of chemically induced "transfiguration."

John Yale, known then as Brahmachari Prema Chaitanya, had been living at the Hollywood Vedanta monastery up on Ivar Avenue for several years. He spent a good part of his time editing the society's magazine, *Vedanta for the West*, and had become close to his predecessor, Christopher Isherwood.[35]

In his memoir, Prema recalled that for a while you could find a copy of *The Doors of Perception* in the bookcase of the reception room in the

Vedanta center. Huxley had inscribed it, "For Swami, This account of a glimpse of reality from an unusual angle, in friendship and admiration, Aldous Huxley, 1954."

However, Swami Prabhavananda was embarrassed by Huxley's book and the way it linked Vedanta and psychedelics. His view on the matter was uncompromising: drugs, even those that produced visions, could cause "spiritual dryness," "disbelief," and even permanent brain damage. The swami saw nothing redeeming in them.[36]

Before long, the inscribed copy of *The Doors of Perception* disappeared, as did the magazine's Editorial Board, which had made good use of both Heard and Huxley to draw readers to the Vedanta Society's magazine.[37]

Huxley wasn't moved by his critics, and if he was, it was only to make his case for mescaline more vigorously, now to the largest possible audience.

Writing in the *Saturday Evening Post* in October 1958, Huxley added lysergic acid diethylamide, or LSD, to the list of substances that cleansed the doors of perception and concluded, with evident satisfaction, that the new mind changers would soon instigate that "famous 'revival of religion,' about which so many people have been talking for so long."

He went so far as to call this imminent, biochemical religious revival a "revolution."[38]

(He also noted that most civilizations have used drugs toward God realization—e.g., the ancient Greeks had their cult of Dionysus—and in so doing placed this imminent revolution squarely in the bounds of accepted history.)

The idea wasn't so far-fetched. Americans in the late 1950s were a pill-popping, drug-loving bunch, consuming sleeping pills, diet pills, pep pills, and "vitamin" pills at alarming rates. The one statistic Huxley cited was grim enough, and it hardly scratched the surface of actual usage: American doctors wrote 48 million prescriptions for tranquilizers in 1957. (According to the most recent census, the *entire* population then numbered about 151 million.)[39]

In celebrating the new "mind changers," Huxley was just promoting a different kind of pill.

This wasn't necessarily good news for yoga. Near instant beatification made the idea of a *sādhana*, a path leading from here to there, at best hilarious, at worst, dangerous and wasteful, and in general rather irrelevant.

As Huxley himself acknowledged, yoga could "change the quality of consciousness." But his long-held belief was that yoga was difficult and its real fruits accessible to the rare and dedicated few.

Mescaline, LSD, and the dozens of mind-changing drugs on the pharmacological horizon would make "pre-mystical and mystical experiences common." They would democratize transcendence, and who could argue with that?

This was, of course, the conundrum that had brought the usually unflappable Prabhavananda near to indignation almost a decade before.

Zen, on the other hand, at least in Watts's rendering, promised instant, chemical-free transfiguration. Awakening to our "'own original inseparability' with the universe seems," as Watts put it, "however elusive, just around the corner."[40]

At the time, it was winning over many more Americans.

"Any book with the word *Zen* on it sells fast here," Sigmund Cohen, proprietor of Sheridan Square Chemists, told Gay Talese in the fall of 1959. "We've sold *The Way to Zen, Zen Buddhism, Buddhism Zen . . . Zen Flesh, Zen Bones.*" The trend was so pronounced, at least in Greenwich Village, that Cohen tore down his soda fountain to make way for more paperbacks.[41]

In the fall of 1960, Dr. Timothy Francis Leary, a lecturer in the Psychology Department at Harvard University, began conducting research on some of the new "mind changers." He had at his disposal office space, research assistants, a pool of willing experimental subjects, and a supply of potent, medical-grade psychedelics.

Leary was trying to scientifically measure the benefits of chemically induced religious revelation without letting on that this was what he was doing. He initially focused his efforts on psilocybin (derived from a species of Mexican mushroom) and soon thereafter on LSD.

Leary's office was in Harvard's Center for Research in Personality in a modest frame building on Divinity Avenue. However, he conducted many of his experiments at a rented mansion full of thick rugs, books, and Moroccan lamps, out in suburban Newton.[42]

Dr. Leary struck many people as personable, serious, and a little naive. Alan Watts's first impression of him was of "an extremely charming Irishman who wore a hearing-aid as stylishly as if it had been a monocle."[43]

Huxley was supportive of Leary's work from the get-go. He sat in on some early planning sessions in 1960 and introduced Leary to religious scholar Huston Smith, then at MIT. Privately, he found Leary, a trim, handsome fellow, and now a single father of two youngsters, a bit square, which he saw as an asset for research into psychedelics.[44]

In early 1962, in answer to one of Leary's questions, Huxley sent him a short reading list on Tantra. Besides Arthur Avalon, he particularly recommended Mircea Eliade's books on yoga, "the fullest scholarly treatment [of Tantra], on a manageable scale."[45]

Like Emerson, Huxley had read all the best books about Indian thought, including yoga, and would recommend these to anyone who displayed the slightest interest, even though he had little interest in the yoga techniques themselves.

He further advised Leary that "LSD and the mushrooms shd be used, it seems to me, in the context of this basic Tantrik idea of the yoga of total awareness leading to enlightenment within the world of everyday experience—which of course becomes the world of miracle and beauty and divine mystery when experience is what it always ought to be."[46]

Here was America's preeminent advocate of mind-manifesting substances exhorting Leary, still employed by Harvard's Psychology Department, to see his project in terms of an antispeculative, body-centered religious movement dating back to fourth-century India.[47]

You have to admire Huxley's audacity. He had a knack for extracting the part of a religion that pleased him and adapting it to his own needs, tapping Tantra, Vedanta, and Zen like so many rubber trees.

That said, Huxley lays perhaps too much emphasis Tantra's promise—the mundane becomes divine, the profane becomes sacred—and not enough on its demands. "The fact is," states Eliade in no uncertain terms, "that the tantric road presupposes a long and difficult *sādhana*."[48]

Around the same time Huxley and Leary were corresponding about Tantra, Leary met Fred Swain, a former air force major, now a monk at the Boston Vedanta Temple.

Swain acquainted Leary with the Hindu pantheon and its scriptures, which, according to Leary, "read like psychedelic manuals," and its myths, which were, in Leary's parlance, "session reports." Swain brought him around to the Vedanta Center on Deerfield Street, a three-story, brick, colonial-revival-style house with small windows and white trim.

Even today, the place retains almost all of its original details—wood-paneled walls, marble fireplaces, transom windows—and you'd hardly know it was a holy place dedicated to an Indian guru save for the shrine set up at the top of carpeted stairs and photographs of past and present swamis on the mantels.

This was about as close to Tantra as Leary could get in Boston in the spring of 1962.

Almost inevitably, given the mutual interest, one morning after a service of chanting and meditation in the temple, Leary was invited to lead a small group of monks and nuns in a psychedelic session, which he memorialized in his book *High Priest*, first published in 1968 and clearly the cornerstone of his own mythmaking.

Incense and candles burned. The LSD was in chalices on the altar.

Leary and a few Vedanta devotees added holy water from the Ganges to the chalices, blessed the "sacrament," and drank it.[49]

The group, Leary, Swain, and the Vedanta devotees, then sat cross-legged on Oriental rugs and chanted. When the acid hit, Leary saw shock and amazement on the "Holy folk," despite their years of practicing Bhakti and Raja Yoga. He himself imagined, briefly, that he was Shiva. A nun crawled over to him and put her head in his lap. Fred Swain was Hanuman, the god who led an army of monkeys in the *Ramayana*, crouching nearby. The statue of Ramakrishna came to life, breathing and twinkling, in comic cosmic affirmation. Even the portrait of Vivekananda beamed his assent, as the "sacred kundalini serpent uncoiled up the bronzed candelabra to the thousand-petaled lotus blossom."

That day, Leary discovered that he was and we all were Hindus "in our essence. We are all Hindu Gods and Goddesses." (He also understood that he was a prophet. The monks and nuns immediately started to treat him as a guru. To them, according to Leary, he was no longer a Harvard psychologist with a staff of research assistants; he was "playing out the ancient role.")[50]

High on acid, Leary was grasping for a symbolic system that could accommodate his visions. Hinduism had a lot going for it: sensual and complex rituals, a densely populated pantheon, an ancient lineage, a bias for seers and visionaries, and in yoga, a whole host of techniques for God realization.

The revelation, though—that Hinduism lay at the core of himself and the mind-stuff of acid—was quite literally foreordained.

Before he had visited the temple, Huxley had convinced Leary that the Yogis were talking about the states induced by LSD. The idea was part of Leary's *set*, his term for your "expectations and predispositions at the start of the [psychedelic] session." Then, prompted by the appropriate *setting*, the temple itself, the incense, the admiring nuns and monks, Leary felt this for himself, he came to know it as the Truth.[51]

More remarkable was that about a year before Leary tuned in to his and our "Hindu essence," Alan Watts had made a similar discovery.

Up in Marin County, in a wooden house with a broad terrace and a garden filled with fuchsias and hummingbirds, Watts imbibed a goodly amount of LSD in several sessions. Under the swaying eucalyptus, he saw, off along the ridgeline, forests of redwood that looked like "green fire" and copper-gold grass "heaving immensely into the sky."[52]

Most strikingly he became aware of the eternal cosmic play—or divine *līlā*—in which that single, original point of consciousness (he called it the Eeenie-Weenie) cloaks itself beneath ordinary reality and then tries to find itself, in an eternal game of hide-and-seek. This discovery of the divine consciousness, whether it's figured as Atman or Self or Brahma, in everyone and everything is exactly what yoga urges the practitioner to make.[53]

Reflecting on a gas station, that most dully prosaic of scenes and also a potent symbol of midcentury America, Watts didn't see (in his mind's eye) dust and exhaust fumes and the "regular Standard guy" in a baseball cap. Instead, he saw people "pretending not to see that they are avatars of Brahma, Vishnu, and Shiva," people who were so good at pretending they're not what they are, they also missed the obvious, to Watts anyway, fact that their bodies were composed of a million cellular gods and that everything that surrounded them, from the gaudy billboards to the dust, was numinous, jeweled, unspeakably holy.[54]

Watts, known at this point in his career primarily as an exponent of Zen, was surprised that the "flavor" of his experience was Hindu, not Chinese. He concluded that "Hindu philosophy was a local form of a sort of undercover wisdom, inconceivably ancient, which everyone knows in the back of his mind but will not admit."[55]

Watts being Watts, which is to say a ceaseless talker and inveterate recorder of his thoughts, he wrote a book about his experiences with LSD—*The Joyous Cosmology*. (He also produced an ecstatic, improvised LP of chanting, drumming, and singing titled *This Is It*.)

Leary and his aide-de-camp, Richard (Dick) Alpert, cowrote the introduction to Watts's book. At the time of writing, January 1962, the two
Harvard employees were still reasonably confident about continued, systematic, scientific research on substances such as psilocybin and lysergic acid.[56]

They were evangelists, their fervor the fervor of the reborn. And Shiva
was now part of their religion.

Timothy Francis Leary had always been something of a renegade. He had
left the Catholic Church, and he had left West Point. For much of his
adult life, he understood himself as "an atheist, a rationalist," an empiri-
cist, allergic to authority, ritual, tradition, and faith.

Then on August 9, 1960, in Cuernavaca, Mexico, he ate some magic
mushrooms. At first he described his experience in psychological and literary terms. "We're all schizophrenics now and we're in our own institution," he remarked. "But I finally understand James Joyce." He later traced
his spiritual rebirth to this particular trip.[57]

From then on, Leary was first and foremost a psychedelic explorer and
only secondarily a researcher and lecturer at Harvard.[58]

Before acid, Richard Alpert had, by comparison, been more eager to
please and on the surface less rebellious.[59]

The son of a railroad executive and a founder of Brandeis University,
Alpert had contracts with four major universities (Harvard, Yale, University
of California at Berkeley, and Stanford) by the time he was twenty-eight.

His main interest was in human motivation.

With a dazzling smile, good salary, and all the toys a young bachelor
could want, including a motorcycle and Cessna plane, Alpert struck people as a typical, if precociously successful, clinical psychologist.

He was devoted to the "scientific method," which in those days meant
conducting studies on rats, in possession of a mostly charming verbosity,
and politically astute.[60]

And after he took acid?

"Now Alpert was sitting on the floor in Perry Lane in the old boho
Lotus hunker down" was how Tom Wolfe began his description of Alpert
at novelist Ken Kesey's place near Stanford, "and exegeting very seriously
about a baby crawling blindly about the room. Blindly? What do you mean
blindly?" This was Wolfe channeling a young woman's memory of Alpert's
chatter. ". . . That baby sees the world with a completeness that you and I

will never know again. His doors of perception have not yet been closed. He still experiences the moment he lives in."[61]

Or as Alpert phrased it later in an interview, on acid, "all that you become is awareness, is a point of awareness. That's all that's left."[62]

At Harvard, Alpert had a five-year fellowship, appointments in four different departments, including Psychology and the Graduate School of Education, two secretaries, and several student assistants.[63]

But the days of unfettered, public, and funded research into "consciousness altering" drugs were numbered, and Leary and Alpert were among the first casualties.

They could not, would not, contain their enthusiasm for the new "consciousness-expanding materials." They took psilocybin or LSD with their subjects (a pox be on objectivity!). They crunched the data and found 69 then 95 percent of test subjects had positive, life-changing experiences, results that they mimeographed and distributed to the Center for Research in Personality staff. They "turned on" divinity students by the dozens.

Undergraduates were intrigued and eventually started experimenting on their own.

When Harvard voted not to renew their terms (they ran out in 1963), Leary and Alpert became even more vocal in their pursuit of "applied mysticism." This caused still more controversy and more awkward publicity for the university.[64]

All along the way, Leary and Alpert were defying the advice of people such as Heard, Huxley, and Watts, the "psychedelic sages," to stay underground or to abide by at least some of the rules of the academic game.[65]

They paid for it too. After its earlier attempts, Harvard successfully and permanently ejected them in May 1963.[66]

Leary and Alpert, along with graduate student Ralph Metzner, continued their investigations in Millbrook, New York, a small town near Poughkeepsie, where Peggy Hitchcock and her brother had an enormous, sixty-four-room Victorian mansion set on vast tracts of wooded land.

To start, about two dozen people lived up there, more or less full-time. (The number swelled to sixty, including fifteen children, by 1966).[67]

Hundreds of others flocked to the mansion, jazz musicians Maynard Ferguson and Charles Mingus, filmmaker D. A. Pennebaker, and photographer Diane Arbus among them. Most dropped acid; some came to attend biweekly workshops where participants explored nonchemical means—including Buddhist meditation and yoga—to expand consciousness.[68]

An air of raunchy bohemianism prevailed.

First because of the squalor.

One reporter for *Look* magazine described the interior as "an amiable but unhygienic shambles," where he himself dined on a kitchen sideboard alongside house cats and where residents lounged on dirty mattresses on the floor. Watts, who was fastidious by nature, couldn't fathom how people so dedicated to expanding awareness could tolerate the unmade beds, grimy floors, and decrepit furnishings.[69]

And second because the place paid gaudy homage to India.

A Kanphata Yogi looked out from one side of the house, each eye about the size of a window, earlobes drooping onto the eaves of the porch. Inside, the walls were decorated with pictures of the subtle body, described by one resident as "garish meta-anatomical diagrams of chakras and ectoplasmic plumbing," and there was a "Hindu room" for meditation, in which cotton, Indian-print bedspreads covered every visible surface.[70]

In the winter of 1964, Leary married Swedish model Nena von Schlebrugge, and they spent their honeymoon in India, where he smoked hashish on the ghats of Calcutta "with a gang of wood-carrying Sivites" and practiced yoga daily under a bamboo grove in Almora. Though their marriage didn't last, several months in the subcontinent had reaffirmed Leary's interest in India's various spiritual traditions.[71]

At bottom, despite the spontaneous nude dances, the experiments with free love, the parade of junkies, celebrities, and reporters, Leary saw Millbrook as a twentieth-century ashram.

"Men have been discovering this experience and developing methods to get high, or to go out of their mind, for thousands of years," he explained in a 1965 Canadian Broadcasting Company (CBC) interview. "And LSD is simply the modern yoga made possible by advances in science which have produced these incredible chemicals which we call psychedelic drugs."[72]

No surprise to anyone, Leary and Alpert's work at Millbrook was the subject of much speculation, among locals and the press. They were priests and gurus if you read underground papers such as the *San Francisco Oracle* or the *East Village Other*, impresarios and leaders of a drug cult if you read *The New York Times* or listened to disgruntled townsfolk.[73]

Leary's aspirations notwithstanding, Millbrook was actually more like Clarkstown Country Club—minus Pierre Bernard's business savvy and De Vries's impeccable taste—than an ashram.

Whether this was a service or disservice to yoga depends on your perspective. Take what happened to Arthur Kleps.

When he first showed up at Millbrook, Kleps was not a popular fellow. A boyish-looking school psychologist, he was seen by many, including Leary and Alpert, as immature and insufficiently tuned in to the cosmic consciousness. He also drank too much.

During the summer of 1965, this seemed as good a reason as any to dose him with a thousand micrograms of LSD (several times the normal dose), administered unbeknownst to him in a glass of brandy. Predictably, Kleps went out of his mind. "I seemed to be inside a whirlwind of electrical plasma which also made two-and-one-half gigantic turns, this time counter-clockwise" was how he described one fragment of the timeless, discontinuous space he occupied. "It seemed as though all the thoughts which had entered the minds of men and beasts in the last million years were going through my mind at the same time and with the same intensity and velocity, resulting in a kind of violent white hum . . . Sweat poured from my forehead, but the rest of my body was dry."[74]

A few months later, Kleps stumbled on Arthur Avalon's *Serpent Power*, the most read exposition of Tantric Yoga, and deduced that up at Millbrook he had experienced the awakening of Kundalini.[75]

Leary and Alpert, by the way, disagreed with his interpretation of events, but who's really to say?

Yoga had made sense of Kleps's trip.

It wasn't long before others worked out, more precisely, the relationship of yoga and mind-changing drugs.

John Bleibtreu made a valiant attempt in *The Atlantic Monthly* in September 1966. He argued that recently discovered neurotransmitters such as serotonin might be the mechanism whereby LSD activated the ājñā chakra, or Third Eye.

His analysis extended to yoga, and if he was right, then the subtle body now lay within the ken of science.

But Bleibtreu's essay was more suggestive than explanatory, and in the end he didn't get too much further than Vivekananda had, in identifying the sahasrāra chakra as the pineal gland.[76]

That winter, Bob Simmons wrote a piece for the *San Francisco Oracle*, titled simply "Yoga and the Psychedelic Mind."

(Allen Cohen had launched the *San Francisco Oracle* in the fall of 1966; the idea for the paper had come to him in a "rainbow dream." And that's what the *Oracle* was like, a Technicolor dream, full of poetry and illogic and naked bodies and ideas that blithely defy physics. It had immediate impact and was a lifeline for Leary and Alpert, making their somewhat dusty philosophy newly, madly, intoxicatingly NOW.)[77]

Yoga, said Simmons, provided a "topographical sketch of the labyrinths of consciousness" for anyone who has tripped, be it on meditation, fasting, sex, or mind-expanding drugs. Specifically and personally, yoga helped him experience both the "depth and power of my own BEING" and "to tune in to all the subtle and astral planes of thought waves that have ever been projected within this universe."[78]

Simmons, who had learned Hatha and Raja Yoga from two Indian swamis now based in the States—Dr. Mishra, who taught yoga in New York City and ran the Ananda Ashram in Monroe, New York (not far from Millbrook), and Swami Vishnu-Devananda, a disciple of the famed Swami Sivananda of Rishikesh, whom Theos Bernard had greatly admired—also held a workshop on yoga at Golden Gate Park. People thought he was giving "yogurt" away for free.[79]

It wasn't that yoga was new to San Francisco. Walter and Magana Baptiste had been teaching Hatha Yoga in San Francisco since the 1940s. And Vivekananda himself had set up the San Francisco Vedanta Society at the turn of the century. Over time, and despite periodic declines, the society, which is still housed in a Queen Anne building topped with minarets, turrets, and onion domes on Webster and Filbert streets, became one of the Vedanta movement's most vital centers.[80]

But this new generation of California seekers had yet to come across yoga or Vedanta. Some were too young to have done much sampling of other cultures (outside of the *Encyclopædia Britannica* or *Ripley's Believe It or Not!*). Many came from somewhere else, the somewhere most often being a community that didn't support a thriving yoga scene. Like the Eaters Anonymous group Indra Devi addressed in the early 1950s, these kids had had so little exposure to the discipline, they didn't know the word for it.

Which just goes to show the reversal that had happened in a generation.

Watts, Huxley, Heard, and even Isherwood had come to psychedelic drugs through their interest in yoga or Eastern religion.

For Leary and these California youngsters, drugs were the gateway to spiritual seeking.

And since acid came late to California—by 1962, it was easy to get good-quality, reasonably priced LSD in Greenwich Village, but high-grade, retail LSD didn't arrive in the Bay Area until 1964—so did, relatively speaking, this youthful zeal for yoga.

And by the time it did, LSD was considered a public scourge.

Some estimated that 4 million people were using the drug in 1966. Critics portrayed these users as hapless youths seduced by Leary and Ken Kesey, whose Acid Tests turned on hundreds at once.

But all kinds of people were turning on—businessmen, editors, lawyers, educators, middle-class housewives, and corporate barons.[81]

Of course, a lot of young people *were* dropping acid because America had become a country of youths. The number of Americans between eighteen and twenty-four years old was roughly 16 million in 1960, about 10 percent of the overall population. A decade later it had shot up to more than 24 million.[82]

Beyond the statistics, LSD made great copy. The headlines capture the general sentiment, which swung between moral panic and fascination: "Drug Disorients," "Damage to Mind from LSD Feared," "Drug-Taking Spreads on Nation's Campuses," and, from *The Washington Post*, "Sex, Poetry, Music; LSD Simulation Session Lures 16 to 'Ecstatic Experience.'"

In 1965, the federal government severely restricted the use, possession, and production of the drug.[83]

The day LSD became illegal in California (October 6, 1966), the heads in Haight-Ashbury celebrated by holding a Love Pageant Rally at San Francisco's Golden Gate Park. As the story goes, almost every one of the five hundred who showed up dropped acid. Janis Joplin and the Grateful Dead played. A good time was had by all.

Starting at about that moment, all eyes turned West. The party became a spectacle. The scene grew exponentially. (More than twenty thousand attended the next gathering, the first Human Be-In, held less than six months later.)[84]

Now that acid was illegal, the *San Francisco Oracle* had a de facto political stance. It wasn't just the voice of consciousness expansion. It was the voice of resistance, of outlawry, of revolution. And yoga was part of the revolution.

(In this, the *Oracle* was linked to *The Atlantic Monthly* of the nineteenth century, which had continued to publish in-depth pieces on various aspects of Asian religion. A curious side effect of the editors' interest and openness to the subject was that, almost immediately, the magazine solidified the link between Eastern philosophy and liberalism. This persisted long after the Civil War.)[85]

The *Oracle's* message was simple. Yoga and psychedelics. Different means, same end. The discipline validated the head's way of life, and the reverse was just as true. But elsewhere an outright blending of the two practices had already begun to displace such cool analogies.

The official marriage of yoga and psychedelics took place in October 1966 on the East Coast and in January 1967 on the West Coast. Dr. Timothy Leary was present at both ceremonies.

Leary, Richard Alpert, and Ralph Metzner had always touted yoga at Millbrook, but there wasn't much in the way of sustained practice or instruction (save occasional seminars).

At Ananda Ashram, on the other hand, which was halfway between Millbrook and New York City, Dr. Mishra was teaching Hatha Yoga, Vedanta, and meditation.

Mishra, known as the "uptown swami," had a Hatha Yoga studio on Seventy-second Street in Manhattan and had been a practicing medical doctor when he arrived in New York. As soon as he had enough students, he gave up his medical practice. By the mid-1960s, he split his time between the city and his ashram in Monroe.

Dr. Mishra also functioned as a sort of liaison for other swamis, new to the States. He'd invite them to lecture and put some of them up until they found their footing in the United States. Most recently, Mishra had hosted Srila Prabhupada, a Bhakti Yogi from Calcutta, who performed "ambrosial," "electrifying" Kirtans and converted some of Mishra's own students.[86]

A circuit developed. It was well traveled by people like Bob Simmons and had as its loci the Paradox macrobiotic restaurant in New York City's

East Village, Mishra's Upper West Side Yoga Society, Ananda Ashram, and Millbrook.[87]

In the fall of 1966, tensions between a small but growing faction of new, younger students and older devotees at Ananda Ashram came to the fore. Young students believed in the efficacy of psychedelics. The older students didn't. These original devotees eventually won the day and gave the pro-drug faction, led by Bill Haines, a bearish World War II veteran, thirty days to relocate.

Arthur Kleps introduced Haines and Leary. The event was highly anticipated with everyone "dressed to kill in the best beads and batik money could buy." The meeting was held in the dining room of the main house at Millbrook, which Leary's acolytes had filled with incense and flowers. Members of the ashram sat on one side of a low table, and Millbrook residents sat on the other.

At one point in their initial conversation, Leary asked Haines how he reconciled yoga and LSD. Haines gave a lengthy reply which, according to Kleps, "stressed the idea that the whole purpose of yoga was to reach Enlightenment and that this could only be done through intense personal experience of the kind psychedelic drugs provided."

Haines had clearly hit the right notes for his audience.

About ten evicted members of Ananda Ashram moved into Millbrook on October 28, 1966.[88]

The West Coast marriage of yoga and psychedelics was the Mantra Rock Dance, held at the Avalon Ballroom in San Francisco on Sunday, January 29, 1967.

The event was in essence a fund-raiser for Srila Prabhupada. After about a year in New York City, Prabhupada, who was also known as Swami Bhaktivedanta, moved to San Francisco, where he opened up a Hare Krishna temple on Frederick Street.

The poster for the Mantra Rock Dance featured a photograph of Prabhupada, crouched and bald save for a tuft of hair on the back of his head. Bent red type, rolling in a gentle sine wave across the page, listed the night's attractions: "Krishna Consciousness Comes West. Swami Bhaktivedanta * Allen Ginsberg * The Grateful Dead * Moby Grape * Big Brother and the Holding Company."

Leary, wearing a Brooks Brothers suit, paisley tie, and bone-carved mandala pendant, is said to have paid the $2.50 entrance fee just like everyone else.[89]

That night, the place was packed, as the Avalon and Filmore were every weekend, with what Hunter S. Thompson called "borderline hippies . . . who don't mind paying for the music and the light show."[90]

At around 10:00 p.m., Allen Ginsberg, long-haired, bearded, and robed, introduced Bhaktivedanta, and then the chanting began.

Bhaktivedanta started slowly. He was doing the maha-mantra—"Hare Krishna, Hare Krishna, Krishna, Krishna, Hare, Hare, Hare Rama, Hare Rama, Rama, Rama, Hare, Hare"—and as his rhythmic chant built, people began to dance.

By the time the swami himself, no young man at seventy, started dancing, arms in the air, the crowd was making a holy ruckus, banging on small drums, shaking rattles, tambourines, cymbals, and whatever other musical instruments they'd brought.

Huge images of Krishna pulsed, as if breathing, on the walls, projected, according to one devotee, in "perfect sync with the beat of the mantra."

When Bhaktivedanta had come to be known, a few months earlier, after an afternoon chanting in Tompkins Square Park, Ginsberg explained that "the syllables force yoga breath control," and this was partly why continuous chanting induced ecstasy.[91]

But that night at the Avalon, in moments, the audience was jacked into a synesthetic, electronic, chemically enhanced swoon.

Before he left the stage, Bhaktivedanta shouted, "All glories to the assembled devotees!" three times.

He had given his blessing to the psychedelic scene.

"We sang Hare Krishna all evening," Ginsberg said sometime later. "It was absolutely great—an open thing. It was the height of the Haight-Ashbury spiritual enthusiasm."[92]

The marriage of acid and yoga was at this point happy, exploited, flaunted, and generally embraced. It could, from a certain vantage point, be justified by tradition. A number of Tantric texts mention cannabis (in various forms, including bhang) or datura. And these were not the only entheogenic (God-manifesting) substances used by Tantric Yogis.[93]

In the account of his final initiation, which would have taken place in 1936, Theos Bernard offered this detail: "After assuming my posture, I went through the rites of purifying my offering, which consisted of the narcotic, Bhang, prepared from the leaves of hemp." He then recites a mantra and drinks the concoction.[94]

Although Theos fabricated this scene, that he bothered to mention bhang at all suggests it was part of what he considered an authentic Tantric tradition and may well have been something his father did experience.

In June 1967, the *San Francisco Oracle* published the (seemingly) definitive piece on the subject, titled "Psychedelic Yoga," written by Sri Brahmarishi Narad. The author's premise was that "psychedelic drugs induce greater sensitivity to subtle spiritual and psychic energies and speed up the influx of impressions from deeper levels of consciousness." By applying "yoga meditation" you can direct these energies.[95]

Narad's lengthy piece was more or less a primer on the subtle body and different kinds of meditation (on the heart center, on the chakras, observing the breath) for those who wished to practice under the influence. Though he referred to the various forms of meditation as Raja Yoga, Narad made no mention of particular texts or the sources of his information. His was an original adaptation of yogic techniques to the psychedelic experience.

Even more powerful and succinct testimony to the union of discipline and drug was a 1967 poster for "Superior Acid."

The text—SUPERIOR ACID, AT YOUR LOCAL DEALER, BLOWS YOUR MIND—frames a picture of a young Indian Yogi, in full lotus. His hands rest, palms up, below his navel. He has long black curls and a mustache. Fat plumes of purple smoke burst from his head. But it's not just smoke. The plumes form the profile of a woman, a staff, and a grinning, gargoyle-like visage.[96]

In late 1967, Richard Alpert found himself in the Kumaon Hills in northern India, at the Bhumiandar temple, one of several temples and ashrams that Neem Karoli Baba inhabited in the area.

The temple was (and remains) a simple structure set in the side of a steep hill. It has vistas of snowcapped Himalayas and, closer in, the piney slopes of the valley.

On this day, Maharaj-ji, which was how devotees addressed Neem Karoli Baba, called for Alpert and asked for his "yogi medicine." Alpert didn't know what he was talking about at first. He thought maybe Maharaj-ji wanted a vitamin B shot. (He was up in years, though no one knew exactly how old.)

But, as soon became clear, Maharaj-ji wanted Alpert's acid.

By this time, not only was Alpert a full-blown psychedelic prophet, "exegeting" in the movement's bible (the *Oracle*), he was also burned-out and a little dispirited about psychedelics since neither he nor anyone else had figured out how to stay high without continuously dosing himself.

So when he got the chance to go to India, he took a bottle of LSD. He thought he'd "meet holy men along the way," give them LSD, "and they'd tell me what LSD is."[97]

If he and Leary hadn't been glossing their movement with yoga and Buddhism, if Alpert himself hadn't already started tilting toward India and its modern avatars, this might have sounded disingenuous.

And it wasn't the whole truth.

Before he gave Neem Karoli Baba the acid, Alpert had already heard— and rejected—the idea that yoga or meditation might be a better way if you wanted to rejoin "the universe spiritually."[98]

In 1966, concerned by the reports of drug use among American youngsters, Meher Baba, a Sufi spiritual teacher then residing in India, had written an antipsychedelic tract called "God in a Pill?"

He had also struck up a correspondence with Alpert, among others.

Now Alpert had deep respect, you could say reverence, for Baba. Still, he wasn't entirely convinced that drugs produced "Perverted Consciousness," as Baba insisted.

"I spent six months without LSD pondering the significance of it all," Alpert told the *Oracle*. "My conclusion after this period was that Meher Baba was further along the path than anybody else I knew but that what he said about LSD just did not stack up with my internal computer's assessment of the Way the World REALLY Is."[99]

Alpert had tried life without acid and had concluded it was no better than life with it.

So he took a whole travel kit full of various mind-manifesters to India.

Alpert had by now grown his hair and lost a bunch on top. Kermit Michael Riggs (then and now known as Bhagavan Das), who had introduced Alpert to Neem Karoli Baba, remembers in particular how big Alpert's head looked and how, to him, Alpert seemed to have two personalities, the lying-down one—feminine, receptive—and the standing-up one—male and compulsive.[100]

But Alpert was also still very much the social scientist, on some level, a note taker, an observer of events.

Once he had figured out what Neem Karoli Baba wanted, Alpert handed him a single pill, which contained 305 micrograms of LSD. Maharaj-ji asked for another. And then another. Maharaj-ji ended up taking almost as much as Kleps had, a whopping dose, even by Alpert's standards.

And then nothing happened.

Alpert saw this. So did Bhagavan Das.

They kept checking to see if Neem Karoli Baba would succumb, show even the slightest sign of the drug's effects. Bhagavan Das remembers that Maharaj-ji would periodically "check in with Siva," moments when the guru would turn inward. This, though, was entirely normal, and he did so no more often on acid than off.

Alpert was astonished.

Maharaj-ji didn't say anything afterward about LSD. It just now seemed more or less beside the point.

But in the United States, the out-and-out critics of mixing yoga and psychedelics were growing in number.

These weren't always your usual suspects either.

Ken Kesey had found the whole atmosphere at Millbrook stultifying and cold. He had chalked it up to the residents' infatuation with Indic religions.

"The trouble with Leary and his group is that they have turned *back*" is how Wolfe rendered Kesey's reaction in the *Electric Kool-Aid Acid Test*, ". . . only with them it's—India—the East—with all the ancient flap-doodle of Gautama Buddha or the Rig-Veda."[101]

The analysis was as simple as it was powerful. Leary and his acolytes said they were starting a religious revolution. But their most revered texts came from Indian Tantra, Tibetan Buddhism, and Taoism, and their practices were (perhaps pale) derivations of yoga techniques.[102]

Even friends challenged easy analogies between the heaving, breathing, merging, multicolored reality LSD delivered and Eastern religion.

Leary "had all the background in psychology but he didn't have all the necessary background in the history of religions," Watts chided in a 1967 interview with the *Southern California Oracle*. "And, therefore, I think he has been uncritical in his acceptance and use of religious imagery."[103]

In practice, the combination of yoga and psychedelics wasn't always harmonious either.

Up at Millbrook, tensions between former ashram members and Millbrook residents had almost immediately arisen. "The people of Millbrook are used to privacy + quiet," noted beat poet and former ashram resident Diane Di Prima in her journal, "—the people of the ashram are noisy + boorish."[104]

But the far bigger problem was that psychedelics tended to displace a sustained yoga practice. At Millbrook, Di Prima, for one, found it difficult to make time for yoga with much regularity, and her favorite yoga teacher had left for California by the late fall of 1966.[105]

Of all the critics, the Indian Yogis opposed the marriage of yoga and LSD most vociferously.

Those who had large American followings almost to a one dismissed psychedelics as a legitimate "yoga" and frowned on any mingling of drug and discipline. After all, they were protecting a tradition.

Srila Prabhupada saw drugs as contrary to his whole endeavor, which was to tune the world in to Krishna Consciousness.[106]

Same goes for Swami Cinmayananda, who told the *Oracle*, "If it is spiritual development and evolution that is in view, then drug use is a dangerous suicidal path."[107]

Even Maharishi Mahesh, that most permissive of gurus, discouraged drug use. And this in no uncertain terms.

At a lecture in Santa Monica in the fall of 1967, "several of the beads, beards, and bells set" asked about LSD. He replied that it was unnecessary and, as the *East Village Other* related, "that anyone who took LSD was (loosely translated) a schmuck."[108]

Mahesh went so far as to require that students be clean of drugs for fifteen days before they learned TM.[109]

The very vehicle that had brought so many to yoga—psychedelics—now stood in the way of it. This would be the second reversal of the decade. Together the social scientists and the drugs had returned yoga to the temple, or had at least restored some of its spiritual import. Now it was left to the swamis to get rid of the drugs without sacrificing this newly divinized yoga.

•

Alpert had ended up staying in the Kumaon Hills for several months. When he came back to the United States, he started preaching a new gospel. At first, he talked to small groups.

"I have three chapters," he told the audience assembled at the Seminar House in Bucks County, Pennsylvania, in the fall of 1968, "each of which . . . led quite naturally into the next."

The first two were social scientist and psychedelic explorer.

And the third?

Student of Ashtanga Yoga, that eight-limbed yoga, expounded in Patanjali's *Sutras*, which takes as its main objective quelling the fluctuations of the mind.

In India, Alpert, like some middle-aged caterpillar, had gone through yet another metamorphosis.

He traded his Western suits for kurtas and churidars.

He walked around barefoot.

He started doing all sorts of austerities. He'd rise at 3:00 a.m., eat simple, vegetarian foods, and do pujas at his own little shrine. The only thing he *couldn't* manage was the cold morning bath.[110]

He also learned asanas and meditation. That is, as he later realized, he had been inducted into both Hatha and Raja Yoga.

Shortly before he left India, Neem Karoli Baba tapped him on the forehead three times, and Richard Alpert became Baba Ram Dass.[111]

The reborn Alpert was tall and gangly, having lost nearly sixty pounds in India. Intense as ever but clearly deeply happy.

In New York, WBAI, the *East Village Other* of radio, started broadcasting his talks. Rotary clubs, universities, borscht-belt hotels, and communes invited him to come share what he had learned in India, and he rarely turned down an invitation.[112]

Now there was no longer an exact analogy between the two—psychedelics and yoga—nor was the thing to do to combine them.

The relationship had become progressive: you graduated from acid to yoga, so to speak.

"I myself have given up pot—and LSD, but not because I think they are bad," explained Baba Ram Dass in a 1970 *Playboy* roundtable. "I quit for personal reasons—first because I'm doing *pranayam* breath control and that doesn't mix with psychedelics and, second, because I don't want to break the law, since that leads to fear and paranoia."[113]

A version of this had been happening all over America.

The psychedelic subculture represented a lot of people looking for God or anyway for something that material abundance—America in the 1960s saw "full employment," and people, in all seriousness, predicted, "The superior man of the future will be the person who can cope with a world without work"—was not supplying.[114]

And when pressed, more than a few of the Indian Yogis who disparaged drugs agreed that acid could give you a little taste of divinity.

Americans "wanted a material for approaching God," said Hari Dass, "and they got it in the form of LSD."

This wasn't all bad, explained Hari Dass, for if you didn't believe in God, then how or why would you bother to seek the divine?[115]

Even Meher Baba allowed for this.[116]

That so many kids had experienced chemically induced transcendence made yoga, whatever form it was, a much easier sell.

Srila Prabhupada's International Society for Krishna Consciousness (ISKCON) was particularly good at turning heads into yogis.

Bhakti Yoga is relatively easy to do, you just chant, and, like TM, it often yielded quick results.

"I started chanting to myself, like the Swami said, when I was walking down the street," one early disciple recounted to the *East Village Other*, ". . . suddenly everything started looking so beautiful, the kids, the old men and women. . . . It was like I'd taken a dozen doses of LSD. But I knew there was a difference. There's no coming down from this."[117]

Plus Prabhupada's "blessing" at the Mantra Rock Dance, despite his objections to drugs, also proved excellent marketing. His San Francisco temple became headquarters for kids who wanted to find another way.[118]

TM also surged in popularity around this time. Some calculated that the Maharishi Mahesh Yogi's following approached 115,000, or even 150,000 people, in up to fifty countries, a fantastically high number for such a relatively young movement.

Students made up a sizable portion of Mahesh's following. Jerry Jarvis, a charismatic and extremely persuasive TM teacher, would initiate one hundred students a day at his Berkeley, California, center, many of whom attended the nearby university. They'd troop to his center on Channing Road, with their offerings, fruit and flowers, and wait patiently to be admitted to the upper rooms, sometimes as long as two hours. With two assistants, working from morning to evening, Jarvis still couldn't keep up with demand.[119]

Christopher Isherwood had his own, rather high-minded, diagnosis of the surge in popularity of TM among college students: Americans had become slaves to their machines. "We—some of us—sense the need for a great psychic advance, so that we are still in a position of control," said Isherwood, who lectured frequently on California campuses. "Kids are the least corrupted part of our society, and they sense this need . . . this creates a great turning toward religion."[120]

This may have created the need, but TM had other advantages, notably its celebrity following. According to Jarvis, the Beatles' adherence to TM almost immediately doubled and trebled attendance at lectures.[121]

Even so, this couldn't entirely explain the numbers of adherents. What TM offered was a simple, undemanding system and near instant results. "It's very easy to live in peace and happiness," Mahesh liked to say. "It is not necessary to live in suffering."[122]

This reasoning opened Mahesh up to critics, especially his competition, who rightly reckoned he was selling yoga the way McDonald's sold hamburgers. "Maharishi says do whatever you want—eat hearty and have free sex—then come and meditate. That cannot work," explained Swami Vishnu-Devananda, who then ran a yoga school on Sunset Boulevard in Los Angeles and ashrams in Montreal and the Bahamas, to the *Los Angeles Times*. "Meditation cannot be treated lightly, for its the seventh, not the first, step of yoga. Most students are ready for it only after they have gained complete self-discipline."[123]

Nonetheless, countless TM students—unschooled in yoga or indifferent to its tradition—concurred with Mahesh.

Take Paul Saltzman, a young Canadian filmmaker who had been in Rishikesh during the Beatles' stay.

Raghvendra, a longtime disciple of Mahesh's, had initiated him.

Saltzman sat on the floor of Raghvendra's quarters on a white futon.

After a short puja and a little practice silently repeating his mantra, Saltzman lost himself in thought. Then he began replacing his thoughts with his mantra. Fairly quickly, he lost a sense of time "and for a moment only the sound of my mantra was in my conscious mind." Once this sound faded, Saltzman found himself in a place "without sound and without thought." He had "transcended," and the feeling it brought was "deeply peaceful" and energizing.[124]

The whole process took less than forty-five minutes.

Fred Smithline, who never fashioned himself a disciple or even a student of TM, experienced something surprisingly similar. In Rishikesh, Mahesh himself had initiated him and his wife, Susan.

Self-hypnosis was how he described TM. He recently said it had brought about "bliss consciousness" and that it had left him in a state "not sleeping, not awake . . . mellow."[125]

This wasn't "gratuitous grace," unbidden, effortless, and it wasn't the clear light void, which you could enter, according to Leary and Alpert, with enough acid and the right frame of mind, but it was close.

After "a three-day course in Transcendental Meditation," Mahesh once boasted, hundreds of young people had ceased to be hippies.[126]

There may have been something to this. In an unscientific poll of a dozen students attending Mahesh's three-month training session in Rishikesh, all except one admitted to having done acid.[127]

In February 1968, the same week *Life* came out with its "Year of the Guru" package, *Look* magazine put Mahesh on its cover and the caption "And Now Meditation Hits the Campus: How Hindu monk Maharishi turns the students on—without drugs."[128]

Allen Ginsberg has been made to stand in for many aspects of the 1960s— "tutelary deity of the flower people," "bohemian prototype," "hairy freak," "father goddam to two generations of the underground"—so it's with some hesitation that I present him, a tragicomic hero, an icon, a metaphor for yoga in the Age of Aquarius. But I'll do it anyway because, as a matter of public record, it was probably Ginsberg who pioneered this graduated approach to psychedelics and yoga and because Ginsberg saw himself as an example.[129]

Back in December 1960, the poet had spent a weekend at Leary's place in Newton, Massachusetts. There, with his lover Peter Orlovsky, he took a large dose (36 mg) of psilocybin. Afterward, he wrote up a testimonial. Psilocybin was "some sort of psychic godsend" that "aids consciousness to contemplate itself." It catalyzed "transcendental or mystical awareness," and "a kind of useful, practical cosmic consciousness."[130]

At this point in his life, Ginsberg had felt compelled to expand his consciousness via psychedelics. (Besides the psilocybin, he had ingested pretty much every variety then available.) And this had negative as well as supremely positive consequences.

On the plus side, Ginsberg was adding new types of perceptions—cosmic ones—and what he described as "new data" to his field of view.[131]

On the minus side, the drugs made him sick, sick with fear (of, he confessed, a serpent, and more broadly death) and quite literally sick to his stomach.

In 1962, off Ginsberg went to India.

Ginsberg's India was a seedy place, a great and wondrous place for a young Beatnik whose dishevelment was a form of protest.

It was not a particularly spiritual place.[132]

He did meet a number of Yogis including Swami Sivananda in Rishikesh, who ran an ashram where you could learn Hatha and Raja Yoga.

The swami told Ginsberg, "Your own heart is your guru." He, along with some other "holy men," pulled Ginsberg out of his mind and back into his body. They said, "Live in the body," Ginsberg recalled in an interview for *The Paris Review* in 1965, "this is the form that you're born for."[133]

It wasn't that Ginsberg gave up drugs. He still used them, but he had found other ways to reach "euphorias, ecstasies of pleasure."

He started chanting as soon as he got back to North America (at a poetry conference in Vancouver in 1963).

Swami Muktananda, a Kashmir Saivite, gave him a mantra, and he worked with that one for a year and half. By the time Prabhupada showed up in New York City in 1966, Ginsberg considered him and his message "reinforcement for me, like 'the reinforcements had arrived' from India."[134]

Soon enough, Ginsberg was using his mantra—his breath and his body—to reach startling and ecstatic states right there in view of all the world and all the TV cameras and hundreds of young, turned-on people assembled to protest the Vietnam War at the Democratic National Convention in August 1968.

Ginsberg had agreed to attend the Festival of Life after its organizers,

Abbie Hoffman and Jerry Rubin, assured him there would be no violence. However, the Festival of Life turned into a carnival of brutality, piped to Americans in color during prime time.

Ginsberg did the only thing he could think of. He started chanting in Lincoln Park.[135]

Ginsberg had begun his chant on Sunday afternoon. This went on for hours. But the way Ginsberg was singing "Om" so irked an Indian listener he or she wrote a note to Ginsberg pleading him to do his mantra "seriously by pronouncing the 'M' in OM properly."

Ginsberg complied, and soon enough his breathing became more regular, and then not too much later he felt a tingling in his feet that spread to his whole body, until it was "one rigid electrical tingling—a solid mass of lights."

The electricity running through his body forced him to straighten his spine. He put his legs in full lotus, something he could rarely do comfortably. People grabbed his trembling hands.

And he kept chanting.

This was American yoga circa 1968.

Its avatar wasn't Krishna. (Watts, impish and lusty, might have made for a decent Krishna.)

It wasn't Shiva. (Though Huxley, who had died the day JFK was shot, had had something of Shiva's austerity to him.)

And it certainly wasn't Kali, who was far too bloodthirsty a deity for American tastes.

It was Ginsberg in his thick, black-framed glasses, his beard and his beads and his stringy, long hair sitting in lotus position in Lincoln Park, Chicago, on a hot August day.

As more than twelve thousand police patrol the streets, he chants.[136]

As the police club unarmed protesters and reporters, he chants.

As people come and go, swelling and shrinking the circle, he chants.

As the sun went down and the city lights went on, Ginsberg chants.

And for all his chanting, Ginsberg didn't bring peace to Chicago, or even to Lincoln Park for long.

What actually happened to him came out only the following spring, in an interview with *Playboy* magazine.

On that August day, Ginsberg turned his body into some sort of divine vessel.

He felt "as if I were breathing the air of heaven into myself and then circulating it back out into heaven."

He felt "cellular extensions of some kind of cosmic consciousness within my body."

He no longer feared death.

"I was able to look at the Hancock Building and see it as a tiny little tower of electrical lights," Ginsberg told *Playboy*, "—a very superficial toy compared with the power, grandeur, and immensity of one human body."[137]

He said, "It felt like grace."

11

HOW TO BE A GURU
WITHOUT REALLY TRYING

Swami Satchidananda was late.

In the middle of August 1969, almost exactly a year after Ginsberg's chant, another helicopter descended into another wooded valley, landing on an expanse of grass as muddy and densely populated as a Maha Kumbh Mela, the pilgrimage and ritual bath that attracts tens of millions to one of India's sacred rivers every dozen years.[1]

This time, one of the passengers filmed the landing.

Four decades later, the black-and-white footage of the event is grainy and degraded. But you can clearly make out a swath of grass and a thick stand of trees, the edges of Yasgur's farm in Bethel, New York, and then all you see are gray and white pebbles filling the frame. These were people, nearly half a million of them.

The helicopter was ferrying Satchidananda, a fifty-five-year-old swami who wore dull orange robes and had a great white beard and ropy strands of gray hair, to the Woodstock Music and Art Fair so he could give the invocation.

After he landed and disembarked from the helicopter, Satchidananda's disciples clustered around him, hugging him gleefully in greeting; most reached only to his shoulders. Satchidananda smiled broadly and, soon after, walked over to a blue tent and bent his tall frame to go inside as though he were a young man.

Satchidananda went onstage second, right after Richie Havens, and sat in lotus position on a raised dais flanked by devotees. Some wore white robes, others flaming ocher.

"America is helping everybody in the material field," the swami told the massive crowd, "but the time has come for America to help the whole world with the spirituality, also."

Satchidananda was not, as Vivekananda had more than seventy-five years before, damning Americans for their materialism. He was exhorting them to redirect their prodigious energies.

He also wanted to make sure the crowd didn't get violent. Defying the producers' expectations, the Woodstock Music and Art Fair had blossomed into something else, something bigger, something far more like a Kumbh Mela or a hajj, with its millions of pilgrims making their way to Mecca, than your typical festival. (At their peak, the Beatles played in front of only fifty-five thousand, at New York's Shea Stadium.) Woodstock was the largest gathering of young people ever in America, and the bloody Festival of Life in Chicago haunted this music fair. "Therefore, let us not fight for peace," he urged the crowd, "but let us find peace within ourselves first," and reminded them that the world was watching.[2]

Satchidananda concluded his brief remarks by chanting, "Hari Om, Hari Om, Hari Hari Hari Om. Hari Om, Hari Om, Hari Hari Om. Rama Rama Rama Rama Rama Rama Rama Ram," and the multitudes chanted along with him.[3]

Earlier in the year, Richard Hittleman had opened up "the largest full-time Yoga College in the U.S.A." in a repurposed banquet hall above New York City's Grand Central Station.

Hittleman was from the Bronx, had short-cropped hair, and starred in a nationally broadcast TV show, *Yoga for Health*.

Advertisements for his Yoga College assured all comers that they would achieve "better health . . . a trimmer figure . . . and extraordinary peace of mind." The six-week class package included showers, a free sauna, dressing rooms, and free mats. It cost forty-two dollars. About forty office workers and housewives enrolled.[4]

They learned the "cobra pose (Bhujangasana)" and the "locust pose (Salabhasana)" and others, some simple breathing exercises, and "sensory awareness," in a large, well-lit, well-ventilated space, just steps from the subways and commuter trains in the heart of Manhattan.

By 1969, yoga was something the hippies had in common with their putative enemies: the middle-class conformist, the corporate drone, the happy housewife. The discipline was to grow hugely among both groups.

The media prognosticator and futurist Marshall McLuhan pointed out, at the time, that television, jets, and computers were creating "a simultaneous 'all-at-once' world in which everything resonates with everything else as in a total electrical field." The "over-all awareness of a mosaic world" was displacing single points of view.[5]

This was true of yoga now and would be for the next decade.

Gurus such as Satchidananda, Prabhupada (of ISKCON), and Muktananda had become so popular that leftists accused them of pacifying young Americans and draining the movement of its most vital political energies.[6]

Even the press was won over. Unlike previous generations of journalists, who had rarely been dispassionate and some number of whom could be relied upon to be downright hostile to yoga, a fair number of reporters were open to the discipline. In some cases, they were eager to dive in.

"Trying the Dance of Shiva" went a headline for a 1973 *Sports Illustrated* article, which detailed its author's attempt at "yoga tennis." Instructor Tim Gallwey, who had been on the Harvard tennis team, explained what yoga could do for his game:

> You have to check the mind, to preoccupy it, stop it from fretting. Look at the ball. Look at the *seams* on the ball, watch the pattern, get preoccupied so the mind can't judge. In between points put your mind on your breathing. In, out. In, out. A quiet mind is the secret of yoga tennis. Most people think concentration is fierce effort. Watch your facial muscles after you hit the ball. Are they tensed or relaxed? Concentration is effortless effort, is *not trying*. The body is sophisticated; its computer commands hundreds of muscles instantly; it is wise about itself, the Ego isn't.[7]

Two adventuresome novices traveled to the Bahamas to endure a week at Swami Vishnu-Devananda's Paradise Island Yoga Retreat, then wrote it up for *The Washington Post*. "As we soon learned," they confessed, "self-discipline is encouraged by the rigid schedule of the ashram," which began with a 6:00 a.m. meditation and concluded by 10:30 p.m., at which point most guests were in bed, despite the proximity of the Nassau casino just yards away.[8]

By 1974, *Time* magazine observed that yoga was "rapidly becoming as much a part of American life as organic apple pie." Like most trend stories, this one extrapolated from scant data. It captured a mood more than a reality for most Americans. Yet the editors were onto something.[9]

Take a look at two movies—the 1967 musical and Elvis vehicle *Easy Come, Easy Go* and the 1979 film *Being There*—and you can see yoga's status shift right before your eyes.

In *Easy Come, Easy Go*, Elvis played yet another straight man, a demolitions expert for the navy, who has just finished his last job and has enlisted artist, beatnik, and heartthrob Jo to help him remove a treasure chest from a sunken ship.

The improbable plot lands Elvis in a yoga class, where Jo and a chorus of lithe, young women are doing some simple poses. Elsa Lanchester, famous for her role as the monster's bride in the 1935 *Bride of Frankenstein*, played yoga teacher Madame Neherina. Dressed in a long, batiked muumuu, she looked like Endora, Samantha Stephens's mother, in the hit television series *Bewitched*.[10]

Here yoga was yet another excuse for comedy as the square Elvis, confounded by the practice, joins the flaky Madame Neherina in a duet, "Yoga Is as Yoga Does." "How did I get so tied up / In this yoga knot," sings Elvis, who doesn't get anything but sore "posteriors" from his attempts at simple postures.

In this classic, though lifeless, fish-out-of-water joke, Elvis couldn't make sense of this weird discipline; participation was pretty much out of the question. Presumably, he stood in for most of America—the millions who would never grow their hair out or drop acid, the millions who would always have a steady job.[11]

By the time *Being There* was released a dozen years later, yoga had become part of the fabric of American culture and media. The movie's hero, Chance, played by Peter Sellers, absorbed the discipline the way he absorbed everything else on TV—the commercials for Gatorade or *The Washington Post*, game shows such as *Hollywood Squares*, the cartoons, the weather reports.

At two moments in the movie, a yoga show so completely distracts Chance, he's oblivious of anything else going on around him: a reporter's urgent call (he's trying to find out Chance's real identity) and, in a later scene, sex. The first scene is mildly amusing, the second outright funny. In it, Chance tries to do a headstand on a four-poster bed, following along with Lilias Folan, a real-life yoga teacher who had a popular TV show at the time. The humor of the scene isn't yoga per se. It's that Chance is trying to do something that takes a good deal of coordination and concentration as Eve (played by Shirley MacLaine) is giving herself an orgasm on a bearskin rug nearby, having failed to seduce him. (Yoga, incidentally, doesn't appear anywhere in the Jerzy Kosinski novel that the movie was based on.)

By 1979, the discipline wasn't necessarily the butt of a joke or a test of hipness. It was just another American pastime.

Look closely though and you can see signs that yoga had begun to react with itself, as if the yoga of Muktananda and Prabhupada and Satchidananda had set off an autoimmune response whereby another set of yoga teachers, like hypertrophied macrophages, were hurriedly ridding the discipline of those very aspects that had prompted its resurgence.

In fact, when *Time* observed that yoga was almost as American as "organic apple pie," the magazine was careful to qualify which type of yoga—mostly the yoga "shorn of incantatory mysticism"—might soon meet this standard.

This had happened before. The Vedanta swamis at the turn of the century battled over which form of yoga was best for Americans. But never had yoga been in conflict with itself on such a large scale for such an extended period, as it was during the so-called Me Decade, when the discipline was drawing so many to its fold.

During this time, tens of thousands of Americans dove headlong into a spiritualized yoga, the kind that took over your whole life, the kind that made you drop everything to follow your guru around, the kind that got you to India, no money in your pocket and you didn't even care.

This was the yoga Swami Satchidananda had brought to the Woodstock Music and Art Fair. Those who made it to Bethel were high or wanted to be high, and they had spent much time and some money getting there. They were after transcendence and endured all manner of inconvenience—traffic, mud, not much food and water—to achieve it. The ordeal involved in being on Yasgur's farm and the sheer numbers of people uttering Sanskrit syllables in unison made Satchidananda's chant all the more powerful.

At the same time, many other Americans had started practicing a totally secular, even clinical Hatha Yoga so devoid of transcendence and so rooted in the body as to appease the most nervous rationalist.

This was the kind you'd find at Hittleman's Yoga College, and it catered to an entirely different, even opposite, set of impulses.

This yoga appealed precisely because of its convenience and its curative potential.

Fitness was achieved in half the time of ordinary calisthenics, promised Hittleman, and if you couldn't attend his college or find a class in
your own town, then you could avail yourself of any number of books or
his television show. You might find a class useful, but the teacher, the
community of students, yoga's metaphysics and rituals, were all second-
ary, if relevant at all, to a set of simple techniques that were fairly easy to
replicate, so Hittleman liked to say, alone in your own living room.

The proponents of this yoga—and especially Hittleman's successors—
behaved more like physical therapists or dance instructors than gurus.
They taught in YMCAs and opened up whitewashed studios across the
country. Their guiding light was B.K.S. Iyengar, who recently said, "The
philosophical teaching [of yoga] came to me only after 1960" (about three
decades into practicing and teaching).[12]

Yet you'd be wrong to think these Hatha Yoga teachers were any less
spiritually ambitious. In fact, they were very self-conscious about their
task. They were saving an ancient spiritual discipline from the excesses of
the hippies. They were making it safe for Middle America. And they too
saw themselves as rebels. But they weren't launching their revolt against
the broader culture per se, as Thoreau or Ram Dass had. They were rebel-
ling against yoga as incarnated by the gurus—though, in an oedipal twist,
they revered many of them—and parodied by pop culture.

Once American yoga became so set against itself, it naturally self-
destructed.

To understand the sway of the Indian guru in the 1970s and how these
men moved so many Americans to choose lives that from the outside look
even more constrictive than corporate jobs and suburbia, you need look no
further than Swami Muktananda.

Among Yogis, Muktananda was a relative latecomer to the United
States, making his first tour here in 1970, after he had already established
a substantial following in India. But his big splash in the States was his
second tour, his "meditation revolution," which had him traversing the
country via Route 66 from 1974 to 1976.[13]

Muktananda came to a changed nation—and not just because we had passed the Civil Rights Act and sent a man to the moon or because Americans were routinely challenging the prerogatives of power generally and the Vietnam War specifically.

In October 1965, President Johnson had signed the Immigration and Nationalization Act into law. The new law may not have affected any single Indian swami's decision to come to America, but by eliminating the quota system, which had for the past forty years sharply curtailed the number of Asians who could settle in the United States, the bill made it much easier for these men to stay.

The effects of this change were immediate and quantifiable. In the first year after the bill's passage, immigration was up by about 9 percent, and twenty-nine thousand more Asians received permanent-resident status than had the year before.[14]

Swami Satchidananda was among those who came to America just as the nation flung its doors wide.

Unprompted, filmmaker Conrad Rooks bought Satchidananda a plane ticket to New York in 1966, and artist Peter Max introduced the swami to his circle of friends. It was a large circle, and the swami's "two-day stopover" in New York lasted five months.

The swami was more impressed by the boorishness of his first American students, who would sit with their feet in his face, blowing smoke rings.[15]

A year after Woodstock, Satchidananda, who like Vishnu-Devananda was a disciple of Swami Sivananda of Rishikesh, claimed hundreds of thousands of followers, and students had established Integral Yoga institutes based on his teachings in Los Angeles, San Francisco, Dallas, and Detroit.[16]

Swami Rama, another Indian who took advantage of the changes in U.S. immigration law, arrived in 1969 and, soon thereafter, began lecturing at liberal churches and in Hindu temples, teaching Hatha Yoga at YMCAs and YWCAs, and giving classes in private homes.

That first fall in the United States, the handsome swami, who claimed an education in the caves of the Himalayas and the halls of Oxford, offered himself up as a research subject to Elmer and Alyce Greene, then conducting experiments in biofeedback at the Menninger Foundation in Topeka, Kansas. Swami Rama demonstrated that he could stop his heart for seventeen seconds at will. The feat made national news.[17]

He went on to set up the Himalayan Institute in Illinois, which advertised a scientific and "modern" approach to yoga and expanded steadily.[18]

Yogi Bhajan also arrived in 1969. A Sikh from Punjab (Pakistan), Bhajan wore the requisite turban and beard. He was forty at the time and already had a wife and family. He taught Kundalini yoga, which was his own synthesis of Sikhism and Tantra, and called his organization 3HO, for "Healthy, Happy, and Holy."

As legend has it, Bhajan gave his first lecture in the United States to an empty high school gymnasium and went on to open more than fifty ashrams in the next two years, with about half in the Southwest.[19]

The young writer Sasthi Brata saw this explosive growth as a great opportunity. Late in 1969, he placed an ad in *The Village Voice*—"Guru Chakravarti Assists Achieve Brahman Thought by Hatha Yoga Phone" and recounted the results of his subterfuge in the Personal Testament section of that same paper, under the headline "How to Be a Guru Without Really Trying."

Twenty people phoned for appointments; one "dazzling 22-year-old" woman dressed in a sari seduced him; and a seasoned female seeker told him she "had a little money stashed away in the bank so [he] wouldn't have to worry about the material side of things." Brata concluded that he could make a living as a guru in New York, and probably a better one than he could as a writer.[20]

In many ways, Swami Muktananda's story ran along the same lines as the other swamis' had—just delayed a few years. He comes, he attracts a small and devoted following. By the time he returns a few years later, his following has grown, then it swells so quickly, he's constantly surrounded by shiny-faced devotees. Creative types, celebrities, and liberal politicians discover him.

But Muktananda didn't look very much like the other swamis already here. He had something hard, something masculine, about him, evident even in some grainy footage shot during his first American tour.

In it, he wears a bright ocher crocheted hat with a pom-pom protruding front and center, a long tailored jacket, a white sweater, and gold-rimmed sunglasses.

His back is straight, and from the gray in his beard, you might have put his age at forty-five. But that would have been nearly two decades shy of it. He was already sixty-two.

Nor did he consider yoga as central to his whole project as most other gurus did. By this point, Satchidananda and Vishnu-Devananda had boiled down their respective techniques to a set of postures, simple breathing exercises, chanting, and mantra-based meditation, and Yogi Bhajan had elaborated his own sequences of postures, chanting, and breathing to raise Kundalini.

To be in Muktananda's presence was enough, too much almost, for many of his devotees. Sure, people who stayed at his ashram in Ganeshpuri, India (about sixty miles north of Bombay), were busy the whole day long. His followers meditated and chanted at regular intervals whether in India or New York. Yet none of it seemed to cause the inner transformation his followers sought, though it aided and abetted it once it was under way.

More than a few of his most ardent devotees claim they hadn't been looking for any sort of transformation in the first place. No, Muktananda drew people in who didn't seem to be the type to fall for a guru, then turned them inside out. Poet, critic, and essayist Paul Zweig was one.

By the time he met Muktananda in 1974, Zweig was thirty-nine years old, happily married, and the author of several well-received books. He was respected in New York literary circles, but fame—and popular success—had so far eluded him. He was also in the throes of a midlife crisis. His first attempt to renew his sense of purpose was a month's sojourn, alone, in the Sahara Desert.

Not long after, and back in New York, an old friend invited him to meet Swami Muktananda, and he consented partly because he didn't have to travel far (about twenty blocks from his apartment in Manhattan) and partly, or so he convinced himself, to please his friend.

Zweig described his first impression of Muktananda in his memoir, *Three Journeys*: "I didn't see the door open. He was simply there, quite suddenly. . . . He wore an orange ski cap, dark glasses, and a gaudy robe." He had a lithe build and a surprisingly large belly, and "he bore a slight resemblance to Dizzy Gillespie."

Zweig was observant, and his description was pleasingly allusive—exactly what you'd expect from a writer of his caliber who fashioned himself a tolerant atheist.

Within about twenty minutes though, things started to shift. Sitting on the floor of a carpeted room along with the other devotees, like nursery-school students at story time, Zweig began to shake with intense feeling. His body "had become buoyant and warm" and the "forms and colors of the room glided" past him like "paper cutouts," and his "jaws felt like hinged gates into a cave full of tears."

Walking home down Broadway after that first encounter, which included a vegetarian lunch at the ashram, some chanting, and another group darshan, Zweig found himself "in a state between dreamy relaxation and pure aerial energy."

He was perplexed. Not by the intensity of emotion he was feeling; this presented itself as an unassailable fact. Nor was the cause of this feeling mysterious. Zweig was certain Muktananda had instigated it. But the mechanism eluded him, especially since Zweig had barely interacted with the man. His friend had introduced him to the swami, who asked Zweig a question about one of his book titles. The whole exchange took place through Muktananda's interpreter, since the swami didn't speak even passable English. Zweig had not done a single yoga posture or breathing exercise. He had not himself chanted or even attempted to still his own mind.

Later, after being so uncannily moved, Zweig had asked a single follow-up question. But mostly the writer had observed Muktananda talk to the other devotees, and, as Zweig himself noted, the swami wasn't very charismatic or even terribly attentive, fidgeting, playing with his fingers, and, at one point, even picking his nose.[21]

During lunch, one of these devotees explained that Zweig had received shaktipat, which is in essence the transmission of energy from guru to student, like "a lamp lighting another lamp." This didn't mean much to Zweig at the time.

Muktananda was famous for his ability to almost immediately awaken Kundalini. Sometimes he'd touch someone's head. He'd brush someone else with a perfumed peacock wand. Many others, such as Zweig, had only to sit in the man's presence. So strong was this power, or siddhi, some people would begin assuming complex asanas spontaneously although never instructed in Hatha Yoga.[22]

Other swamis had a similar effect.

Yet many people who experienced some sort of transmission, call it shaktipat, call it grace, experienced the source as at once oddly impersonal and utterly compelling.

Zweig concluded that Muktananda had "no character in the way that we normally mean," rather he had "many characters: every mood and mannerism is exhaustive and wholly articulated."

Zweig was more able to grab on to Muktananda's physical form—"his graceful busy toes; his smooth shins with little scars on them" and "above all, his wonderful stomach swelling under the gauzy shirt he wore"—which he described with the detail and precision of a lover.[23]

This intensity of feeling and the slipperiness of its object usually led people to conclude they had found *their* guru, which is to say not much volition was involved at all.

Robert Moses, formerly Swami Sankarananda, a disciple of Vishnu-Devananda, remembers meeting his guru for the first time in 1972. "Suddenly this energy came bursting up the stairs, and this man burst into the room. He seemed to me about three or four feet high, and he was dark, a really dark Indian man dressed in a brown raincoat and pants—not like a swami at all." By this point, Vishnu-Devananda was four hours late to a party celebrating his arrival.[24]

When the swami grabbed both of Moses's hands in his, it felt as if "his hand was pulsating," and as if he were seeing Moses's "past, present and future through his hands, and everything was known to him." And then he was off to chitchat "with the ladies."[25]

Like falling in love, these feelings could be rationalized, since many of these swamis had impressive backgrounds. (Vishnu-Devananda had played a key role in Sivananda's Rishikesh ashram, heading up the Hatha Yoga program. And Muktananda was one of the very few disciples of Bhagwan Nitayananda of Ganeshpuri, famous for his potbelly and his massive darshans.)[26]

The reverse wasn't true; you couldn't reason yourself into this feeling.

These, in essence, are conversion experiences triggered by Muktananda and any number of Indian gurus. Many young Americans were having them. Not all were so dramatic at Zweig's. Sometimes someone would be attracted to a guru and his technique for one reason, say because yoga "helped chronic backache," then would stay for another, "to be one with our Lord; to share, love, live gracefully and righteously."

But even this more gradual induction had similar results—a thorough-going commitment to a new lifestyle centered around a guru and his movement.

As a two-year veteran of 3HO, Yogi Bhajan's organization, put it, "I originally just got high from the yoga, and that's still true, and now I feel strongly about creating a New Age society."[27]

In May 1975, a group of seven Californians, including Rama Vernon, Judith Lasater and her husband, Ike, and William Golden (then William Staniger) put out the first issue of *Yoga Journal*. Volunteers staffed it, the editors didn't pay for submissions, and the magazine was distributed by a Bay Area company that specialized in gay pornography.[28]

Among its other goals, the founders hoped to "convince people that [yoga] wasn't weird. . . . It was not voodoo."[29]

They had taken it upon themselves to counter a whole host of misconceptions about yoga, and their task seemed more urgent than ever.

Judith Lasater, one of the founders, served first as *Yoga Journal*'s copy editor and then its associate editor.

In 1970, she had stumbled on yoga at the YMCA in Austin, Texas. Lasater, then twenty-three, had got a job at the YMCA, and as an employee she could take any class for free. She took a one-hour Hatha Yoga class taught by Sally Elsberry, a slim and friendly student of B.K.S. Iyengar.[30]

Iyengar, like Indra Devi, is a disciple of Hatha Yogi T. Krishnamacharya. His method emphasizes the postures and pranayama. He is famous for his insistence on correct alignment and having students hold poses for long periods.

During the first class, Lasater learned some simple poses and pranayama. Lasater felt as if she were praying with her body. She continued to practice, and soon the arthritis that had plagued her for two years disappeared.

At the Y, Lasater had had a conversion experience as real and as true and as earth-shattering as the one Zweig had sitting in a Manhattan apartment, jaw unhinged, before Muktananda.[31]

Soon after, she moved to San Francisco with her husband, Ike, where she earned a degree at the California Asian Academy, a successor to the American Academy of Asian Studies, which had foundered under Watts's leadership.

There she quickly became part of a small but growing community of American Hatha Yoga teachers. They socialized, they shared information, and some banded together to form the California Yoga Teachers Association. It was avowedly nonsectarian; however, in its earliest days, CYTA teacher training was in the style of B.K.S. Iyengar.[32]

The CYTA newsletter, originally called *The Word*, became *Yoga Journal*.

This was the missing media link: a publication by insiders that, like *Runner's World* or *Popular Mechanics*, would give this subculture a voice but not limit itself to a single teacher or technique.

Dozens of books about yoga had been published in the last two decades.

Swamis Satchidananda and Vishnu-Devananda, along with B.K.S. Iyengar, all wrote popular ones that detailed their teachings and included photographs of each author demonstrating various asanas. Of these, Iyengar's *Light on Yoga* (1966), which provided detailed information on about two hundred postures and more than six hundred photographs of his own demonstrations, soon became the standard text for anyone with a serious interest in Hatha Yoga.[33]

American yoga students and teachers had also continued to write books on the subject, with far more success than Theos Bernard had had. In *Yoga, Youth, and Reincarnation* (1965), Jess Stearn had documented his own transformation from stiff, slightly overweight, middle-aged divorcé to virile yogi under the tutelage of a lithe Hatha Yoga teacher in Concord, Massachusetts. His appendix included an illustrated home course.[34]

More significant, yoga was now a staple of daytime TV. These shows were a pretty good indicator of how you'd have to address Americans if you hoped for a mass audience—or, in the case of *Yoga Journal*, an audience large enough to sustain it. TV, that icon of "middle class non-identity" (as Jack Kerouac had put it in *Dharma Bums*), which would tune all American minds to a single way of thinking, demanded maximum assimilation.[35]

As early as 1960, nine out of ten American households owned a TV set.

The three big networks—ABC, CBS, and NBC—scheduled national programming during the afternoon and prime time, but they ceded week-day mornings, from 7:00 a.m. to 10:00 a.m., and the five-o'clock news slot to local affiliates. (The exception being CBS, which ran *Captain Kangaroo* from 8:00 a.m. to 9:00 a.m.)[36]

In 1961, KHJ Channel 9 in Los Angeles started airing *Yoga for You*, featuring Virginia Denison, a dark-haired beauty, on weekday afternoons. By fall the station had moved the show to a late-morning slot, alongside game shows such as *Your Surprise Package* and *Concentration* and the sitcom *Our Miss Brooks*, starring Eve Arden, which were also geared toward a female audience.[37]

Alan Watts, a notorious flirt, called Denison the Yummy Yogi. Only Blanche De Vries impressed him more when it came to executing complex asanas.[38]

Competition arrived almost immediately in the form of Hittleman's *Yoga for Health*, which took over Jack LaLanne's morning slot, airing at 9:30 a.m. on KTTV in Los Angeles.

Hittleman had already devoted much of his life to yoga. He had run a successful yoga school in Miami and authored several yoga books. Once in California, he taught at various locales around the city, including the American Legion Hall in Hollywood, and studied with Watts up at the AAAS.[39]

On-screen, an attractive young woman (who would become his first wife) assisted the dark-haired and trim Hittleman. Both demonstrated the simple poses, he wearing tight-fitting trousers, ballet slippers, and a purple shirt that looked dark gray on TV, and she in a leotard and tights. The show ran a half hour, during which Hittleman moved viewers through a set of poses, breathing exercises, and simple meditations.[40]

As Hittleman often repeated, "The physical dimension of yoga" was "a wonderful way of reducing the tensions and fatigues of missile-age living." It also increased "vitality, mental alertness, and general well-being."[41]

A fun-loving, cigar-smoking guy who become deeply committed to Zen as well, Hittleman would "play it straight" when he was teaching yoga. Like Devi, he kept mum on the complete transfiguration yoga could effect, although he believed "pure bliss consciousness" was the whole point of practicing.[42]

Hittleman had never studied in India and had no guru on the order of Krishnamacharya. He had only his own experience, and since starting to teach yoga in the late 1940s, he had learned a powerful lesson about the discipline: Americans didn't really relate to yoga. They related to "exercise, sports, health." He felt he had to keep its esoteric elements—pesky and possibly untoward details about the subtle body and Kundalini—to a minimum if he was to reach Americans "en masse."[43]

By Hittleman's reckoning this was a good bargain, and one he was happy to make. His *Yoga for Health* quickly became a "smash hit." At least that was what its producers thought, and the numbers they publicized suggested a decent and devoted audience. Hittleman typically received six hundred letters a week from viewers, and when he mentioned that he'd give private instruction to anyone who wrote in, "he got over 1,500 reservations the first day."[44]

His converts included such stars as Carolyn Jones, Jennifer Jones, and Olivia de Havilland (the latter two had also studied with Indra Devi), as well as *Los Angeles Times* gossip columnist Joan Winchell, who mentioned Hittleman when she had the least excuse.

Even his production crew in Hollywood tried out Hittleman's yoga. When asked by a *Herald Tribune* reporter how he felt afterward, one "old timer" said, "Lousy but not as bad as when I used to do [Jack] LaLanne's exercises. . . . Then I felt lousy and tired."[45]

Thirteen years after *Yoga for Health* aired nationally, Lilias Folan debuted her own Hatha Yoga show on Cincinnati's public TV station, WCET-TV.

Folan had been a housewife and mother of two who had turned to psychotherapy to relieve a growing sense of dissatisfaction and malaise. Then she discovered Hatha Yoga at her local YMCA.

Besides losing her belly flab and tightening her thighs, she regained a sense of purpose. Soon she began teaching. One of her students, who was married to a producer at WCET, urged her to do a show, and Folan was intrigued. The biggest challenge, she said, "was convincing Public Television that yoga wasn't peculiar, strange and un-American, that it *isn't* a religion—that was the big one."

And of course it was, since this was the exact moment gurus such as Satchidananda, Muktananda, and Prabhupada were amassing large followings. Certainly what these gurus offered had all the markings of a religion, and a religion that was far more consuming than mainline American Judaism or Christianity.

Folan convinced public TV that yoga could be educational, and *Lilias, Yoga and You!* launched on WCET in early 1974.

Within a few days of airing, the show received more than 150 letters, and by October of the same year, 124 PBS stations had picked it up.[46]

In her late thirties at the time, Folan was quite pretty but not haughtily beautiful. She was trim but not skinny. She had long, dark hair that she tied into a loose ponytail or braid. She wore a matching long-sleeved leotard and tights, in pink or red, with a racing stripe down one side and an Om symbol in a lotus tastefully appliquéd just below the neckline.

The set was simple, and as Folan moved through a sequence of postures, she'd parse each one into intelligible segments, explaining what it was good for and how to do it. She insisted on using the Sanskrit names but otherwise hewed to the postures and their physical benefits.[47]

As *Time* put it, "With a persuasive manner that can drive any executive to lock his office door and stand on his head, Lilias promises to become the Julia Child of yoga."

Consciously or not, the founders of *Yoga Journal* had learned many of these lessons well.

The magazine favored the language of science and physiology, of diet and blood pressure, running such articles as "Yoga and the Endocrine System," "How to Choose a Yoga Method: From Psychological Research," "Pranayama and Physiology," "Yoga as Pychotherapy," and even "Aluminum and Plastic in Food" alongside such discussions as "Symbology of the Om," "Effects of Mantra," and "The Mystique of Enlightenment."[48]

Yoga Journal wouldn't necessarily inspire you to start practicing yoga—it was too earthbound and technical to seduce the uninitiated—but once you had begun, it would arm you with more information than you could possibly take in to reassure you that this was a scientifically sanctioned and entirely rational course of action that would inexorably lead you to vitality and health. When the magazine did cover more mystical topics, such as "Yoga, Sexuality, Matter and Energy," it did so using highly clinical-sounding language ("The energy which causes the illumination of a house through turning on a light switch . . . is the same energy based on the same principles which 'lights up' the nervous system") and often illustrated these pieces with line drawings that—save for their actual subject—would fit right into to any high school science textbook.[49]

This stress on the therapeutic value of yoga, issue after issue, set the magazine apart from such periodicals as *New Age Journal*, which in documenting the arrival of a totally new consciousness, covered yoga and its proponents.

"It was this revolutionary idea," recalls Lasater, "that you could use yoga to help with your lower back."[50]

Of course, starting in the late 1940s, Indra Devi and Richard Hittleman and most of their celebrity students had assiduously promoted the idea that yoga could cure all manner of physical and emotional ills.

Golden, Lasater, and many of the teachers profiled in *Yoga Journal* were clearly their pedagogic heirs. Many read their books, and the CYTA hosted Indra Devi for a weekend workshop in June 1975.

("From the moment [Devi] entered in saffron sari, with a lightness of step which belies her 75 years," began the magazine's write-up of the event, "it was evident that she is most deserving of the title 'First Lady of Yoga.'")[51]

In *Yoga Journal*, founding editor Golden and his colleagues had constructed a new vehicle for promoting a version of yoga that Devi and Hittleman had already popularized.

Still, Lasater *felt* as if she were fomenting a revolution because in the mid-1970s this version of yoga was far less visible than it had been in the 1950s.

Lasater wasn't up against the history of yoga in America—though it certainly informed some of the stereotypes—so much as the present state of affairs.

And here's where things stood:

Swami Vishnu-Devananda had greatly expanded his reach in the United States during these years. By 1970, he had set up the Sivananda Yoga Vedanta Center in Manhattan, as well as centers in Washington, D.C., Chicago, and Fort Lauderdale.[52]

Yogi Bhajan was drawing ever-larger crowds as well. His summer solstice retreats, such as the one held in the Jemez mountains of northern New Mexico in 1973, would attract upward of a thousand young men and women, most of them white, who'd eagerly submit themselves to a grueling schedule of yoga, chanting, and meditation.

They'd wake up at 4:00 a.m. to assemble, "eyes closed, palms pressed together at the center of their chests," by 5:00 a.m. for the opening chant, followed by an hour of vigorous Kundalini yoga—"catching hold of the toes with the legs outstretched and bringing the forehead down to the knees and up in a rapid pumping motion," "lying on one's back and raising one's legs, for thirty seconds at a time, to six inches from the ground, then twelve inches, then two feet, then to a forty-five-degree angle, then sixty degrees, and finally ninety degrees, all the while maintaining the breath-of-fire"—and so on.

They had still more chanting and meditation before the vegetarian breakfast, available no earlier than 8:00 a.m., then just an hour of free time, before another class (this one on child-rearing in 3HO), and later maybe a session of Tantric Yoga for couples. (Yogi Bhajan himself would direct the couples to hold certain positions for such long periods that they'd feel "great pain," either physical or emotional.)[53]

Unlike the Acid Tests of the 1960s, such retreats demanded commitment. And some number of Americans were willing to step up. They had been moved enough by yoga to change every aspect of their lives—from their dress to their work to their friends and intimates—to be near their guru if not in physical space then in the spiritual, psychic, emotional continuum provided by his organization. And you couldn't dismiss all of these people as psychologically dysfunctional or credulous or naive.

A case in point was Sally Kempton, who was *New York Post* columnist Murray Kempton's daughter and a journalist in her own right; in 1974, she became one of Swami Muktananda's most devoted disciples.

Kempton first met the swami at a house in Pasadena, California. She didn't speak to him at all directly. Rather, much like Paul Zweig, she listened to other people's questions and the swami's answers. She found him casual to the point of insouciance. Afterward, she drove home feeling ecstatic and charged with a fantastic energy. When she lay down and closed her eyes, she found herself floating in a "pool of soft air," which turned out to be the most "intensely sensual feeling" she had ever had. So good was this feeling, she felt immediately guilty for having it. The more she saw of Muktananda, the more she had this feeling.

Kempton, who struck many as icily beautiful, had rattled the literary world four years earlier with her essay "Cutting Loose," in which she detailed the mental, emotional, and sexual compromises she had made as a woman born and raised after the war and before women's liberation. The piece appeared in *Esquire*, and in it Kempton admits to the fantasy of bashing in her husband's head with a frying pan.

She had begun her own journalism career in the late 1960s. Soon enough, she was writing essays for *Esquire* and book reviews for *The New York Times*.

But once married, she had semiconsciously assumed the "classic housewife's position" and more or less given up writing, which made her economically dependent on her husband, the successful Hollywood producer Harrison Starr. Now Kempton was expected to "subordinate [her] needs to his."[54]

Not long after her brilliant, angry confession, Kempton divorced Starr and started writing again. She dabbled with Arica, a movement led by an elusive, middle-aged Bolivian that combined yoga, encounter groups, and numerology and, because participation was expensive (six hundred dollars for forty days of training and three thousand dollars for the three-month course), tended to attract a wealthy following.[55]

Then, after her 1974 encounter with Muktananda, as she put it, "one thing led to another." Kempton stopped smoking (though she had loved to smoke), stopped getting irritated by the things that usually irritated her, and within three months began touring with the swami. She had only a few hundred dollars to her name and ended up staying on, eventually making his ashram in upstate New York her home base. The devotees had taken over an old borscht-belt hotel in South Fallsburg, about sixteen miles from the Woodstock Music and Art Fair site.

The reason was simple. Now Kempton had only to sit and close her eyes and she'd "feel her consciousness expand until it encompassed everything."

She continued to write some, but Muktananda had become the central fact of her life, the special needs she had lamented not fulfilling while married to Starr seemingly evaporated.

Certainly, she had no time or inclination to fulfill them. She, like Muktananda's other disciples, was up at 5:00 a.m. every morning, spent three to four hours a day chanting, and worked a lot, mostly doing publicity for Muktananda and his fast-expanding organization. Her ambition, she confessed in an autobiographical piece in *New York* magazine, was "to become a saint" like her guru.

What's so striking about Kempton's experience—which she recounted in *New York* magazine in 1976 as her last act of journalism for more than two decades—is how quickly she shed the vocabulary of feminism. Certainly choosing Muktananda as her guru was an exercise of free will, over and against any societal expectations. But you could also say Kempton had just traded one patriarchal relationship (her marriage) for another (her discipleship).

The main difference was that dozens of men had also submitted to Muktananda's authority as unreservedly as Kempton had. By 1976, three hundred people lived at the swami's South Fallsburg ashram.[56]

And of course, Kempton had told her story as one of uplift and transformation: she had shucked a number of bad habits and found a blissful alternative to both the life of a housewife and the life of a journalist.

But by this time, a darker side was beginning to surface too, stories of coercion and duplicity. It was hard to know what to make of these, but they were informing any conversation you had about yoga.

They centered for the moment on ISKCON.

Since the late 1960s, Prabhupada's followers had expanded their outreach efforts way beyond the burnouts in Haight-Ashbury. Now they went door-to-door and handed out flowers in airports.

They preached Bhakti Yoga and the power of Krishna Consciousness. (Read the *Gita* properly, said Prabhupada, with the real understanding that only a spiritual master can grant you, and you'll recognize Krishna as the Supreme Personality of the Godhead and become his devotee.) Much like Muktananda's organization, ISKCON's identity revolved around the goal, Krishna Consciousness, not the method for achieving it—yoga.[57]

Meanwhile, Ted Patrick, nicknamed Black Lightning, had developed a methodology for reversing religious conversions particularly among young people when such conversions displeased relatives.

Parents, confounded by their kids' decisions to join the Hare Krishnas, the Jesus Freaks, Sun Myung Moon's group, or the Children of God, would hire Patrick to retrieve them and bring them to their senses, which meant abandoning any and all new beliefs and habits and readopting the worldview and lifestyle of their parents.

To do this, Patrick would waylay the kids, spirit them away from the offending "cult," and spend hours talking at them, until the sleep-deprived and emotionally assaulted youth "snapped" and admitted he or she had been "brainwashed."

Patrick called his method deprogramming. His success rested on his ability to limit the reality available to his charges (they were often captives in their former homes), and then to physically exhaust and psychologically overwhelm them.[58]

Originally from Tennessee, Patrick was not a trained psychologist or counselor of any sort. His methods were dubious, even illegal, and he went on trial several times for kidnapping and infringement of constitutionally guaranteed freedom of religion.

But Patrick had a lot of public sympathy. All along his work had been supported by a loosely coordinated anticult campaign and a number of vocal experts, including doctors and psychologists.[59]

Support also came from ex-"cult" members, such as Randy Sacks and Scott Berner, successfully disaffiliated by Patrick and steered to reporters.

Sacks had spent four years, from age fourteen to eighteen, as a Hare Krishna. A smart kid, he abandoned his studies and rose quickly in the organization, heading book distribution and altar worship. He excelled in sales and eventually became treasurer of his local temple.

Sacks believed that he, like many other young, smart kids, had been brainwashed by the Hare Krishnas—he became "a robot"—and this is what he told the *Chicago Tribune*.

Sacks further insisted that any attempt to connect with one's past was strongly discouraged and any doubts brushed away as a matter of the novice's own impurity. "The Hare Krishnas are good," says Sacks, "they are the reality. They are right and everyone else is wrong."[60]

Berner had had a similar experience, though he hadn't risen so high in ISKCON's ranks, and now felt that living as a Hare Krishna was a form of mind control. "Everything was so structured: rise at four a.m., cold shower, meditate, class, meditate." On this schedule, he lost a sense of time and had no time to think. Said Berner, "It's like being high but worse."[61]

This is why it seemed like a "revolutionary idea," as Lasater had put it, "that you could use yoga to help with your lower back." To imagine yoga ameliorated pain but didn't overwhelm your entire consciousness or dictate much else about your life was to wrest it back from the swamis.[62]

But Lasater and her colleagues wouldn't have succeeded had they not been students of a man as stubborn, exacting, and knowledgeable as B.K.S. Iyengar.

Iyengar was no less a guru to them than Muktananda or Yogi Bhajan or Satchidananda was to his students; however, his influence would ultimately be felt far more widely. For he was an Indian Yogi, and so had all the credibility and authenticity his ethnicity conferred, who had, in effect, stripped the religion out of yoga.

In class, he forbade instructors to teach meditation and chanting. Instead, they were to focus only on poses and pranayama.[63]

Anyway, these other aspects of Hatha Yoga would be redundant. Iyengar saw the asana practice as a meditation unto itself, and this meant his classes were slow, methodical, and physically demanding (at least at the upper levels). The greatest attention was paid to one's anatomy and placement of limbs, fingers, toes, and the oppositional energies of the body.

He had also developed a set of props—wooden blocks, ropes, pulleys, and strategically placed blankets—to help students assume challenging poses more easily.

A fully equipped Iyengar studio has at least one wood-paneled wall to which pulleys are fastened, which makes it look a lot like an old-fashioned gymnasium, where endless sets of push-ups and climbing ropes were the order of the day.

Of course, Iyengar had his critics too. In an interview with Vishnu-Devananda in the November/December 1975 issue of *Yoga Journal*, Judith Lasater asked the swami, "Did Sivananda think of the asanas as a meditative thing, or did he teach that they were just something you did to keep your body healthy and your mind calmer?"

"No, they are a part of the spiritual life, because discipline is essential," answers the swami. "Without discipline you will live a haphazard life and meditation won't come."

Asanas, in the Sivananda Yoga system that Vishnu-Devananda taught, were essential to meditation; however, they didn't themselves constitute meditation. They remained a single limb in a multilimbed system transmitted and adapted by the guru.[64]

In their bid to warm up their audience to yoga, particularly those Americans leery of the swamis and their organizations, teachers such as Lasater went even further, contending that Hatha Yoga itself could take on "elements of the other Yogas, such as Mental (Jnana) and Devotional (Bhakti) Yoga."

Their message was that you need not chant or meditate before a ravishing plaster deity or prostrate yourself before your guru. The physical practice was sufficient and would transmute itself and you.[65]

12

MARSHMALLOW YOGA

Yoga was nothing if not plastic. It was a cure for back pain, a beauty regime, and a route to God. And now, yoga seemed to be everywhere: it was on TV, in paperbacks, in movies, magazines, newspaper articles, the cities and the suburbs.

The discipline seemed more popular than it had ever been. Statistically speaking, this was true. According to a 1976 Gallup poll, about 3 percent of those polled participated in yoga, which translated into roughly 5 million Americans, and another 2 million participated in "Oriental Religions." Interestingly, the researchers distinguished between yoga and TM, and the number of Americans involved in TM outflanked yoga by about a million. Young people (ages eighteen to twenty-four) were still the most likely to be involved.[1]

Yet yoga was nowhere near a mass phenomenon. The discipline had about as many adherents as *Time* magazine had readers—4.5 million in 1976—but far fewer than *TV Guide*, which, with a weekly circulation of more than 20 million, had recently outstripped *Reader's Digest* as the top-selling magazine in the nation.[2]

A number of scholars and journalists believed that even these relatively modest figures amounted to a "new religious movement," one that could "no longer be taken as a transitory cultural aberration." Their implicit argument was that the absolute numbers didn't capture the level of influence yoga had on American culture.

Yoga's power lay in its potential and pliability. Just as it had been reduced to a health tonic, it had lately been expanded to contain all our wishes and hopes about how things could be different. Cast this way, yoga was no mere technique. Yoga was a complete ideology, a ready-made antidote to modernity itself, which amounted to all the unappetizing elements of that particular moment—whether soot-belching factories, as in Thoreau's time, or traffic jams or nuclear warheads or pesticides or Dexatrim or Watergate. Yoga, as historian Theodore Roszak put it in 1977, offered a "conception of human potentiality to challenge the adequacy of our science, our technics, our politics."[3]

As an idea, yoga was incredibly potent. Just as *The Joy of Sex* shaped the way a whole generation of Americans *thought* about sexuality, yoga shaped the way they *thought* about spirituality.[4]

So appearances didn't entirely match reality. Because as a practice in America, yoga was quite fragile. Not that many people devoted more than an hour or two a week to it, if that. And some of its most respected proponents disagreed about its very nature, with this one insisting yoga was not a religion and that one demanding total fealty to Krishna.

These were the seeds of yoga's self-destruction.

In November 1976, George Harrison and Paul Simon appeared as guests on *Saturday Night Live* (then still called *NBC's Saturday Night*). In the opening sequence Simon runs into Chevy Chase, who's singing for spare change near the elevators of Rockefeller Plaza, and Harrison calls Lorne Michaels "pretty chintzy" for reducing Harrison's fee. Later in the show, wearing a turkey costume, Simon sings "Still Crazy After All These Years."

That was in some ways where things stood for the icons of the 1960s and early 1970s. They were still with us and still crazy, and now they were easy targets for comedy (though Simon and Harrison spared themselves to an extent by making the joke first).

That same month, a piece titled "Egg on My Beard" appeared in *Yoga Journal*. It was less an article than a long-winded confession by Ram Dass, and it gave Americans the first really good glimpse of how a movement consumes itself.

Unlike Patrick and his colleagues, Dass wasn't on an anticult crusade. He wasn't out to undermine yoga or Hinduism or any other category of spiritual wisdom. He wanted to clear his name, and in so doing he tried to show how easily the wish for self-transformation at the root of the Me Decade could lead you down a rabbit hole.

At the time, Ram Dass was considered "the most popular guru in the spiritual movement in America." Yoga still informed his teachings, but he no longer described himself as a student of the discipline. He had become a sort of pan-spiritual teacher as eager to expound on the *Bhagavad-Gita* as on psychic powers, and really it all boiled down to Neem Karoli Baba's injunction to "love, serve, and remember" God.

Dass's confession in *Yoga Journal* began with an account of his life since Maharaj-ji's death in 1973. He had been set to go back to India, but got waylaid by a Brooklyn housewife, Joyce Greene, who now called herself Joya Santayana and lived, surrounded by disciples, in Queens. Dass came to believe she channeled Maharaj-ji as well as other spiritual masters. (Perhaps she was really Helena Blavatsky's reincarnation.)

Dass stayed with Joya for a year and became her spiritual partner. Many of his followers showed up in Queens too, including Bhagavan Das (Kermit Riggs).

The sadhana there was like an encounter group on speed.[5]

For twenty out of twenty-four hours of the day, they chanted, practiced pranayama, and listened to Joya, who under normal circumstances spoke with a heavy Brooklyn accent but when in a trance spoke in eloquent, unaccented poetry and "shared great truths."

But by November 1976, Dass had broken with Joya. According to Dass, to be with Joya was to "surrender" completely to her, and this included accepting many events that defied common sense, such as her propensity to bleed in great quantities. (Joya claimed she had "manifested the stigmata," though Dass never personally witnessed this.)[6]

When Dass resisted or withdrew, he claimed Joya would bully him out of his resistance, and he'd surrender even further. Sleep deprivation and the consuming hours of sadhana edged out any other reality.

At a certain point, their relationship turned sexual. Dass, who was bisexual (and now publicly admitted as much), felt that Joya would help him to "see the world as the Mother," whereby, Maharaj-ji had assured him, he would "know God," something Dass had always had a hard time with. He saw, or tried to see, Joya as Tara, a Tantric deity.

Meanwhile, Joya, and by extension or at least implication Dass, expected her followers to be celibate.[7]

Here's where the guru-disciple relationship—between the two and between the pair and their followers—went even more disastrously wrong.

According to tradition, your guru is your most direct route to liberation, a channel, if you will, for the divine, and so complete faith in your guru is absolutely necessary.

As the scriptures put it, "The *guru* is the demiurge Brahma, the *guru* is Visnu, the *guru* is Siva, verily, the *guru* is the Absolute made visible, obeisance to that *guru*." (Harrison included the prayer, in Sanskrit, in his single "My Sweet Lord," which topped the *Billboard* charts in December 1970.)[8]

But gurus are not gods. They are men and sometimes women, which is where it gets confusing, particularly since the gurus themselves seemed to encourage complete obeisance.[9]

Muktananda once said that a real guru should produce change in the disciple's outlook; the disciple should begin to get unitive awareness. But he added, "It isn't enough for the guru to be a true guru. The disciple also has to be true."[10]

Ram Dass and Joya Santayana both excited this kind of devotion— Dass because he had done it all and done it before anyone else and made a profession of his spiritual quest, and Joya not the least because she, like other gurus, was both there, in her fake eyelashes, white bell-bottoms, and heavy makeup, and not there—she'd easily drop into a trance state with no perceptible pulse or heartbeat and take leave of her waking personality.

Dass admitted culpability, up to a point. His defense was his own credulity. He claimed he had been taken in by Joya and her theatrics, and in his *Yoga Journal* confession, he pointed to the "similarities between" what he experienced with Joya, and "the stories about other movements" such as the "Reverend Sun Myung Moon's Unification Church, and the Krishna Consciousness scene. Once you are in them, they provide a total reality which has no escape clause."[11]

Try as he might to put a contemporary spin on his downfall, Dass's tale updated a trope familiar to any reader of Western literature. Joya was Dido to Dass's Aeneas (or Bianca to Mick Jagger). He had succumbed to her wiles and lost sight of his original purpose, only to escape her clutches after a suitable lapse of time.

Still Dass's tale begged a real and pressing question: Where's the line between surrender and psychic suicide, sādhana and abuse, Tantric ritual and carnal love? And who's at fault when it's crossed?

Dass and Joya were just the first casualties of Americans' disillusionment.

Major news outlets across the country began printing tales of sexual hypocrisy and other abuses of power by the most popular gurus—a run of bad press that lasted more than a decade. (Some allegations dated back to the early 1970s; most had swirled around the gurus' organizations for years before being made public.)

You'd be right to wonder if reporters hadn't simply come to their senses. Wonder and admiration don't typically become the image of a reporter, especially in the post-Watergate era. Skepticism and a certain immunity to personal charisma, these were the traits that defined the heroic newsman or newswoman.

This time around though, the takedown stories were more true than not. The moralists hadn't won the day. Reporters began to accrue evidence that the gurus had gone bad.

In 1977, just as President Jimmy Carter and the nation were drifting into an era that *Time* described as "what well might pass for 'normalcy,'" the magazine ran an unsympathetic profile of Yogi Bhajan, head of 3HO.

Apparently, the married Yogi was served "by a coterie of as many as 14 women, some of whom attend his baths, give him group massages, and take turns spending the night in his room while his wife sleeps elsewhere." The source of this information was Colleen Hoskins, who spent seven months working at his New Mexico residence.[12]

A year later, the very notion of the guru's spiritual authority was even more severely tested.

In the fall of 1978, the Reverend Jim Jones moved the flock of his People's Temple, which had been headquartered in San Francisco, to a remote jungle retreat in Guyana. That November, nearly all of his followers drank cyanide-laced Flavor Aid. More than nine hundred people died. About a third were children.

Studies done in the 1980s show that from that moment on, the media stopped distinguishing one "new religion" or group from another. Overnight, "movements" became "cults," which were, de facto, "sinister" and "bizarre."[13]

This suspicion about new religions, including those centered on yoga, was soon fueled by more revelations. In 1983, with the memory of Jim Jones still fresh, several of Muktananda's former devotees aired their own grievances, alleging that their guru, who had died the year before, had had sex with numerous devotees (even raping one) and, making matters worse, that his minions threatened anyone who left the ashram or criticized his behavior.

Victims, who spoke out anonymously, claimed that Muktananda would describe these encounters, most of which took place with very young women, as Tantric initiations (a line Joya had used as well).

But as matter of policy, the swami had always insisted on strict celibacy for both himself and those followers staying at his ashram. Indeed, he saw this as the source of his own spiritual authority. A true guru, he once said, was "not an individual, but the divine power of grace flowing through that individual." This power was "Shakti," and it depended on the guru's own discipline. "He follows strict celibacy."[14]

The former devotees levied their charges in the Winter 1983 issue of *CoEvolution Quarterly*, the successor to *The Whole Earth Catalog*, and bigger outlets, such as the *Los Angeles Times*, picked them up in their coverage of Muktananda's successors—a brother and sister team.[15]

(Sally Kempton, who was initiated as a swami in 1982 and given the name Durgananda, at first insisted the allegations were "ridiculous" and later equivocated.)[16]

More headlines followed, and they went from bad to worse: "Culture Clash in Oregon; After 27th Rolls-Royce, Town's Curiosity About Guru's Disciples Turned into Shock" (*Washington Post*, 1983), "Good Hustle, Dial Om for Murder: The Case of the Krishna Killers" (*Rolling Stone*, 1987), "The Case Against Swami Rama of the Himalayas" (*Yoga Journal*, 1990), "Ex-Followers Say Swami Demanded Sexual Favors" (*Richmond Times-Dispatch*, 1991).

In the *Richmond Times-Dispatch* article, Susan Cohen summed up her experience. In 1970 at the age of eighteen, Ms. Cohen became a student of "one of the best-known gurus in this country," Swami Satchidananda, and moved into an Integral Yoga institute in Connecticut. She said the swami "called us his spiritual daughters." Cohen eventually became Satchidananda's secretary, at which point she claims he "sexualized the relationship." While the shift made her uncomfortable, she didn't at first protest, explaining that "part of the teaching is obedience." But she eventually concluded the swami's actions amounted to "abuse."

The accounts of sexual misconduct by other gurus were eerily similar. The gurus repeatedly seduced a succession of very young female disciples, many of whom first believed they were participating in a sacred ritual and then, when they discovered otherwise, were too scared to come forward (or in some cases did, to no effect). Other disciples went to great lengths to protect their guru, heaping blame instead on the women or denying their version of events outright.

By the early 1990s, the affection and reverence Americans had shown these men over nearly two and half decades looked like a graver mistake than the reflexive distrust of earlier generations.

In stark contrast, if you were to attend one of Judith Lasater's classes in the Bay Area in 1979, you would not, like Randy Sacks, find yourself immersed in an all-consuming reality. Class took place in a rented space, a single photograph of B.K.S. Iyengar affixed to its white walls. You'd pay the class fee, which in 1979 was about three dollars. (Lasater pegged her fees to the cost of a movie.) Women outnumbered men. Most of the women wore black leotards and tights, which had stirrups. Some students would cut the feet off their tights until companies started marketing footless ones in the early 1980s.[17]

Once on your mat, Lasater would guide you through a variety of the more challenging poses—such as "Marīchyāsana (pose dedicated to the sage Marichi)," "Natarājāsana (Lord of the Dance pose)," and "Ūrdhva Dhanurāsana (back bend)"—a simple pranayama, and then end with "Śavāsana," or "corpse" pose.

Lasater remembers that her student body grew fairly steadily from the mid-1970s through the 1980s.

The key for Lasater and other Hatha Yoga teachers had been dispensing with any religious elements and distinguishing her offerings from those of gurus such as Muktananda (though many personally respected these men, and *Yoga Journal* would run favorable articles about them).

Yoga Journal's circulation tracked with the growing enthusiasm for Hatha Yoga. The founders had distributed three hundred copies of the first issue in 1975; by 1990, *Yoga Journal*'s circulation had increased to fifty-five thousand.

American Hatha Yoga teachers didn't fall as spectacularly as the swamis because they hadn't risen to such heights. Still, they too suffered, and they were partly to blame for their own setbacks. They had convinced even more Americans that yoga was a highly beneficial, primarily physical discipline, accessible to average, middle-class folks. In their hands, yoga was exercise or therapy, a salve that healed the body and soothed the mind.

But this repositioning had its risks. Presenting yoga as indebted to religion but no longer of it caused the discipline to almost immediately lose the depth and complexity that makes it so compelling. It's like taking all the sad or troubling passages out of a novel. Imagine *The Great Gatsby* without Jay Gatsby's shame-fueled ambition, without Daisy's ennui, without Nick's ambivalence and acuity. You'd have the lovely view of Long Island Sound, the vivid descriptions of Jazz Age decadence, and a few plot twists. But Tom wouldn't have betrayed Daisy, his mistress wouldn't have died at Daisy's hands, and in all likelihood Gatsby wouldn't have managed to purchase a mansion on East Egg, Long Island, in the first place. Take away the darker shades, and you lose human motivation, which is intimately connected to our propensity for suffering. True yoga seeks to alleviate this suffering. Still, it's effective precisely because it so clearly identifies the source—our own minds—and the difficulty of escaping our self-made hells.

Here's how psychologist and author James Hillman identified the problem: "In the East the spirit is rooted in the thick yellow loam of richly pathologized imagery—demons, monsters, grotesque goddesses, tortures and obscenities." You remember, Krishna consuming bodies by the thousands after giving Arjuna the gift of divine vision, bloodthirsty Kali. "But once uprooted and imported to the West it arrives debrided of its imaginal ground, dirt-free and smelling of sandalwood."[18]

Harvard theologian Harvey Cox saw this as part of a pernicious "psychologizing" of yoga and related spiritual technologies.

And over the decades since yoga's arrival in America, this habit had intensified. No longer did psychology seem a useful vocabulary for conveying *some* aspects of yoga; it seemed more than adequate to describe the discipline in its entirety.

Take the phrase *self-realization*, which Paramahansa Yogananda and others had used as shorthand for that experience of the identity of Atman-Brahma at the base of much (some might say *all*) yoga practice and theory. (Yogananda found this formulation of yoga's purpose so useful that he officially changed the name of his entire organization to the Self-Realization Fellowship in 1935.) Said one seeker in 1971, when asked what she was looking for, "Well, I was seeking integration, psychologically. Realization of myself. I'd never thought about enlightenment. That's just recently come into the picture."[19]

This shift toward a purely psychological conception of yoga had begun with such teachers as Vivekananda, who encouraged connections between yoga and the emergent field of psychology, was then intensified in Carl Gustav Jung's 1932 lectures on the psychology of Kundalini yoga (first published in English in 1975 and 1976), and cemented at such places as Esalen Institute in Big Sur, California, the hotbed of the Human Potential movement, which drew heavily on yoga, meditation, and a whole panoply of Asian spiritual technologies, often as interpreted by Americans.[20]

And so, by the mid-1970s, the term *self-realization* had taken on the cast of Abraham Maslow's "self-actualization," which posits that an individual has an essential purpose, and to discover and attune oneself to this purpose is to live spontaneously, happily, and free of neuroses.

It was this impulse and its expression—the primal screams, the encounter sessions, the skyrocketing divorce rates, the *tripling* (a Midwestern term for a ménage à trois) and wife swapping, and the rampant spiritual experimentation—that Tom Wolfe had so aptly captured and satirized in his famous essay "The Me Decade."

The Self, that God spark in everyone, had been demoted to the "self," the attuned individual. The shift in case is a small alteration, yet you have to take it seriously, and if you do, well, then the lowercase *s* is quite insistent. It insists, for instance, that yoga surrender its claim to transcendence. It nullifies the idea of Brahman.[21]

It wasn't that venues such as *Yoga Journal* denied the possibility of transcendence or ignored the gurus. Rather, such notions, and their proponents, were overwhelmed by the other options, which they reported assiduously: "Yoga: A Cure for Depression" (March/April 1980), "Getting Clear on Relationships: An East-West Approach" (March/April 1981), "Reducing Stress with Yoga" (October 1982).

Ultimately, though, presenting yoga as a kind of exalted (and ancient) "psychotherapy" proved most a problem for purists and scholars, pace Cox. It wasn't a problem for many Americans. It made sense of the discipline for them and drew them to it.

Presenting yoga as physical fitness had far more deleterious effects. What had at first seemed a tactically savvy move—yoga was no longer threatening and foreign—had made the discipline quite vulnerable. Now people were just as apt to compare yoga to jogging or aerobics as they had been in an earlier generation to compare it to Zen. Soon enough yoga's stature shrank. Like Lily Tomlin's Incredible Shrinking Woman, a toxic combination of aerobics and Jazzercise melted it to near invisibility. In their effort to sell the discipline to Americans, Hatha Yoga teachers had inadvertently reduced it out of existence.

"An effective workout," remarked Jane Fonda in her 1981 *Workout Book*, "requires the vigorous and sustained use of your entire body for at least 20 to 40 minutes." Or, as she also put it, and countless aerobics teachers repeated, you have to "go for the burn."[22]

In 1984 *Sports Illustrated* reported that the fitness business had become a $1.4 billion industry, up by more than 33 percent from a year before. Because this number included only fitness "products" (everything from jump ropes to Nautilus machines) and "apparel" (Flexatards, leg warmers, Day-Glo sweatshirts, New Balance, Nike, and Reebok) and didn't account for books and videos, it was low.

At the time, the leading fitness trend was aerobics. *Jane Fonda's Workout Book* sold 1.25 million hardcover and a half million paperback copies in the first nine months of 1984 alone.

To be fit was to sweat—in an aerobics or Jazzercise studio or on the streets of your neighborhood. (By 1986, about a quarter of Americans jogged or ran.)

While it was a colossal flop, the movie *Perfect* (1985) seared the image in our memories: Jamie Lee Curtis, lean and androgynous, leading dozens of men and women as they swing their arms and grind their hips to the rhythm of synth-pop; everyone is sweating under the neon lights, and the mirrored walls repeat the scene in triplicate.

And now to be a fit *woman*, in its most idealized form, meant having a body sculpted out of muscle. This was the very moment that feminism as an idea became passé but that women were flocking into the workforce. By the mid-1980s, most mothers of preschool-age children worked. Women were visible in almost every profession you could think of (though hardly equally represented), from medicine to the military, from politics (Geraldine Ferraro was Mondale's running mate in 1984) to television (the *Oprah Winfrey Show* launched nationally in 1986).[23]

Aerobics emphasized power and strength, as women climbed career ladders and started competing more directly with men in much greater numbers. Its benefits were, in a word, masculine. To practice yoga was to move slowly and deliberately, being careful not to strain or overexert yourself. Yoga was gentle, relaxing, and safe, qualities not likely to help you break through the glass ceiling. It was comparatively soft and stereotypically feminine.

Even male Hatha Yoga teachers, such as Alan Finger, one of the most sought-after teachers in Los Angeles, spun the practice this way. In his 1983 video *Yoga Moves*, Finger advised, "Don't strain. It doesn't give you enlightenment. It gives you sore muscles."[24]

By 1986—the year the *Challenger* exploded on live TV, the year the Clash disbanded, the year the nuclear reactor at Chernobyl melted down, and the year that Apple Computer introduced the Macintosh Plus (priced at twenty-six hundred dollars)—about 2 percent of Americans practiced yoga. This represented a relatively slight dip, in absolute numbers, since Gallup's 1976 poll.[25]

However, its cultural relevance had precipitously dwindled. The gurus had been discredited, and Hatha Yoga no longer synced with the zeitgeist.

For nearly a century, yoga had contracted or expanded to meet the needs of succeeding generations. The discipline's capaciousness and complexity—the dozens of different types of yoga, the countless gurus and Yogis who had lived over the centuries, the thousands of texts, with their Talmudic commentaries—had been the secret of its longevity in America. If you just found the right lineage (Krishnamacharya, say, in the 1940s and 1950s or Muktananda in the 1970s), you'd find the right type of yoga for Americans of that moment.

But in the 1980s the tempo changed. And yoga, particularly Hatha Yoga, couldn't keep up. Music got faster; the folk bands that had managed to keep a foothold alongside disco faded away; people sweated to Madonna's chirpy beats in aerobics classes, they danced to the Go-Go's or the ska of the English Beat at the Roxy in L.A. Even drugs sped up. Cocaine displaced marijuana and psychedelics and quickly destroyed any number of celebrities, most famously John Belushi.

And in 1982, the CDC named a cluster of related disorders AIDS. Now sex could kill you.[26]

To come of age in the 1980s was to embrace the synthetic, the manufactured, the unreal, and the apocalyptic. A certain segment of Americans wore a sort of death mask: pale skin, black-rimmed eyes, dark hair teased up with Tenax gel, and shoes so pointy you could spear a small dog. British bands—the Cure, the Smiths, Tears for Fears—wrote our dirges.

Yoga, with its promise of physical-psycho-spiritual transmutation, was far too hopeful an endeavor for this generation. It emblemized the 1960s— its false starts, its misplaced idealism, its kindly but illusory Mother Nature. Reaganism and cocaine, the Berlin Wall and Madonna, South African apartheid and Basquiat, aerobics and AIDS. Those were the facts at hand. Jacking yourself into cosmic consciousness might be nice, but it couldn't mend our present reality.

And no type of yoga was up to the task.

Now that Hatha Yoga is routinely described as a multibillion-dollar *industry*, it's hard to appreciate its relatively recent obscurity. But by 1986, the discipline had become far too modest a proposition to be of any use to younger Americans. So we ignored it. And Hatha Yoga, like hula hoops and waist-reducing machines, drifted into the cultural wilderness, where it would remain for the better part of a decade.

"In the United States, or especially on the East Coast, what has become popular is what some of us call the marshmallow school of yoga," lamented Judy Brick Freedman, a certified Iyengar yoga instructor. "You sort of lie on the floor and exhale a whole lot and it's good for puffy ladies. But that really isn't what yoga is."[27]

13

THE NEW PENITENTS

The first thing you notice when you walk into a Bikram Yoga studio is the heat: 105 degrees. It feels as if you were walking into a sauna, which triggers mild anxiety since you have yet to exert yourself at all.

The second thing you'll note are the mirrored walls—at least two walls, and often three, are covered, floor to ceiling, in reflective glass. On the floor, instead of the usual hardwood, you'll find carpeting, a short, tight weave in neutral colors, and above, usually fluorescent lights.

A typical Bikram Yoga school doesn't coddle the senses. It looks like a newsroom without the desks or an aerobics studio. It makes similar demands: you must stay alert, you will have little time for breaks or self-reflection, you will be working your body as hard as you'd work in any aerobics class, and you must use nearly every ounce of energy at your disposal to make it through a ninety-minute practice, which never varies: students perform twenty-six poses (each twice) and two breathing exercises.[1]

As you try to fold yourself properly into "Eagle Pose (Garudasana)" or "Triangle Pose (Trikonasana)," you fix your gaze on your reflection. You'll quickly see how well or badly you're doing each pose and, ideally, make the necessary adjustments. Because classes are usually full, it's more than likely an instructor won't be nearby to help.

"The mirror gives you feedback, we give you instruction," says Emmy Cleaves, a student of Bikram Yoga for forty-five years and currently the most senior teacher in the United States. "So the mirror is there to teach you to take responsibility for your body."[2]

Jarring as they are if you have studied other types of yoga, the mirrors in Bikram Yoga studios serve a clear pedagogic purpose.

Before class, though, the mirrors are simply mirrors, into which students, many wearing only bikini-like shorts and skimpy sports bras, gaze.

They turn this way and that. They take a few poses. They fix their hair or tug at their shorts. They study themselves like beauty contestants and rarely smile at their own reflections.

Hatha Yoga's resurgence in America first became visible in the mid-1990s, but it had begun a full decade before the discipline had even fallen out of favor. (Evolution of anything—whether a species or a culture—is rarely sequential; as the environment shifts, so does the relative advantage of any single trait.) Two signs of things to come were easy to miss: a certain subset of yoga students began to sweat as they practiced, and more men started taking up yoga. These changes were largely the work of Bikram Choudhury and Sri K. Pattabhi Jois. They had come to America in the 1970s, and each had brought a more arduous kind of yoga with him, directly from India.

Shortly after Bikram Choudhury (known by all as Bikram) arrived in the United States in 1971, he began teaching at spas and health resorts, including the Ashram in Calabasas, north of Los Angeles, run by Anne Marie Bennstrom.

A few years later, two students, Bennstrom and Shirley MacLaine, who had tracked him down in Bombay in the early 1960s, encouraged him to strike out on his own. With the two women's help, Bikram opened his first Los Angeles school at number 9441 Wilshire Boulevard, in the basement of a bank building. For a while, he slept there too, in one of the adjacent conference rooms.

He was then in his late twenties, and he'd teach shirtless, waist wrapped in a gaudy piece of fabric, which, said Bikram, was the kind worn by hookers in Calcutta. Something about his face, his full lips, a certain wayward sensuality, prompted reporters to dub him an Indian Paul Anka.[3]

As a teacher Bikram was irreverent and unforgiving, and his classes were more physically demanding than almost any other Hatha Yoga class you could find in the United States at the time.

"Yoga works on muscles I never used in dancing," the legendary Hollywood dancer Marge Champion told the *Los Angeles Times* in 1974. "I mean, my upper inner thighs are really tight now. You couldn't get that tautness no matter how many barre pliés you do." Another student said she went "from a size 6 to a size 4 in Anne Kleins in one month."[4]

More than one student described himself as addicted to Bikram's yoga, and many showed up five or six days of the week.

Champion was just one of many entertainers who frequented Bikram's school.

Bikram's show business connections almost immediately yielded more publicity than most yoga teachers receive in a lifetime. In August 1974, he appeared on the *Tonight* show, guest-hosted by the *M*A*S*H* star McLean Stevenson, to demonstrate part of his sequence in the air-conditioned studio.[5]

Soon, Beverly Sassoon, wife of hairstylist and beauty mogul Vidal Sassoon, began taking Bikram's classes (fully made-up), as did Keir Dullea, who starred in *2001: A Space Odyssey*, Candice Bergen, Martin Sheen, Susan Sarandon, and Raquel Welch, to name just a few. Hollywood's demands on the body had increased over the decades, as fashions got flimsier and the films more risqué. Many actors and actresses found Bikram's classes kept them at an ideal weight (or helped them get back to it quickly), and Bikram was unabashed about publicizing their interest, however fleeting, in his yoga.[6]

But Bikram didn't immediately know how to turn all of this interest into a financially sustainable yoga school.

At first, as was customary in India, classes were free. Bikram put out a small box, assuming this alone would encourage students to make a small donation for each class. No one checked students in or managed these fund-raising efforts. Worse still, according to Cleaves, Bikram's operation was so disorganized that students took towels and dishonest volunteers occasionally stole donations, which were meager to begin with.[7]

Apparently, MacLaine took the young Bikram aside and, as he relates it, told him, "You cannot run a yoga school the Indian way."

Bikram began charging for classes, and, much as Mahesh had experienced in the 1960s, attendance quickly *rose*.[8]

Within a few years, Bikram's school was self-sustaining.

By 1984, he had done something few had been able to do: he had gotten rich teaching Hatha Yoga. And unlike Pierre Bernard, he didn't primarily depend on the patronage of wealthy students. No, his money came from selling yoga retail.

A decade after opening his first school in the basement of a bank, the price of a Bikram Yoga class had shot up from five dollars to twenty dollars (about forty dollars today). A ten-class package cost one hundred dollars, and his Beverly Hills school was taking in roughly one thousand dollars per day.[9]

These numbers were another sign of Hatha Yoga's eventual resurgence. As Hatha Yoga, broadly speaking, was fading from view, Bikram was amassing considerable personal wealth by teaching it.

A number of factors contributed to Bikram's success. His celebrity connections obviously helped, as did his pedigree, for Bikram comes from a lineage of famous and prosperous Yogis.

Starting at the age of four, Bikram practiced yoga—sixteen hours a day, he claims—for fifteen years under the tutelage of Bishnu Chandra Ghosh.[10]

Ghosh was Paramahansa Yogananda's youngest brother and a famous physical culturist. He used Hatha Yoga primarily for healing and health. He also took much from weight lifting and the earliest bodybuilders, and he wrote two books, *The Key to the Kingdom of Health*, and with Keshub Ch. Sen Gupta, B.A., *Muscle Control and Barbell Exercise* (1930).[11]

Ghosh had helped develop Yogananda's Yogoda method and set up his own College of Physical Education in 1923 in Calcutta. In the late 1930s, he toured the United States, demonstrating poses to astonished audiences. Later, in India, Ghosh inaugurated yoga competitions.

Bikram was All-India National Yoga Champion at twelve years of age and retained his title three years running.[12]

But at least one person who has watched his career closely believes his success rests almost solely on the force of his personality. "The one thing that you must really remember . . . ," says Cleaves, is that "the man possesses an absolute truckload of charisma. An unbelievable amount of charisma. And that is really what accounts for a lot of his success."

He's the kind of person who can contest a traffic ticket, says Cleaves, "and the judge will let him off—every single time."[13]

And still others point to his results, testified to already by Champion and others.

These explanations are all valid, but there was something else Bikram did that was key to his success, something that he had in common with Jois, even though they trained in different parts of India, under different gurus, and possessed entirely different (you might even go so far as to say, opposing) worldviews.

The two men put the religion back in Hatha Yoga.

Sri K. Pattabhi Jois made his first visit to the United States in 1975, a year after Bikram opened his yoga school in Beverly Hills. When he arrived, Jois was already sixty years old; he was bald and trim, wore thick, black-framed glasses, and while teaching favored white boxer shorts and a simple, sleeveless undershirt.

The middle son in a devout Brahman family, Jois grew up in Kowshika, a small village in the southern-Indian state of Karnataka. When he was twelve years old, he witnessed a demonstration by Yogi Krishnamacharya (Indra Devi's and Iyengar's guru). At the time, despite inroads by Kuvalayananda and Yogendra, many Indians, and certainly Jois's own family, regarded yoga as an esoteric practice best suited to monks and sadhus. Defying his own tradition, Jois tracked Krishnamacharya down and began his training, which lasted for twenty-five years.[14]

If Bikram was Paul Anka, Jois was Arthur Miller.

He taught Ashtanga Yoga (the name is a direct reference to Patanjali's *Yoga Sutras*), and he claimed he taught this system as he had been taught by his guru, though how much he altered or even invented aspects of the method is hard to know.

The way the postures are linked to each other and to the breathing (a multilayered synchronization called vinyasa) distinguishes Ashtanga Yoga from Iyengar's style of teaching and Bikram's.

Once you begin, you move continuously, pausing only to hold a posture for five to eight deep breaths, and even then you are working hard to maintain certain internal locks, or bandhas.

Jois taught six series of postures, each more difficult than the first. (Few ever learn all six; the vast majority of students never make it past the second series.) Even in the primary series some of the poses are as intricate as any you'd find in Theos Bernard's book, and you don't have much time to assume each one as you must keep the postures synced with the breathing.

The sequence (of any of the six series), starting from the first sun salutation to the last pose, looks like some sort of slowed-down, slightly repetitive, possibly exhausting gymnastic routine.

Tim Miller, one of Jois's early American students and a longtime Ashtanga Yoga teacher, remembers stumbling on an Ashtanga Yoga class in an abandoned church in Encinitas, California, in 1978.

"There was no electricity in the building or anything, so when I arrived, it was kind of dark inside and people were lighting candles and this gentleman walked over to me and asked me if I was there to take some classes," recalls Miller.

(American Ashtanga Yoga studios tend to be as austere as any Iyengar studio, save a small shrine with incense and pictures of any number of gurus, or poster-size photographs of Jois in various poses taken when he was a young man.)

Miller arrived dressed in a pair of jeans and a flannel shirt. He had expected just to watch the class. But the teacher started to teach him then and there.

"He started showing me Surya Namaskara [sun salutation] . . . and so I proceeded to become very hot and wet within a few Namaskaras."[15]

That Miller could walk in and receive one-on-one instruction wasn't unusual (though you do usually have to watch one class first). Ashtanga Yoga classes are taught Mysore-style. There's no teacher at the front calling out poses to everyone present. Instructors teach each student a pose or two at a time, based on individual aptitude. Once you learn the poses, you practice on your own, pacing yourself and your breathing. This means you might be doing a different sequence from the person on the mat next to you, and you can't necessarily look to your neighbor or the teacher (who may be helping someone else) for guidance.

Put simply, Ashtanga Yoga classes aren't user-friendly.

If you were interested in Jois's philosophy, you faced even greater hurdles. Jois didn't speak English well, and the most important book he wrote on the practice of yoga, *Yoga Mala*, wasn't translated into English until 1999, nearly four decades after Jois wrote it.[16]

The purpose of yoga, according to Jois, is "internal cleaning," not "external exercise," and "self-knowledge." He boils down his approach: "99% practice, 1% theory."

It's a pithy nugget that makes yoga less intimidating to Westerners. At the same time, the formula belies Jois's own scholarship (he taught yoga at the Sanskrit College in Mysore and earned the title Vidvan, roughly equivalent to our Ph.D.) and abiding commitment to Advaita Vedanta.

In Jois's view, the only purpose of yoga, even a yoga as physically demanding as his, is to fix the mind in the Self, to realize one's true nature—
supreme peace, eternal bliss.[17]

You could say that Jois's deep scholarship and piety made him and his
yoga quite another order of thing from Bikram's. The only specific feature
they have in common is that each demands a near daily commitment.

But they shared something much more potent: to practice either type
is to make a sort of physical penance.

When Jois and Bikram made their first inroads into the American yoga
scene, Americans were just beginning to discover jogging for exercise.
Runner's World had launched in the early 1970s, and the first line of Nike
shoes came out in 1972. (That year, the Grant Boys store in Costa Mesa,
California, advertised the Nike Marathon running shoe for $9.99, about
$50 in today's dollars.)[18]

Over the next decade both jogging and aerobics exploded. Endurance,
sweat, and performance were the guiding principles of these activities,
principles that echoed a whole cultural ethos.

By the time Bikram relocated his Yoga College of India from the bank
building to the mezzanine of a nearby high-rise, Drexel Burnham Lam-
bert had opened offices on the same nondescript stretch of Wilshire Boulevard, not far from the Beverly Wilshire Hotel and a stone's throw from
Rodeo Drive.

There, from an X-shaped desk on the fourth and then fifth floor, between 1979 and 1989, Michael Milken materialized huge sums of money
by selling high-yield bonds, also known as junk bonds. Rumor had it that
Milken could raise a billion dollars over the phone in a single hour. All of
this money funded then new ventures such as MCI Communications and
Turner Broadcasting, among others, and helped Drexel and its clients gain
control of companies such as Unocal and Beatrice on the mere threat of a
leveraged buyout.[19]

Few outside of trading circles knew of Milken before 1984. By then,
he was making so much money that he became impossible to ignore.

In short order Milken became an icon for the 1980s, first its financial
wizardry, then its excesses, and finally its demise (though he was not, as
commonly believed, the inspiration for Oliver Stone's Gordon Gekko).

But before Milken became mired in scandal, the most interesting fact to surface about him was that he worked harder than almost anyone else. He had moved his office from New York to Beverly Hills partly to add hours to his already long day.

"We get up at four a.m., and we don't go out to lunch, we don't take personal calls, don't tell jokes, don't talk about the ball game," boasted one trader on Milken's team. "No one in America works as hard as we do."[20]

There was nothing frivolous or even fun, so these traders wished us to believe, about their lives. They were ascetics, in their way, so singularly focused on transactions, they had time for almost nothing else.

At first glance, these three men—Bikram, Jois, and Milken—had little in common. By now Bikram taught his classes in a black Speedo, hair pulled into a topknot, and restored Rolls-Royces for fun; Jois still woke before dawn to do pranayama and wouldn't eat his first meal of the day until he had finished teaching, bathing, washing his laundry, and performing certain pujas, which was usually around one or two in the afternoon; the "Junk Bond King" was slim and sallow and wore European-tailored suits, but otherwise kept his real wealth out of view. However, all three subscribed to the idea that with no pain, there was no gain.

In Bikram's case, this philosophy made for highly entertaining in-class patter—"I don't say I love you," Bikram told one student in 1982 as a reporter for *Yoga Journal* looked on. "I am a butcher and I try to kill you. . . . But don't worry, yoga is the best death. Don't forget, this is Bikram's torture chamber!"[21]

Jois didn't focus much on the pain; he was always more matter-of-fact: "You do!" But his son Manju, who accompanied him on his first visit to the United States, seemed to relish it. According to David Swenson, one of Jois's first dozen Western students, when Jois introduced Manju as "swami," Manju quickly corrected him: "I am no swami—my name is Manju, and we have come to break your backs."[22]

In Milken's universe, Bikram's, and to an extent Jois's, winners pushed harder. Winners submitted to punishing routines for their dreams. Winners were not smarter or more creative or "team players." Winners were tougher.

In 1984, *Sports Illustrated*'s Jack McCallum observed a class at Bikram's Los Angeles Yoga College. Sitting on blue satin cushions at the front of the room, Bikram heartily abused his two dozen students: "You have money! You come to me for pain, you Beverly Heels people! You pay me to hurt you!"

They responded like eager cadets.

McCallum singled out one student, a particularly beautiful and able woman, to capture the effect: "Perspiration is running off her gloriously chiseled face, down her elegant neck and onto a skintight leotard."

The religiosity that Bikram and Jois brought to Hatha Yoga had little to do with the usual rituals. They didn't reintroduce its deities or ask that you learn the symbolic circuitry of the subtle body (though this would certainly be helpful) or that you sit long hours in meditation, though Jois's students do recite a Sanskrit prayer before each class.

Bikram and Jois each taught a form of Hatha Yoga so vigorous and relentless that it quickly unsettled most of your usual routines and called into question the most basic assumptions about your life.

From a practical standpoint, anyone who sampled either type of yoga quickly figured out why both Bikram and Jois insisted their students practice ninety minutes, six days a week. If you veered from that schedule, you usually paid in injuries or slow progress.

The stringency of the Bikram or Ashtanga yoga practice had another, more far-reaching result: most students weren't, for the most part, fitting their practice into their lives in hour-long sessions a few days a week. They were orienting their lives around their practice, which often meant giving up drinking, late nights, and even jobs if the hours were too long, and this meant taking a leap of faith since few Americans spend ninety minutes a day, six days a week, doing anything besides driving, working, or watching TV.[23]

By the time Milken went to jail for securities fraud, in 1991, a good number of American students of Bikram's and Jois's had reoriented their lives around this daily penance and made a complete religion of bodily purification with its own rituals, vestments, and language.

Female students of Ashtanga Yoga would wear tight-fitting, footless leggings, sports bras, and tiny tank tops; the men would often practice shirtless in long shorts. The outfits were stripped down versions of aerobics gear—the Ashtanga students got rid of the sweatshirts, leg warmers, skinny belts, and headbands, for good reason too. You needed maximum mobility; even an extra eighth inch of fabric might affect your ability to bind in a tricky pose, such as "Marichasana C" (sit with your left leg extended, right knee bent up, straighten the chest, turn the waist toward the right, bring the left arm around the front of the right knee, twisting the left hand and arm around toward the back, bring the right arm around the back and grasp the left wrist with the right hand, then straighten up your spine).[24]

Most Ashtanga Yoga students forswore meat. Many of the more committed ones studied Sanskrit, and a good number—of all levels—would travel to Mysore, India, each year, to study with Jois and later his grandson Sharath Rangaswamy.

Bikram Yoga students were less particular about diet. (Bikram insisted that his yoga was so powerful, diet made little difference, and to prove it, he'd eat Junior's burgers and munch on See's candies during class.)[25]

As for dress, many favored the skimpiest of clothing—spandex shorts that covered only the essentials, sports bras that could pass for bikini tops—the only sensible attire given the intense heat. Seasoned students always arrived prepared, with a clean cotton towel and a large bottle of water.

To practice Bikram or Ashtanga Yoga was to assume an entire identity (one that you might keep secret if necessary from coworkers, but not from close friends and family). But it stood almost in direct opposition to the Hatha Yoga lover of the 1960s. This identity revolved around sweat and commitment. There was nothing pleasant about Bikram or Ashtanga Yoga. There were no accommodations nor even much encouragement as you struggled along, and that made it feel truer, more authentic.

Yet secreted away in the pain was intense pleasure. For those who could bear the schedule, the physical demands, and the verbal abuse, there came a deep feeling of vitality, a feeling of pure energy, an unbowed posture, and mental acuity.

That the ecstasy, if it came at all, was hard-won made it feel deserved. We couldn't trust "a new morning in America"; we couldn't trust our banks or our bankers; we couldn't trust our pop stars to be who they said they were (you remember Milli Vanilli winning a Grammy for lip-synching?) or our sports heroes (Pete Rose was caught betting on games and banned from baseball in 1989, and Mike Tyson was convicted of rape three years later); we couldn't even trust sex anymore; but we could trust this.

Bikram and Jois had tapped directly into that deep, pulsing vein of American puritanism, and for this they evoked the kind of veneration usually reserved for gurus such as Muktananda or Vishnu-Devananda. Bikram isn't one for formalities, but whenever Jois received his students after one of his classes, especially when giving workshops in the United States, they would approach him and prostrate. Crouching on their shins, they'd press their foreheads to the ground near his feet.

To be fair, many of Iyengar's students treated their practice and their guru as reverently as students of Jois's and Bikram's, and many claimed this type of yoga had transformed their lives; however, proponents of Iyengar Yoga—whether in videos, classes, books, or in places such as *Yoga Journal*—had always emphasized its therapeutic value, how it might improve your flexibility, straighten your spine, help you relax, or strengthen your core muscles; that is, how it might heal your particular complaint. This feature is particularly evident in the workshops American Iyengar teachers routinely offer. If you're so inclined, you might sign up for the intensive course "Hip Joint Agility," "Asanas for Emotional Stability," or "Yoga for Scoliosis."[26]

In contrast, both Bikram and Jois presented their versions of yoga as an unvarying whole, not to be tailored to the particulars of an individual or illness. You had to adapt to it, not adapt it to you.[27]

This then marked a sort of healing of yoga, and, you could say, something truer to the Hatha Yoga tradition, for both Bikram and Jois expected a level of devotion far greater than most teachers at the Y had. Their demands might seem ludicrously modest—to practice almost every day for ninety minutes—and yet to make that simple commitment required a whole host of choices that almost invariably changed many aspects of your life.

The last time Hatha Yoga had insinuated itself this deeply into the lives of Americans was during the 1920s up at Clarkstown Country Club, and this had been among a comparatively small group.

But to most outsiders, this new religiosity was almost imperceptible. The press giddily reported not that yoga required new levels of sacrifice and piety but that yoga had become athletic.

In 1994, *U.S. News & World Report* declared, "Yoga Goes Mainstream." This almost exactly twenty years after *Time* had done the same.[28]

U.S. News was either decades late or premature, depending on how many people need to participate in any movement to qualify it as "mainstream."

What the magazine had picked up on was the waning of one fitness trend and the waxing of another.

New York City aerobics studios were closing faster than the peep shows in Times Square, and Jane Fonda had released yet another installment in her video series: *Jane Fonda's Yoga Workout*.[29]

Yoga had always been a word that defied easy explanation. No longer. When people talked about yoga, almost to a one, they were talking about Hatha Yoga, and only one or two limbs of Hatha Yoga—asana and pranayama. They were talking about exercise. No one mentioned "Oriental religion" much anymore or worried about their kids joining the Hare Krishnas.

Bikram had encouraged this view. He hadn't, for instance, made much of the subtle body until he began his teacher-training program in 1994. Then his wife and other lecturers began teaching the "subtle anatomy" and "chakra systems" along with "allopathic physical systems" such as the skeletal, muscular, and endocrine systems.

While Jois hewed more closely to traditional Hatha Yoga and its spiritual physics, he didn't explicitly mention the subtle body in his most thorough text, *Yoga Mala*. Instead, he liberally quoted from the *Hatha Yoga Pradipika* and the *Yoga-Yajnavalkya*, both of which detail the nadis and chakras and the mechanics—and necessity—of raising Kundalini for spiritual realization. His wasn't a secularized yoga, but it was easy enough to get this impression if you didn't have the stamina to learn Sanskrit or the wherewithal to make a trip to Mysore, where Jois would sometimes lecture about yoga theory in the evenings. Many of his American disciples were reserved when it came to yoga philosophy, parroting Jois himself, "99% practice, 1% theory!," which made it easy to overlook the complexity of his teachings.

Conventional wisdom had it that the boomers, who had burned out on aerobics, were now flocking to yoga because it was a kinder, gentler fitness regimen. ("As people age, they slow down and incorporate more practical routines into their lives," explained former aerobics star Kathy Smith, who released her own yoga video in 1994 as well.)[30]

Some anecdotal evidence suggested that injuries and even the stress of aerobics had soured some people on it. But this was only half the story.

The bigger story, and the one that would be repeated almost ad nauseam starting at this moment, was that yoga had become aerobic.[31]

In its 1994 trend piece, *U.S. News & World Report* noted, "A class in Urban or Power Yoga will really get your heart rate up." A number of yoga teachers and students as well as a cardiologist from Cedars-Sinai in Los Angeles helpfully testified to this. Of all the different types of yoga now available—for students of both Iyengar, Jois, and Bikram had taken their teachings and crafted a number of new derivatives—Ashtanga Yoga and its offshoots (Urban and Power Yoga, neither of which had been sanctioned by Jois himself) were considered the most aerobically demanding. "After thirty-five minutes of yoga," explained Richard Villella, who taught at Yoga Zone in Manhattan, "people are sweating like crazy."[32]

Two years later *Cosmopolitan* magazine recommended yoga as one of the ways to get off the treadmill and still "get a real workout." The health reporter Linda Dyett assuaged readers' fears: "For anyone who thinks yoga consists of chanting om while seated in the lotus position, sweat-inducing, butt kickin' Ashtanga yoga will come as a shock."[33]

By now the line had become a cliché, but it signified a fairly major development. In just a decade, Bikram and Jois had inadvertently helped yoga catch up to the Reagan era and its commitment to individual achievement, at any cost.

Other yoga teachers had also realized that to make yoga marketable, they'd have to make it tougher.

Mark Becker had even trademarked *Yogaerobics*. "One day I went running on the beach with some friends. I'd been doing two hours of deep breathing, but still that running made my lungs burn and left me tired," Becker, who had previously been known as Dharmamark, told *The New Yorker* in 1984. (The item about Yogaerobics appeared just below one on Robert Bly, headed "Wild Ones.") "And then it hit me! Yes, yoga is five thousand years old, but it *lacks cardiovascular activity*." By adding aerobics moves and music—"Michael Jackson is one of the highest beings on the planet"—Becker believed he had made up for yoga's fatal defect.[34]

Ashtanga Yoga accomplished the same thing without the corny sound track. When Jois and his student Ray Rosenthal put together a video in 1987, they called it *Astanga Yoga, an Aerobic Yoga System: Sequential Movement Synchronized with Breathing*. Shot on a windy day in Santa Cruz, California, the video was simple and unembellished, just a notch or two above a home video. However, watching Chuck Miller (no relation to Tim) and Rosenthal demonstrate the primary series under Jois's direction, there was no denying that Ashtanga Yoga required tremendous strength, agility, and stamina.[35]

Perhaps the most convincing evidence that yoga had toughened up was that so many men were practicing it, and any number of them were willing to step forward to testify to their involvement as if they had been touched by Jesus at a revival meeting.

Here's Mike Tharp reflecting on his first Bikram class on New Year's Day 1994: "By the time we had finished four postures and begun the 'standing-head-knee' pose, I was drenched in sweat. And I was scared— the way I used to be at the end of a three-hour basketball practice in college, just before we ran wind sprints. To do the 'standing-knee-head' pose properly, I would have to lace my fingers around one foot, extend that leg straight out in front of me while balancing on the other leg, knee locked, and touch forehead to knee for one minute. . . . Forget peaceful, this was *serious*."[36]

Jivamukti Yoga marked the apotheosis of this moment, when yoga became sweaty and religious again.

Founders Sharon Gannon, a gamine woman with long, glossy, dark hair, porcelain skin, and a delicate, pierced nose, and David Life, a lithe fellow who often wears a topknot and whose forearms are tattooed with snakes and Sanskrit script, crafted physically challenging Vinyasa classes, then grafted onto these a number of symbols, practices, and rituals they had learned from their gurus—Pattabhi Jois, Swami Nirmalananda (the Anarchist Swami), and Shri Brahmananda Sarasvati (also known as Yogi Mishra, who ran the Ananda Ashram).

They also drew much from people such as Ram Dass and Alan Watts and the green hair and piercings of the musicians and artists, punks and freaks, still flocking to New York's East Village, where Life ran an eponymous café.

In 1989, the pair opened their first yoga center, on Second Avenue and Ninth Street, not far from the Life Café. They painted the walls purple and turquoise, when most yoga studios were still austerely white. They put up pictures of deities, which they took to include Krishna and also Saint

Teresa of Avila and Glinda the Good Witch from *The Wizard of Oz*. They had students chant Om. And they played music—Bhagavan Das and also Van Morrison and Stevie Wonder.

As legend has it, Gannon and Life met with some seasoned yoga teachers as they were getting their school off the ground. The yoga veterans weren't supportive, insisting that to put up "pictures from India" or make any gesture that smacked of psychedelic hippies was to court bankruptcy. Recalled Gannon, "They warned us, above all, 'You can't talk about God.'"[37]

I've always thought of Sharon Gannon as Blanche De Vries's heir. She has a similar theatricality and artistry, a similar coquetry and strength. (Life, though, is no Pierre Bernard. As others have observed, he looks a lot like Iggy Pop.)[38]

Encouraged by their Indian gurus and discouraged by their American competitors, Gannon and Life pursued their vision even more avidly. They believed they were restoring an ancient scriptural tradition to modern yoga, and in so doing they might "bring spiritual substance into the Western lifestyle of shallow materiality."

Whether or not they achieved this part of their vision, by 1998 they had become wildly successful.

They moved their once small East Village center to nine thousand square feet of space above a Crunch gym on Lafayette Street, a location much more convenient to subways and offices.

According to *New York* magazine, Gannon and Life conceived of the new space as both the "biggest yoga studio in America" and "an interdisciplinary, interfaith gathering space." You could take classes in yoga or the *Bhagavad-Gita*, see a dance performance, or buy yoga T-shirts, pants, and tchotchkes.

A yearly membership cost twelve hundred dollars (more than most gyms at the time), and about four hundred people, most of whom were young and white, took classes there each day. As you waited in line to sign in, it wasn't unusual to see one of a number of celebrities—Sting, Sarah Jessica Parker, Mary Stuart Masterson, Willem Dafoe, or Christy Turlington—who had become regular students.[39]

One student, the writer Lynn Darling, referred to Jivamukti's expanded center as "that pink yuppie pleasure palace." The school was the real successor to the yoga institute that De Vries had run up on Fifty-third Street seven decades earlier.[40]

And something was similar about America in the late 1910s and early 1920s, when it shook off the horrors of the First World War and wealth momentarily exploded, along with a culture of decadence, and this moment, when the Internet dematerialized our economy, the wars fought— Bosnia, Somalia, Rwanda—were relatively small and not our own, and we were, as a nation, far more preoccupied with our president's sexual peccadilloes than any number of real and pressing injustices.

De Vries's blend of artistry and asceticism had been surprisingly profitable. So too was Jivamukti. In merging overt spirituality, the chanting, the deities, and the sacred music, with vigorous asana classes, Gannon and Life had created a multimillion-dollar business.

This wasn't all, though. Twenty years after the Beatles' misadventure in Rishikesh, yoga was influencing pop culture again.

In 1998, Madonna, whose music had been a staple of aerobics classes, released her album *Ray of Light*. (She also turned forty.)

The album included several Sanskrit chants and an entire song called "Shanti Ashtangi," based on the prayer that Pattabhi Jois and his students recite at the beginning of each class.[41]

"Yoga has changed my outlook on life," said Madonna. She had started practicing yoga during her first pregnancy. After she gave birth, she began studying Jois's Ashtanga Yoga in Los Angeles.[42]

Though Madonna had become a fitness icon, even she found this type of yoga challenging. "I had this notion that it was going to be easy," she explained, "but it wasn't. And I also got really infuriated with my teacher because she would only teach me a little bit every time. That was a huge lesson for me. I'd only get to learn the sun salutes, then the next day I could only learn one position."[43]

The "Material Girl," now semi-incarnate, had become, as *Entertainment Weekly* put it, the "Ethereal Girl," which proved just as savvy a career move as her invocation of her Roman Catholic upbringing had been. *Ray of Light* received three Grammys and within two years went quadruple platinum (that's 4 million CDs sold).

As more than a few pointed out, Madonna's album was "unbearably trend-conscious," rather than trendsetting. But pioneers rarely popularize anything; Madonna, like the Beatles, who arrived in India years after

Ginsberg and Leary had made their own pilgrimages, set off a tsunami of acculturation.[44]

By the new millennium yoga—namely this reinvigorated Hatha Yoga—was not just mainstream, it was inescapable. Almost all at once, the advertising industry began to exploit the symbolic potential of the discipline. A Hyundai ad featured a limber yogini in several familiar poses (tag line: "Suggested daily routine for achieving inner peace"). Tylenol, Kellogg's, Oil of Olay, Absolut, and Hormel, among countless other companies, inserted people, mostly beautiful young women, in yoga postures into their print campaigns or commercials.

Yoga no longer connoted a life of privation and discipline. It conveyed leisure and control. It sparked our most primal desires—for beauty, for youth, for wealth. In so doing, the marketers believed, it would compel us to buy things we didn't need.

This was a genuinely novel development. In the past, Hatha Yoga teachers had worked hard to link yoga to celebrities and trends in health and fitness. The onus had been on them to sell yoga to a wary public. Now marketers were using yoga to sell other goods.

Of course, Hatha Yoga and its more traditionally minded proponents hold that raising Kundalini is the only route to genuine happiness, and if taken seriously, this notion undercuts the very idea of consumerism.

Such details were irrelevant since Americans had, in about a century, turned this esoteric spiritual discipline into a robust industry. By 2002, between 15 and 18 million Americans practiced yoga, up from 6 million in 1994, and a feature writer for *Yoga Journal* estimated that this represented roughly $27 billion in revenue. While that was certainly an inflated figure (the writer assumed that everyone who practiced spent over one thousand dollars per year on yoga-related goods and services), no one doubted that the discipline, in aggregate, had become big business, or that the Americans who took yoga classes had ample disposable income, which not even the post-9/11 recession had imperiled.[45]

All of which was perfect fodder for the parodists.

In a 2002 *New Yorker* cartoon, two women are sitting in lotus position on yoga mats. The caption reads, "I just found an Eastern philosophy that's very accepting of S.U.V.s."[46]

•

Over this same period, the swamis and their organizations had changed quite a bit too. While Hatha Yoga became more religious, these organizations became less so. They had to or risk total collapse.

Much like the Catholic Church, at the upper levels movements such as ISKCON and Muktananda's organization, now known as the Siddha Yoga Dham of America Foundation, or simply SYDA, were, by all accounts, hermetically sealed, authoritarian, dysfunctional, and corrupt. Yet, to the broader public, the local ISKCON or Siddha Yoga centers were like spiritual oases, unsullied by the machinations above. You could dip your toe in, wade into them, or even dive in for a time. But you need not partake of the organizational ideology.

SYDA in particular weathered more than its share of bad press and internal dissent. Having revolved around Muktananda and his famous ability to awaken Kundalini, it was hard to fathom how it would survive his death and the allegations of sexual misconduct.

The secret of SYDA's success was that most of Muktananda's devotees had not, as Kempton had, given up their day jobs and moved to his ashram. Most had kept their lives more or less intact and visited their local Siddha Yoga center on weekends. And if they did make their way to the South Fallsburg ashram, it would be an occasional event, say for a week of *sevā* (selfless service) or a brief retreat.

Muktananda's most ardent disciples, people such as Kempton, formed a sort of molten core of energy. They threw themselves into their tasks, whether this was cooking a meal or fielding press queries. They kept everything humming, and in the organization's earliest days, they worked for free. (Disciples even had to pay a modest fee, which covered room and board, to live at the ashram.)[47]

But in the decade between Muktananda's death and *U.S. News & World Report*'s pronouncement about yoga, much had changed. Besides the unsavory allegations by former disciples, there was a growing rift in SYDA leadership. By 1985, Muktananda's cosuccessors, Gurumayi Chidvilasananda and her younger brother, Swami Nitayananda, had messily parted ways.

For a while, these events were known only to insiders and those in their extended circle. Then, in her 1994 *New Yorker* piece "O Guru, Guru, Guru," Lis Harris confirmed much of what had been reported in *CoEvolution Quarterly* (although at least one of the women who had been involved told Harris that Muktananda's attentions had been a gift of grace that "had nothing to do with sex") and detailed the succession battle, which had at one point turned violent and was still boiling nearly a decade later. Harris also discovered that people who left SYDA continued to feel threatened. One ex-swami told her, "I left [in 1987] because of the growing stultifying atmosphere of fear, of informers, of public confessions and Big Brotherness." SYDA and its leadership were badly compromised.[48]

In response, the organization professionalized. Managers took over many of Muktananda's functions, and the Programming Department began to run SYDA's religious and outreach programs. Over time, public events became highly scripted. The SYDA leadership, based in South Fallsburg, also began to dictate even more aspects of daily operations at both the main ashram in South Fallsburg and local Siddha Yoga centers around the country.

Margaret Parkinson, an ex-devotee, recalls, "The appearance of the [South Fallsburg] center became more 'yuppie,' and a great deal of emphasis was placed on the style of dress worn at programs. Women were supposed to wear skirts and men were to wear shirts and ties." Once a woman wearing a sari told Parkinson that her embroidered skirt was "too ethnic" to wear there.

According to Parkinson, SYDA officialdom also began to stress the paid courses and intensives as well as selling items in the bookstores.[49]

Harris witnessed much of this firsthand. Gurumayi presided over events like the queen. She attended the last day of a yajna (fire ceremony) held in commemoration of Muktananda's death. As acolytes garlanded sixteen priests who had been flown in from India to conduct the weeklong ritual, Gurumayi sat some ways away. You could see her, and later you might shuffle past her and receive a quick tap from her peacock-feather wand, but she remained a distant figure.

Perhaps more tellingly, she, or at least her organization, wouldn't let Harris have a single conversation unobserved. Instead, any number of handlers, usually Kathy Nash, the SYDA spokesperson, who had been a news anchor for a Monterey, California, TV station, trailed Harris, recording her every exchange.

The effect might be chilling for a reporter, but for a weekend visitor SYDA still had much to offer.

The South Fallsburg ashram encompassed three rehabilitated prewar hotels and manicured grounds. Devotees could come for weekend intensives, where they'd chant in large, carpeted halls or sometimes even under the stars, take Hatha Yoga classes, eat vegetarian food, and enjoy the broad lawns and peace and quiet. Or you could do a weeklong retreat at a local Siddha Yoga center (in Boston, say, or Oakland).

Moreover, professionalization had proved highly lucrative. In 1989, the *bookstore* of Muktananda's South Fallsburg ashram had grossed well over $4 million! Five years later, a weekend intensive cost four hundred dollars; thousands would attend.[50]

SYDA's other assets were substantial as well. The estimated market value of its Catskills complex was between $15 and $17 million.[51]

SYDA's success was a little paradoxical. Its leaders weren't particularly attuned to broader cultural forces—the aging baby boomers, the first Iraq War, the Internet boom and its sybaritic rituals. Instead, most of the changes made between Muktananda's death and the turn of the century were the result of internal power struggles, dissenting devotees, and the financial exigencies of running a sprawling physical center.

Such changes alienated Parkinson. Even Kempton felt it was time to move on (with Gurumayi's blessing, she disrobed and officially left the organization in 2002). However, SYDA was still good at catering to the loosely affiliated, the weekenders, and casual seekers.[52]

Similar dynamics were at work in ISKCON. Almost as soon as Prabhupada passed away, ISKCON had to defend itself against serious and, in its case, substantiated charges of wrongdoing.

The organization was divided among eleven gurus, the Governing Body Commission, each of whom had authority over a different region. Many of these gurus ruled more like autocrats than enlightened leaders, and ISKCON couldn't keep their failures out of the press.

In the late 1970s, two dissident ISKCON members were murdered; in 1980, police discovered a cache of (legal) weapons at a northern-California ISKCON ranch and a garage full of ammunition and bullet-making equipment in the Bay Area; a few years later, rumors that Prabhupada had been poisoned were reinvigorated; and by the end of the decade, allegations that children had been physically and sexually abused at ISKCON gurukulas (boarding schools) began to surface. (ISKCON confirmed many of these charges in 1998.)[53]

To counter the continued onslaught of bad press and legal actions, ISKCON created a professional PR department, headed by one of Prabhupada's early devotees, which put out a newspaper (*The World Review*) and tried to steer reporters to its version of events. Like PR departments everywhere, ISKCON's routinely downplayed unsavory facts.[54]

The organization also reached out to scholars and, more successfully, diaspora Indians living in America. It fashioned itself a local temple for expatriate Hindus, who would come on Sundays, holy days, and special occasions to chant and sing and feast on vegetarian food.[55]

In 2002, just two years after a Dallas attorney sued ISKCON for $400 million on behalf of hundreds of children who claimed to have been sexually abused at the boarding schools, the Hindu community was flocking to a new center in Chandler, a suburb southeast of Phoenix. "There was no room to stand during the arathi [services]," Bhakta Raj Das, the center's director, told the *Los Angeles Times*. Apparently, the center drew Hindus from as far away as Flagstaff, and nearly two hundred people, a mix of Americans and diaspora Indians, regularly attended Sunday meditation services.[56]

A Portland, Oregon, ISKCON center had this same festive quality, seemingly untouched by any of the organization's turmoil, legal troubles, and criminality. A reporter described the scene: "In a quiet corner of Southeast Portland, just two blocks from a Dairy Queen . . . the Hare Krishnas are chanting. They rock back and forth, saying Krishna's name." If you happened to walk by the ISKCON temple, he went on, "you might hear the soft cling of finger cymbals or the beat of a drum. You might smell the drifting sticky-sweet incense or hear the incantations." The reporter also noted a mix of Indians (one came for a "little slice of his homeland") and Americans, all of whom seemed cheerful and hopeful, especially after the free feast.[57]

Over thirty years or so, ISKCON centers had become more churchlike. They were quiet during the week and bustling with activity on the weekends. They didn't require too much of their devotees, and they performed a social function as much as a religious one; they were places to commune with others regardless of the depth of your own convictions or the consistency of your own practice. Conversions such as Kempton's or Zweig's began to seem almost anachronistic, another relic of the 1970s.

At the same time, Hatha Yoga studios around the country became more like roadside Hindu temples, with devotees shuffling in, slipping off their shoes, and making their daily prostrations.

This reversal says a lot about Americans. We could tolerate worshipping foreign gods, up to a point. We could accept intense religiosity as long as it was directed at something concrete and universal: our bodies. It was easy enough to forget that these two modes, chanting of "Om Namah Shivaya" at a Siddha Yoga center or, say, practicing the primary series in an Ashtanga Yoga studio were designed to effect the same thing—what Muktananda described as "sublime intoxication, inner rapture," and what Jois called the dissolution of the mind into "the Supreme Self whose nature is bliss."[58]

On May 18, 2009, Sri K. Pattabhi Jois died in Mysore, India. A month later, a memorial service was held in New York City at Donna Karan's Urban Zen Center on Greenwich Street, nine thousand miles away. Four hundred people came that cool evening; they came on bikes, on foot, by subway, and by town car. They streamed through doors that had been pulled open wide and mounted a few broad, whitewashed steps. Before entering, most paused in front of a white wall decorated with a single, black-and-white photograph of Jois, taken near the end of his life. In it, he wears a white linen cloth wrapped skirtlike around his waist, the sacred thread of the Brahman, and, around his neck, a string of rudraksha beads. Three white stripes, which mark his devotion to Shiva, encircle his forearms, and the design is repeated on his biceps and forehead.

After putting your shoes in a cubby, you found yourself in a large, open space filled to capacity. You had to thread your way through the crowd to find a spot on the concrete floor where you could sit, cross-legged or on your shins, like everyone else. Slide projectors cast pictures of Jois with his family, among his students, and on various tours onto every wall. To the right of the stage, a garlanded close-up of Jois stared out from above vases of flowers and neat rows of candles. Ocher scrims hanging from the rafters floated in the late-spring breeze.[59]

Early on, Eddie Stern, a longtime student of Jois's, the master of ceremonies, and one of the event's organizers, called out the names of about ten yoga teachers—Dharma Mittra, James Murphy, Carlos Menjiva, and Hari Kaur Khalsa among them—and handed each a small gift. (The organizers had invited Bikram, who sent a note with good wishes in his stead.) Each represented a different lineage of yoga: Mittra is a disciple of Yogi Gupta (also known as Swami Kailashananda), and Murphy, of B.K.S. Iyengar; Menjiva represented Jivamukti Yoga, and Hari Kaur Khalsa, Golden Bridge (Kundalini) Yoga. The event was one of the most ecumenical yoga gatherings you'd be liable to find, outside of a *Yoga Journal* conference.⁶⁰

Jois, though, had drawn us here; Jois had helped resuscitate yoga in America. "When a great person is born into the world, he affects everyone," remarked Stern, "regardless of whether they follow his teachings or not."⁶¹

Despite the gravity of the event, the atmosphere was festive, as if we had gathered for an elaborate and somewhat overdone birthday party. Many of the women wore dresses or delicate blouses and skirts. A few wore saris. Many of the men had put on dress shirts. New students and longtime devotees had come to pay homage. There were teenagers, mothers, fathers, and grandparents. But the attendees were almost to a one slim and fit-looking, and a disproportionate number were strikingly beautiful.

When a handful of Jois's most dedicated students paraded onto the stage to share their memories, most related humorous anecdotes—Jois wouldn't let one woman forget the only time she had missed his birthday party in Mysore (she had a good excuse: she was getting married); another was so eager for credentials, she demanded a special seal. Jois complied, but she later realized the joke was on her: he had used an ordinary and meaningless rubber stamp.

Throughout the reminiscences, a line snaked from the far right side of the space behind the stage to a dim anteroom, lit only by looping videos of Jois teaching. Here, several Hare Krishnas were serving steaming plates of samosas, curried chickpeas, rice, and spanakopita. They didn't say much. But they smiled a lot as they handed out paper plates heaped high.

If anything of significance can be drawn from this single event, it's this: Americans have made some sort of peace with yoga in almost all of its permutations.

This acceptance is in some ways merely a symptom of broader forces. After all, we recently elected a black president who admitted he inhaled when he experimented with marijuana.

And more than 2.7 million Indian nationals are now living in the United States.⁶²

The discipline has got a further boost from the medical community. Over the past few decades, studies have shown that Hatha Yoga helps reduce the severity and frequency of asthma attacks, depression, and anxiety, and that regular practice aids in weight loss and can (along with changes in your diet) reverse heart disease.[63]

Meanwhile, in addition to flattening the world geographically, the Internet has flattened it *temporally*. Every moment of history that has been recorded is now (or will soon be) immediately and almost eternally available. You can watch a clip of Swami Muktananda from his first U.S. tour in 1970 or one of the Beatles in Rishikesh in 1968 or even grainy footage of Sri Krishnamacharya practicing yoga in India in 1938 as easily as you can watch Stephen Colbert's most recent interview.

Being so readily available, these moments seem less exotic, less subversive. This is exactly what proponents of yoga—from Vivekananda to Bikram, from Swami Satchidananda to Judith Lasater—would have you believe. They've spent the last century and a half convincing us that this ancient, Indic, and half-tamed spiritual discipline doesn't contravene our most sacred beliefs. They may actually be wrong on this point. It's hard to reconcile the subtle body and the possibility of experiencing divinity for yourself by methodically following a program of exercise, breathing, and meditation with Judeo-Christian notions of God and the afterlife, but we seem willing to ignore the discontinuities.

Maybe it's a sign of maturity that we can tolerate the paradox: yoga is both an indulgence and a penance. It will tone your thighs, and it might crack open your reality.

The morning after Jois's memorial many of us will see each other again. It's a strange intimacy because it's forged in near silence. We'll march up a set of maroon stairs, put our shoes in a different cubbyhole, strip out of our street clothes, and unroll our mats, our rubber prayer rugs, in a room painted bubble-gum pink. At first the room will feel chilled; the radiators have been off for months but it has been a cold, rainy spring. Bare feet planted together, facing a Ganesha shrine—the elephant-headed god is said to remove all obstacles—we'll put our hands together and chant, "Vande Gurunam charanaravinde / Sandarshita svatmasukhavabodhe" (I worship the guru's lotus feet / Awakening the happiness of the Self revealed). Then the unity will dissolve. Some will practice for ninety minutes, others only forty-five. Some will jump back into Chaturanga Dandasana (which looks like a modified push-up) between every pose, others will step daintily into this position. A few will manage such feats of strength—curling their lotus-bound legs up into their armpits and then into a full handstand—that you feel compelled to pause and discreetly watch. The room will get hot. After an hour or so, a whole row of people will be lying flat on their backs near the doorway; by the time you finish your practice and join them, your thin rubber mat feels like the softest mattress, and the clanking of garbage trucks, the squeal of buses braking, and the hum of a distant jackhammer make the sweetest of lullabies. As the city wakes up, the street sounds and the deep, noisy breathing of the next batch of yoga students will rock us to sleep, if only for a little while.[64]

NOTES

SELECTED BIBLIOGRAPHY

ACKNOWLEDGMENTS

INDEX

NOTES

ABBREVIATIONS

BANC MSS 2005/161z	Theos Bernard Papers, BANC MSS 2005/161z, Bancroft Library, University of California, Berkeley
Bull Curtis Papers	Sara Bull Papers, 1830–1910; Brinkler Library, Cambridge Historical Society, Cambridge, Massachusetts
HSRC	Bernard Collection, Historical Society of Rockland County, New City, NY
HYP	*Hatha Yoga Pradīpikā*
LJ MS	Llellwyn (Cheerie) Jackson Manuscript at HSCU
Swanson Papers UTA	Gloria Swanson Papers (TXRC93-A8), Harry Ransom Humanities Research Center, University of Texas at Austin
TCB	Theos Casimir Bernard
VWB	Viola Wertheim Bernard
VWB Papers, HSCU	Viola Wertheim Bernard Papers, 1918–2000, Archives and Special Collections, A.C. Long Health Sciences Library, Columbia University
VWB tr.	Viola Wertheim Bernard, transcripts of taped interviews at HSCU
Wilson-McAdoo Collection UCSB	Wilson-McAdoo Collection, Bernath MSS 18, Department of Special Collections, University Libraries, University of California, Santa Barbara
Wilson-McAdoo Papers LOC	Eleanor Randolph Wilson McAdoo/Margaret Woodrow Wilson Papers, Manuscript Division, Library of Congress, Washington, D.C.

INTRODUCTION

1. Official 2009 White House Easter Egg Roll page, www.whitehouse.gov/easteregg roll/ (accessed July 17, 2009).
2. Transcript, "The Obamas' Remarks at the Easter Egg Roll," *New York Times*, April 13, 2009, www.nytimes.com/2009/04/13/us/politics/13eggroll-text.html (accessed July 6, 2009).

3. Michelle Legro interview with Leah Cullis of Zuda Yoga, June 23, 2009.
4. The quote is from Christina Bellantoni and the item appeared in Lynn Sweet, "White House Easter Egg Roll Preview," *Chicago Sun-Times*, April 12, 2009, blogs.suntimes.com/sweet/2009/04/white_house_easter_egg_roll_pr.html (accessed July 7, 2009).
5. *HYP*, 4:2; *Gherand Samhitā*, 7:1–23.
6. Some consider the sūkṣma-śarīra identical to the prâna-maya-kosha, mano-maya-kosha, and vijnâna-maya-kosha, three of the five sheaths that make up the body according to Vedanta. Georg Feuerstein, *The Yoga Tradition: Its History, Literature, and Practice* (Prescott, AZ: Hohm Press, 1998, 2001), 132.
7. *Woodstock: Three Days of Peace and Music (Director's Cut)*, directed by Michael Wadleigh (Warner Bros., 1994).
8. Spiros Antonopoulos, e-mail correspondence, July 6, 2009.
9. William Ward, *A View of the History, Literature, and Mythology of the Hindoos*, 3rd ed. (London: Black, Parbury, and Allen, 1817), 1:viii–x.

1. BRAHMA?

1. Ellery Sedgwick, *The Atlantic Monthly, 1857–1909: Yankee Humanism at High Tide and Ebb* (Amherst: University of Massachusetts Press, 1994), 35. Sedgwick, a descendant of the *Atlantic*'s eighth editor, has lucidly laid out the early days of the magazine, and I have relied heavily, though not exclusively, on his account in my brief recapitulation here and elsewhere in chapter 1. See also *American Renaissance Literary Report (ARLR)*, ed. Kenneth Walter Cameron (Hartford: Transcendental Books, 1988), 2:166, for the timing of the distribution of *Atlantic* 1, no. 1.
2. Sedgwick, *Atlantic*, 36.
3. Ibid., 29–35.
4. Moreover, the distinction between the two words used was often both subtle and unique to each translator. In his three-volume work on Hindu mythology and culture, for example, William Ward renders the Absolute as Brŭhmŭ, and the creator deity as Brŭhma; while, in his translation of the *Bhagavad-Gita*, Charles Wilkins spells them *Brăhm* and *Brăhmā*, respectively. In part, these variations reflect Sanskrit grammar. William Ward, *A View of the History, Literature, and Mythology of the Hindoos*, 3rd ed. (London: Black, Parbury, and Allen, 1817), 1:iii, 1:xvii; *The Bhagavat-Geeta* (1785), trans., with notes by, Charles Wilkins, a facsimile reproduction with an introduction by George Hendrick (Delmar, NY: Scholars' Facsimiles & Reprints, 1959, 1972), 43, 45, 94. See also H. T. Colebrooke, *Essays on the Religion and Philosophy of the Hindus* (London and Paris: Williams and Norgate, 1858), 29, 32. The contemporary definitions come from Georg Feuerstein, *The Shambhala Encyclopedia of Yoga* (Boston and London: Shambhala, 2000), 61–62.
5. *New York Times*, November 12, 1857, 4, col. 6; Kenneth Walter Cameron, "Emerson's 'Brahma': Early Explications and Commentary," *ARLR*, 2:197–223.
6. Some of these actually tickled Emerson; according to his son, Emerson "never failed to be completely overcome with laughter" when he heard the first lines of one that began, "If the grey tom-cat thinks he sings, / Or if the song think it be sung, / He little knows who boot-jacks flings / How many bricks at him I've flung." Robert D. Richardson, Jr., *Emerson: The Mind on Fire* (Berkeley: University of California Press, 1995), 523.

7. Ibid., 418–19, 524.

8. Ibid., 530.

9. Apparently quartos of Jones's work were "so splendid and ponderous" that the editors believed no more than a few editions existed in the whole country. *Monthly Anthology and Boston Review* 2 (July 1805): 360; Kenneth Walter Cameron, *Indian Superstition: A Dissertation on Emerson's Orientalism at Harvard* (Hanover, NH: The Friends of Dartmouth Library, 1954), 15. Robert Love's article "Fear of Yoga" also mentions the Reverend William Emerson's translation, referring to this text as a "scripture." *Columbia Journalism Review*, November/December 2006, 81.

10. Shanta Acharya, *The Influence of Indian Thought on Ralph Waldo Emerson*, Studies in American Literature 38 (Lewiston, Queenston, and Lampeter: The Edwin Mellen Press, 2001), 51–52.

11. The Reverend William Ward was one of the first to address the topic, and he visibly grapples with his own impulse to explain "Hindoo Religion" as a single system and the impossibility of doing so; hence his first footnote, which complicates the relation of matter to spirit, is about four times the length of his explanation of "Hindoo theology." Ward, *View of the History*, vol. 1, a.

12. Richard King, *Orientalism and Religion: Postcolonial Theory, India, and "The Mystic East"* (London and New York: Routledge, 1999), 67–69, 82–90.

13. *Two Brahmin Sources of Emerson and Thoreau*, ed., with an introduction by, William Bysshe Stein (Gainesville, FL: Scholar's Fascmiles and Reprints, 1967), xv.

14. Ward, *View of the History*, vii–x.

15. Richardson, *Emerson*, 23–25.

16. Arthur Christy, *The Orient in American Transcendentalism: A Study of Emerson, Thoreau, and Alcott* (New York: Columbia University Press, 1932), 65–66.

17. *Sacotalá; or, The Fatal Ring: An Indian Drama*, by Cálidás, translated from the original Sanscrit and Pracrit by Sir William Jones (1789), online version prepared by FWP, January 2004, www.columbia.edu/itc/mealac/pritchett/00litlinks/shakuntala_jones/00_preface.htm (accessed April 23, 2009).

    In his seminal essay *India and Europe*, Wilhelm Halbfass contends Wilkins, along with William Jones and H. T. Colebrooke, pioneered "a tradition of exploring Indian thought in its original sources and contexts of understanding," which "led to the establishment and institutionalization of a research tradition—the tradition of modern Indology. W. Jones's founding of the Asiatic Society of Bengal in 1784 is exemplary in this respect and points in the direction which later developments were to take." *India and Europe: An Essay in Understanding* (Albany: State University of New York Press, 1988), 62.

    Edward W. Said, *Orientalism* (New York: Vintage Books, 1979, 2003), is the ur-text of postcolonial theory. However, for those interested in India specifically, King's *Orientalism and Religion* is essential reading, see pages 88–89.

18. Christy, *Orient in American Transcendentalism*, 70, 283–84; see also Cameron, *Indian Superstition*, 16, 20–21.

19. Barbara Stoler Miller offers one of the most succinct explications of "Hinduism": It is "not based on the teachings of a founder, such as Buddha, Christ, or Muhammed. [Hinduism] has evolved over centuries through the continual interplay of diverse religious beliefs and practice: popular local cultures; orthodox tradition, including the ancient Vedic hymns, the ritual texts of the Brahmans, and the mystical Upanishads; as well as heterodox challenges from Buddhist and Jain ideas and institu-

tions. Even the word *Hindu* is a foreign idea, used by Arab invaders in the eighth century A.D. to refer to the customs and beliefs of people who worshipped sectarian gods such as Vishnu and Shiva." Barbara Stoler Miller, introduction and translation, *The Bhagavad-Gita: Krishna's Counsel in Time of War* (New York: Columbia University Press, 1986), 2.

20. King, *Orientalism and Religion*, 100, 121; Stein, *Two Brahmin Sources*, 2, 4–6; J. N. Farquhar, *Modern Religious Movements in India* (Delhi: Munshiram Manoharlal, Oriental Publishers and Booksellers, 1915, 1967), 32–34.

21. Ward, *View of the History*, 1:vii–xiii.

22. Stein, *Two Brahmin Sources*, 102.

23. Ibid., 75. See Patrick Olivelle for a corrective to Roy's reductionism. He argues the *Upanishads* do *not* express a single philosophy or even theology, and that even though the equation between Ātman, the essential I, and Brahman, the ultimate real, is at the crux of Advaita Vedanta and played a significant role in later developments of Indian theology, "it is incorrect to think that the single aim of all the Upaniṣads is to enunciate this simple truth."

Olivelle notes that the *Upanishads* "came to be considered the section of the Veda containing salvific knowledge . . . whereas the other sections contained information about rites . . . As the revealed source of knowledge, therefore, the Upaniṣads became the basic scriptural authority for most later Indian theological traditions." Patrick Olivelle, introduction and translation, *Upaniṣads* (Oxford, UK: Oxford University Press, 1996), xxxiii, lvi.

24. *Journals of Ralph Waldo Emerson with Annotations*, ed. E. W. Emerson and W. E. Forbes (Boston and New York: Houghton Mifflin, 1909–14), 1:157, cited in Christy, *Orient in American Transcendentalism*, 69; William Jones, "A Hymn to Narayena," from *The Works of Sir William Jones* (Published by, printed for, J. Stockdale and J. Walker, 1807), v. 13. Original from Harvard University, digitized September 6, 2007.

25. Lawrence Buell, *Emerson* (Cambridge, MA: Belknap Press of Harvard University Press, 2003), 165.

26. *Who Was Who in America: Historical Volume, 1607–1896* (Chicago: The A. N. Marquis Company, 1963), 278, 410; *The Harvard Graduates' Magazine* (Boston: The Harvard Graduates' Magazine Association) 8, no. 29 (1899, 1900): 393.

27. Alexis de Tocqueville, *Democracy in America*, trans. Henry Reeve (New York: D. Appleton and Company, 1904), 2:594; John Pickering, "Address at the First Annual Meeting," *Journal of the American Oriental Society* 1, no. 1 (1843): 5–6, 48.

28. Pickering, "Address," 47–53. By 1842, Pickering's *On the Adoption of a Uniform Orthography for the Indian Languages of North America* had earned him a reputation abroad, and his 1815 compendium of Americanisms has fixed him in American literary history. Ward and Trent et al., *The Cambridge History of English and American Literature* (New York: G. P. Putnam's Sons, 1907–21; New York: Bartleby.com, 2000), www.bartleby.com/cambridge/ (accessed September 28, 2009).

29. Carl T. Jackson, *The Oriental Religions and American Thought: Nineteenth Century Explorations* (Westport, CT: Greenwood Press, 1981), 180–84. In this, the Americans were following the German model, which focused intently on philology and translation, at the expense of ethnography.

30. Ibid.

31. Emerson read Thomas Colebrooke's translation of the *Sánkhya Káriká*. Richardson, *Emerson*, 335. Lawrence Buell, *Emerson* (Cambridge, MA, and London, England: Belknap Press of Harvard University Press, 2003), 172; Rick Fields, *How the Swans Came to the Lake: A Narrative History of Buddhism in America* (Boston and London: Shambhala, 1992), 61.

32. Christy, *Orient in American Transcendentalism*, 290. Richardson believes this moment arrived in the mid-1850s (*Emerson*, 522). However, you can see the effect these books had on Emerson's thinking in his chapter on Plato in *Representative Men*, which was published in 1850 and presumably written in the late 1840s. That essay includes several florid paragraphs about the idea of Unity. "Friend and foe are of one stuff; the ploughman, the plough, and the furrow, are of one stuff; and the stuff is such, and so much, that the variations of form are unimportant," he says, and then quotes the *Bhagavad-Gita* at length. Ralph Waldo Emerson, *The Works of Ralph Waldo Emerson* (New York: The Caxton Society, 1900), 4:43–44.

33. Quoted in Christy, *Orient in American Transcendentalism*, 387, from David Lee Maulsby, *The Contribution of Emerson to Literature* (Ph.D. diss., Medford, MA: Tufts College Press, 1911; digitized March 6, 2008), 122–23.

34. George Hendrick, introduction, *Bhagavat-Geeta*, trans. Charles Wilkins, vi.

35. Georg Feuerstein, *The Yoga Tradition: Its History, Literature, Philosophy, and Practice* (Prescott, AZ: Hohm Press, 1998, 2001), 188.

36. Ibid. These may have been interpolated later, but nonetheless are accurate descriptions of the *Gita*'s contents. See for example *Śrīmad Bhagavad Gíta: The Scripture of Mankind*, trans. Swami Tapasyananda (Mylapore, Madras: Sri Ramakrishna Math, 1984), 34.

37. A brief description of yoga is in the *Katha Upanishad*, which Roy rendered this way: "That part of life wherein the power of the five external senses and the mind are directed towards the Supreme Spirit, and the intellectual power ceases its action, is said to be most sacred; and this steady control of the senses and mind is considered to be *Yog* (or withdrawing the senses and the mind from worldly objects)." Rammohun Roy, *Translation of Several Principal Books, Passages, and Texts of the Veds, and of Some Controversial Works on Brahmunical Theology* (London, 1832), reprinted in Stein, *Two Brahmin Sources*, 78.

38. Wilkins, *Bhagavat-Geeta*, 67.

39. Ibid., 138.

40. Acharya, *Influence of Indian Thought*, 179; Wilkins, *Bhagavat-Geeta*, 36, 80, 100.

41. Ralph Waldo Emerson, *The Journals and Miscellaneous Notebooks of Ralph Waldo Emerson*, ed. Ralph H. Orth and Alfred R. Ferguson (Cambridge, MA: Belknap Press, 1971), 354. The brackets and arrows reflect Emerson's edits to these lines.

42. *The Journals and Miscellaneous Notebooks of Ralph Waldo Emerson*, ed. Susan Sutton Smith and Harrison Hayford (Cambridge, MA, and London, England: Belknap Press of Harvard University Press, 1978), 14:101–6.

43. Ronald A. Bosco, introduction to "Notebook Orientalist," *Topical Notebooks of Ralph Waldo Emerson*, ed. Ronald A. Bosco (Columbia and London: University of Missouri Press, 1993), 37. Ralph H. Orth, general introduction, *Topical Notebooks of Ralph Waldo Emerson*, 2:1.

44. Bosco, *Topical Notebooks of Ralph Waldo Emerson*, 135, 138.

45. Sedgwick, *Atlantic*, 29–30.

46. Phillips later wrote to his niece of the dinner, "Leaving myself and 'literary man' out of the group, I think you will agree with me that it would be difficult to duplicate that number of such conceded scholarship in the whole country besides." Ibid., 30–31.

47. Ibid., 31, 34.

48. Frank Luther Mott, *A History of American Magazines 1850–1865* (Cambridge, MA: Harvard University Press, 1938), 495.

49. He also called Whitman's masterpiece "the best piece of American Buddhism that anyone has had the strength to write, American to the bone." Richardson, *Emerson*, 527.

50. Ibid., 193; Frederic Ives Carpenter, *Emerson and Asia* (1930; repr., New York: Haskell House Publishers Ltd., 1968), 30.

51. "Every piece must have something sterling, some record of real experiences," Emerson wrote of the nascent magazine, looking forward to the day when a discerning minority of readers discovered "the Book is right." In Emerson's fantasy, these discriminating Americans would then "abandon themselves to this direction, too happy that they have got something good and wise to admire and obey." Sedgwick, *Atlantic*, 27.

52. By the third issue, even *The New York Times* was won over. "The *Atlantic* has now made its third voyage, and it brings us a richer freight than it ever has done before; its literary forces have been organized, and we begin to perceive what they are capable of doing, and how they mean to do it." "New Books," *New York Times* (1857–current file), January 1, 1858, ProQuest Historical Newspapers, *New York Times* (1851–2005), 2. Below the Mason-Dixon Line, however, the monthly's politics put off readers, as was to be expected. In the view of the *Southern Literary Messenger*, the *Atlantic* was nothing less than "a systematic defamation of everything Southern." Sedgwick, *Atlantic*, 39–42.

53. Of the more than two dozen parodies written shortly after the poem's publication, two of the most popular and often reprinted were "Bacchus" ("If the red drinker thinks he drinks / Or if the drunk thinks he is drunk") and "Damn Ah!" (Iffe ye gray Tomme catte thynkes he synggs / Or iffe ye songe thynkes itto be sunge"). *ARLR* 2:173, 185.

54. "Tell them," he said, "to say 'Jehovah' instead of 'Brahma' and they will not feel any perplexity." Ralph Waldo Emerson, *The Complete Works of Ralph Waldo Emerson* (Boston and New York: Houghton Mifflin Company, 1903–1904), 9:467, cited in Paramahansa Yogananda, *Autobiography of a Yogi* (Los Angeles: Self-Realization Fellowship, 1946, 1998), 32n.

55. James Russell Lowell, review of Emerson's "Conduct of Life," *Atlantic Monthly* 7, no. 40 (February 1861), reprinted in *ARLR*, 2:202.

56. In a sense, the *Gita* can be read as "a call to active life to those who have been divorced from it by asceticism," a veiled reference to Patanjala Yoga. *ARLR*, 2:208.

57. *Journal of the American Oriental Society* 6 (1858–60): 608, and 11 (1882–85): cvi–cvii.

58. *The Genius and Character of Emerson*, ed. F. B. Sanborn (Boston: James R. Osgood and Company, 1885), cited in Christy, *Orient in American Transcendentalism*, 263.

59. Oliver Wendell Holmes, *Ralph Waldo Emerson* (Boston: Houghton, Mifflin and Company, 1885), 397, 338, 179. As Holmes somewhat cynically suggested, several of Emerson's poems weren't much more than translations of "Indian models," which only sounded as if they were original. Christy, *Orient in American Transcendentalism*, 170–

75. Even Christy (p. 6) believed Emerson may have retracted some of his affection for Indian philosophy, noting a journal entry written more than a decade after "Brahma": "I want not the metaphysics, but only the literature of them." However, the phrase referred to Hegel and German philosophy: "Well we have familiarized that dogma, and at least found a kind of necessity in it, even if poor human nature still feels the paradox. Now is there any third step which Germany has made of like importance? It needs no encyclopaedia of volumes to tell. I want not the metaphysics, but only the literature of them." Emerson and Forbes, *Journals of Ralph Waldo Emerson*, 1:248.

2. THOREAU'S EXPERIMENT

1. *The Carlyle Encyclopedia*, ed. Mark Cumming (Cranbury, NJ: Rosemont Publishing and Printing Company, 2004), 102–3; John d'Entremont, "Conway, Moncure Daniel," *American National Biography Online*, February 2000, www.anb.org/articles/16/16-00345.html (accessed September 29, 2009); Moncure Conway, "Thoreau," *Fraser's Magazine*, reprinted in *Eclectic Magazine*, August 1866, 180.
2. Conway, "Thoreau," 184.
3. Robert D. Richardson, Jr., *Henry Thoreau: A Life of the Mind* (Berkeley: University of California Press, 1986), 144–47.
4. Richardson says Walden was "in no sense a retreat or withdrawal," and that Thoreau saw it as a "step forward, liberation, a new beginning." *Thoreau*, 148–53.
5. Diogenes, the most renowned of the Cynic philosophers, lived in a tub in ancient Athens, "where Alexander would be sure of seeing it," to protest prevailing social conventions, including the notion that one needed a house. See Charles Frederick Briggs, "A Yankee Diogenes," *Putnam's Monthly*, October 1854, and "An American Diogenes," *Chambers's Journal*, November 21, 1857, both reprinted in *Pertaining to Thoreau* (Detroit: Edwin B. Hill, 1901).
6. Moncure Daniel Conway, *Emerson at Home and Abroad* (first edition, Boston: J. R. Osgood and Co., 1882; repr. Read Books, 2008), 280; Catherine L. Albanese, ed., *The Spirituality of the American Transcendentalists* (Macon, GA: Mercer University Press, 1988), 290.
7. Catherine L. Albanese, *A Republic of Mind and Spirit: A Cultural History of American Metaphysical Religion* (New Haven: Yale University Press, 2007), 348–49; Walter Harding, *Thoreau's Library* (Charlottesville: University of Virginia Press, 1957), 17.
8. H. H. Wilson, *Religious Sects of the Hindus*, ed. Ernst R. Rost (Calcutta: Susil Gupta Private Limited, 1958). It's worth noting that Wilson mentions *eighty-four* postures where as Patanjali's *Yoga Sutras* says only that posture should be steady and comfortable. His description implies that Hatha Yoga and Patanjala Yoga were bound up with each other and, furthermore, those Yogis who practiced breath control and asana, even under the rubric of Patanjala Yoga, were particularly reviled or feared (115–22). Thoreau may have come across some of these ideas, if not Wilson's text itself, then in Colebrooke's *Miscellaneous Essays*, one of the volumes in Emerson's library. And later, he'd find a discussion of Patanjala Yoga in the introduction to J. Cockburn Thomson's translation of the *Bhagavad-Gita*. Christy, *Orient in American Transcendentalism*, 288, 297–98.
9. Philip F. Gura, "Thoreau's Maine Woods Indians: More Representative Men," *American Literature* 49, no. 3 (November 1977): 366–84, www.jstor.org/stable/2924988 (accessed July 5, 2009).

10. Christy, *Orient in American Transcendentalism,* 188–89.
11. Thoreau's love of these works was deep and abiding. About a decade after his re-treat, he received forty-four volumes "almost exclusively relating to Hindoo literature and scarcely one of them to be bought in America" from Thomas Cholmondeley, an English friend and admirer. By this point, Thoreau had already read many of these books. Still this "royal gift" was so precious to him, he sent news of it to one friend "as I might the birth of a child." Henry David Thoreau, *The Transmigration of the Seven Brahmans: A Translation from the* Harivansa *of Langlois,* with an introduction by Arthur Christy (New York: William Edwin Rudge, 1931), xi–xx.
12. Henry David Thoreau, *A Week on the Concord and Merrimack Rivers, Walden; or Life in the Woods, The Maine Woods, Cape Cod* (United States: The Library of America, 1985), 115.
13. Thoreau, *Walden* (New York: Thomas Y. Crowell and Company, 1910; digitized June 27, 2007), 39–45, 56–59, 102, 201.
14. He's quoting Roy's *Translation of Several Principal Books, Passages, and Texts of the Veds, and of Some Controversial Works on Brahmunical Theology* (London: Parbury, Allen, and Co., 1832); Thoreau, *Walden,* 206.
15. Richardson, *Thoreau,* 179.
16. Mott, *History of American Magazines,* 87; Richardson, *Emerson,* 381–82.
17. Wilkins, *Bhagavat-Geeta,* 64.
18. Carl T. Jackson, *The Oriental Religions and American Thought: Nineteenth Century Explorations* (Westport, CT: Greenwood Press, 1981), 65; Thoreau, *Walden,* 3–6.
19. Thoreau, *Walden,* 105–6.
20. *Compendium of the Enumeration of the Inhabitants and Statistics of the United States, as obtained at the Department of State from the returns of the sixth census* (Washington: Thomas Allen, 1841), www2.census.gov/prod2/decennial/documents/1840b-01 .pdf (accessed May 12, 2009).
21. Wilkins, *Bhagavat-Geeta,* 63–65.
22. Followed by controlling the vital airs (pranayama)—and Wilson's footnote details how you actually do this, i.e., exhaling through the right nostril while you close the left one with your right hand and so on. Wilson, *Religious Sects of the Hindus,* 509–13.
23. *The Journal of Henry Thoreau,* ed. Bradford Torrey and Francis H. Allen, 14 vols. (Boston: Houghton Mifflin, 1906), vol. 4, cited in Richardson, *Thoreau,* 271.
24. Thoreau, *A Week,* 113.
25. Thoreau, *Walden,* 502–3.
26. In his chapter "A Pond in the Winter," he describes a sort of model day at Walden. On waking, he'd read the *Bhagavad-Gita,* but this was no ordinary perusal of words on a page. He'd bathe his "intellect in the stupendous and cosmogonal philosophy of the Bhagavat-Geeta." And in this frame of mind, Thoreau would go to the well, where he'd meet "the servant of the Brahmin, priest of Brahma and Vishnu and Indra, who still sits in his temple on the Ganges reading the Vedas, or dwells at the root of the tree with his crust and water jug. I meet his servant come to draw water and our buckets as it were grate together in the same well. The pure Walden water is mingled with the sacred water of the Ganges." The passage suggests Thoreau transformed the most quotidian tasks into revelations, collapsing time and space. He comes just short of achieving divine congress, though the moment is no less sacred for it. Arthur Versluis, *American Transcendentalism and Asian Religions*

(New York: Oxford University Press, 1993), 83–84; Thoreau, *Walden*, 580. The quote is from *Walden* and is cited in Arthur Christy's introduction to *The Transmigration of the Seven Brahmans*, xix.

27. Christy, *Orient in American Transcendentalism*, 201; Henry David Thoreau, *Letters to a Spiritual Seeker*, ed. Bradley P. Dean (New York: W. W. Norton and Company, 2004), 49–51.

28. Thoreau, *Letters to a Spiritual Seeker*, 48–51.

29. *The Writings of Henry David Thoreau*, ed. Bradford Torrey and Franklin Benjamin Sanborn (Boston and New York: Houghton, Mifflin and Company, 1906; digitized November 28, 2007), 8:191.

30. "Ainsi l'yogin, absorbé dans la contemplation, contribue pour sa part à la création: il respire un parfum tout divin, il entend des choses toutes merveilleuses. Des formes divine le traversent sans le déchirer, et, uni à la nature qui lui est propre, il va, il agit comme animant la matière originelle (pradhâna)." *Harivansa ou histoire de la famille de Hari: ou, Histoire de la famille de Hari*, trans. Simon-Alexandre Langlois (printed for the Oriental Translation Fund of Great Britain and Ireland, 1835; digitized November 21, 2008), 2:327.

31. Wilkins, *Bhagavat-Geeta*, 64–65.

32. Thoreau, *Letters to a Spiritual Seeker*, 48.

33. Agehananda Bharati, "The Hindu Renaissance and Its Apologetic Patterns," *The Journal of Asian Studies* 29, no. 2 (February 1970): 287.

34. Thoreau, *Letters to a Spiritual Seeker*, 38.

35. Thoreau, *A Week*, 110.

36. Ibid., 97.

37. Robert F. Sayre, *Thoreau and the American Indians* (Princeton, NJ: Princeton University Press, 1977), 173–87; Richard Bridgman, *Dark Thoreau* (Lincoln: University of Nebraska Press, 1982), 240.

38. Ralph Waldo Emerson, "Thoreau," *Atlantic Monthly* 10 (August 1862), excerpted in *Thoreau: A Century of Criticism*, ed. Walter Harding (Dallas: Southern Methodist University Press, 1954), 33. It was left to Fanny Hardy Eckstorm, daughter of a Maine lumberman, to put Thoreau's abilities in perspective. Thoreau was neither a woodsman, nor a very good naturalist, in Eckstorm's estimation. He did have more knowledge of his environs than most Concord townsfolk, though. Fannie Hardy Eckstorm, "Thoreau's 'Maine Woods,'" *Atlantic Monthly* 102 (August 1908), in *A Century of Criticism*, 107–9.

39. Henry David Thoreau, *Maine Woods* (New York: T. Y. Crowell, 1909; digitized April 17, 2008), 238–39.

40. Frank Macshane, "Walden and Yoga," *The New England Quarterly* 37, no. 3 (September 1964): 335. The Bhakti Yogi is able to divinize his reality. As Krishna puts it, "The man whose mind is endued with this devotion, and looketh on all things alike, beholdeth the supreme soul in all things, and all things in the supreme soul." Wilkins, *Bhagavat-Geeta*, 64.

41. Sedgwick, *Atlantic*, 59.

42. Thoreau, *Letters to a Spiritual Seeker*, 94–95.

43. Thoreau, *Walden*, 582–83. Alan D. Hodder notes that Thoreau favored the *Gita*'s descriptions of Karma Yoga over and above its theology or its devotional elements. However, at least in his own life, Thoreau very much cherished the fruits of his

actions (as all artists do), making him an imperfect practitioner of this type of yoga. *Thoreau's Ecstatic Witness* (New Haven and London: Yale University Press, 2001), 174–217.

44. Thoreau, *Transmigration*, 5n.

45. David T. Y. Ch'en, "Thoreau and Taoism," in *Asian Response to American Literature*, ed. C. D. Narasimhaiah (Delhi: Vikas, 1972), 406–16. http://www.vcu.edu/engweb/transcendentalism/roots/hdt-tao.html.

46. Thoreau, *Letters to a Spiritual Seeker*, 34.

3. THE GURU ARRIVES

1. Pravrajika Prabuddhaprana, *Saint Sara: The Life of Sara Chapman Bull, the Mother of Swami Vivekananda* (Dakshineswar and Calcutta: Sri Sarada Math, 2002), 91.

2. Ibid., 88–91; Anne Gordon Atkinson, Robert Atkinson, Rosanne Buzzell, Richard Grover, Diane Iverson, Robert H. Stockman, and Burton W. F. Trafton, Jr., *Green Acre on the Piscataqua* (Eliot, ME: Green Acre Baha'i School Council, 1991), 19.

3. Marie Louise Burke, *Swami Vivekananda in the West, New Discoveries: His Prophetic Mission* (1959; repr., Calcutta: Advaita Ashrama, 1992), 2:143.

4. Ibid., 2:146–47.

5. Burke, *Vivekananda*, 2:146–55.

6. Ibid., 2:146. Emma Thursby wasn't present; she copied Locke's notes and saved these. See Prabuddhaprana, *Saint Sara*, 95.

7. Burke, *Vivekananda*, 1:468.

8. Ward, *View of the History*, 1:xii, xxxix.

9. Bernard Stern, "American Views of India and Indians, 1857–1900" (Ph.D. diss., University of Pennsylvania, 1956), 17.

10. Caleb Wright and J. A. Brainerd, *Historic Incidents and Life in India* (Chicago: J. A. Brainerd, 1869), 56–57.

11. Jackson, *Oriental Religions*, 125–27.

12. Ibid., 85–91.

13. Harold R. Isaacs, *Images of Asia: American Views of China and India* (New York: Capricorn Books, 1962), 262–65. Originally published as *Scratches on Our Minds* (Cambridge, MA: MIT, 1958).

14. Burke, *Vivekananda*, 1:467–68.

15. Erik Larson, *The Devil in the White City* (New York: Crown Publishers, 2003), 14–15.

16. *A Museum of Faiths: Histories and Legacies of the 1893 World's Parliament of Religions*, ed., and introduction by, Eric J. Ziolkowski (Atlanta: Scholars Press, 1993), 7.

17. *Dream City: A Portfolio of Photographic Views of the World's Columbian Exposition, with an Introduction by Halsey C. Ives* (St. Louis, MO: N. D. Thompson Co., 1893–94), columbus.gl.iit.edu/ (accessed December 23, 2004); Hubert Howe Bancroft, *The Book of the Fair* (Chicago and San Francisco: The Bancroft Company, 1893), Digital History Collection, columbus.gl.iit.edu/ (accessed November 5, 2004), 53.

18. Larson, *Devil in the White City*, 218–54; Bancroft, *Book of the Fair*, 399–425; "A Vision of Fairyland" was how one photographer captioned an image of the fairgrounds. Neil Harris, *The Land of Contrasts* (New York: G. Braziller, 1970), 302. Caption from original photograph book. This is part of an online exhibition of Co-

lumbian Exposition photographs, curated by the History Project of the University of California, Davis. historyproject.ucdavis.edu/imageaphp?Major=SY&Minor=C &SlideNum=12.00 (accessed October 29, 2004).

19. Bancroft, *Book of the Fair*, 136.
20. Ibid., 305–40, 411.
21. Burke, *Vivekananda*, 1:69–70.
22. Ziolkowski, *Museum of Faiths*, 9.
23. Ibid., 9–11.
24. Abandoning any pretense of religious comity, Barrows insisted, "We believe that Christianity is to supplant all other religions, because it contains all the truth there is in them and much besides." Burke, *Vivekananda*, 1:70–72.
25. Narasingha P. Sil, *Swami Vivekananda: A Reassessment* (London: Associated University Press, 1997), 91, 98. See Gail Collins, *America's Women: 400 Years of Dolls, Drudges, Helpmates, and Heroines* (New York: William Morrow, 2003), 238–48.

    More and more young women went to work outside the home, in urban centers such as Chicago, before they settled into domestic life. This might sound like a rather grim sort of freedom; still, it meant women had income and time at their discretion. The trend was so pronounced, Jane Addams, reformer and founder of Chicago's Hull House, opined, "Never before in civilization have such numbers of young girls been suddenly released from the protection of the home and permitted to walk unattended upon the city streets and to work under alien roofs." Donald Miller, *City of the Century: The Epic of Chicago and the Making of America* (New York: Simon & Schuster, 1996), cited in Larson, *Devil in the White City*, 11. Her alarm wasn't entirely misplaced. During the exposition, a man who went by the name of Dr. H. H. Holmes took advantage of the influx of "unattended" women. Holmes built a hotel near the fairgrounds and lured many of his victims with a promise of employment. Before he was caught, the "doctor" brutally killed at least nine people and confessed to killing eighteen others, most of them women. Larson, *Devil in the White City*, 256–57, 337–70.
26. Ziolkowski, *Museum of Faiths*, 8–9.
27. Burke, *Vivekananda*, 1:79, 102–3.
28. Ibid., 1:110. However, he was not the most popular Asian delegate, which is the impression he gave his fellow monks in India. According to recent scholarship, Vivekananda was no more or less popular than any other Asian delegate, with the possible exception of the Ceylonese Buddhist monk Dharmapala, who received favorable front-page coverage in the *Chicago Tribune*. "Creed of Buddha Expounded," *Chicago Daily Tribune* (1872–1963), September 11, 1893, ProQuest Historical Newspapers, *Chicago Tribune* (1849–1986), 1; Sil, *Vivekananda*, 159; P. C. Mozoomdar, *Lectures in America and Other Papers* (Calcutta: Navavidhan Publication Committee, 1955), ix, 20–21; Sunrit Mullick, "Protap Chandra Majumdar and Swami Vivekananda at the Parliament of Religions: Two Interpretations of Hinduism and Universal Religion," in Ziolkowski, *Museum of Faiths*, 219–20, 227–28.
29. Vivekananda, *The Yogas and Other Works*, chosen and with a Biography by Swami Nikhilananda (New York: Ramakrishna-Vedanta Center, 1953), 63, 192. Vivekananda sounded many of the same notes as his colleague Mozoomdar. Both pointed to the universal basis of all religion and described an omnipresent God. The common ele-

ments of their respective worldviews had a single source. Vivekananda had begun his spiritual career with the Brahmo Samaj, then directed by Keshub Chandra Sen, who emphasized "the unity of the Godhead." Sen's reformulated Brahmoism, which was popular among Westernized Bengalis, had been well received in America. About a decade before Vivekananda's arrival, *Littell's Living Age* had reprinted a lengthy article explaining Brahmoism's basic tenets, among them a "Garland of a Hundred Names" for God. (Besides the most obvious ones—God, Lord, etc.— these included more pantheistic-sounding phrases such as Primary Force, Ocean of Love, and Abode of Beauty, among others.) Even though Vivekananda claimed another teacher, Sri Ramakrishna, as his guru, Sen's universalism had deeply affected him. See Sil, *Vivekananda*, 44–52; Burke, *Vivekananda*, 1:166.

30. Bancroft, *Book of the Fair*, 835, 876.
31. Vivekananda, *Yogas and Other Works*, 183,192.
32. Burke, *Vivekananda*, 1:78.
33. Sil, *Vivekananda*, 140.
34. Burke, *Vivekananda*, 1:86, 139; Sil, *Vivekananda*, 67.
35. Burke, *Vivekananda*, 1:113; Vivekananda, *Yogas and Other Works*, 183–97.
36. P. C. Mozoomdar, *The Oriental Christ* (Boston: Geo. H. Ellis, 1883), 13, 31.
37. Mozoomdar, *Lectures*, 5–14.
38. Burke, *Vivekananda*, 1:102.
39. Sil, *Vivekananda*, 151.
40. Rajagopal Chattopadhyaya, *Swami Vivekananda in the West* (Houston, TX: 1993), 11, 16.
41. Atkinson et al., *Green Acre*, 4, 6–7, 11.
42. Burke, *Vivekananda*, 2:136; Prabuddhaprana, *Saint Sara*, 82–85. See also bahai -library.com/essays/greenacre.html (accessed June 6, 2003).
43. ". . . and I realized, too, how much good would come from a summer vacation if instead of being burdened with the effort of finding amusement for leisure hours, one's mind and soul could be refreshed by helpful thoughts, under spreading pines, in green pastures, beside still waters." Atkinson et al., *Green Acre*, 13.
44. Bancroft, *Book of the Fair*, 411. Moses reputedly lit up "a house in Cambridge with forty incandescent lamps in multiple circuit" on his daughter's twelfth birthday, which was ten years before Edison invented a marketable lightbulb. Atkinson et al., *Green Acre*, 3–5. See also "An Intro to the History of the Green Acre Baha'i School in Eliot, Maine," bahai-library.com/essays/greenacre.html (accessed June 6, 2003).
45. Prabuddhaprana, *Saint Sara*, 10–15, 44–45, 81–82.
46. Ibid., 85–87.
47. Ibid., 87–89.
48. Farmer read Dr. Bonney's letter of support to the assembled. Slavery was no longer the issue exercising religious liberals; now it was the "fierce conflict between Capital and Labour." Like Bull and Farmer, Bonney believed Green Acre would promote spiritual brotherhood; political and economic reform would be its natural outgrowth. Ibid., 89.
49. The campers displayed their mettle when an electrical storm blew in off the Atlantic. "The Dude and Dudines are in the Hotel, but iron-bound nerves of triple steel and spirits of fire are in the camp," wrote Vivekananda, in a letter to Chicago friends

shortly after the storm. "If you had seen them yesterday, when the rain was falling in torrents and the cyclone was overturning everything, hanging by their tent strings to keep them from being blown down . . . it would have done your hearts good." Burke, *Vivekananda*, 2:152.

50. *The Complete Works of Swami Vivekananda* (1956; repr., Mayavati Memorial Edition, Calcutta: Advaita Ashrama, 1989), vol. 7, www.ramakrishnavivekananda.info/vivekananda/volume_7/vol_7_frame.htm (accessed November 17, 2004).

51. Burke, *Vivekananda*, 2:152–53.

52. Ibid., 2:146–49.

53. Mabel Potter Dagget, "The Heathen Invasion," *Hampton-Columbian Magazine* 27, no. 4 (October 1911): 410.

54. ". . . to listen while the Hindu Vivekananda rolled forth the solemn poetry of the Vedas." Burke, *Vivekananda*, 2:151.

55. Emerson, *Journals and Miscellaneous Notebooks*, 9:98.

56. Prabuddhaprana, *Saint Sara*, 37.

57. Ibid., 9–10.

58. Ibid., 61–63, 87–88; Celia Thaxter letter to Sara Chapman Bull, April 27, 1886, Bull Curtis Papers, Cambridge Historical Society.

59. Prabuddhaprana, *Saint Sara*, 61–63.

60. Burke, *Vivekananda*, 2:143.

61. Thomas Wentworth Higginson was particularly impressed by Sara's choice of Janes to direct the conferences. Prabuddhaprana, *Saint Sara*, 183–84.

62. Ibid., 106–7. Dr. Janes, as Bull well knew, agreed wholeheartedly. "To my mind, a lapse into astrology and certain other extreme views held by some doubtless very excellent people," wrote Janes as he was organizing the program for the second year, "is a lapse into the Dark Ages." May 9, 1895, Bull Curtis Papers.

63. Burke, *Vivekananda*, 2:234–35; Prabuddhaprana, *Saint Sara*, 112.

64. Lanman's influence endures: his Sanskrit reader is still used today. Prabuddhaprana, *Saint Sara*, 109–10.

65. Ibid., 118.

66. Ibid., 87, 504.

67. Burke, *Vivekananda*, 2:229–32; *Complete Works*, vol. 8, www.ramakrishnavivekananda.info/vivekananda/volume_8/vol_8_frame.htm (accessed November 11, 2004).

68. In an extended footnote, Wilkins refers to a "metaphysical work called *Patanjal*," in which God is represented as "the great man or prime progenitor" along with a female principle—nature. Wilkins, *Bhagavat-Geeta*, 140ff.

69. Stein, *Two Brahmin Sources*, 113; Ward, *View of the History*, 2:9–10. Still, it would be nearly another two decades before an American ventured a translation of the *Yoga Sutras*.

70. Christy, *Orient in American Transcendentalism*, 288; H. T. Colebrooke, *Miscellaneous Essays VI* (1873; repr., Kessinger Publishing, 2006), xiii–xiv.

71. Colebrooke, *Miscellaneous Essays VI*, 149, 160; Feuerstein, *Yoga Tradition*, 234.

72. Richard King, *Indian Philosophy: An Introduction to Hindu and Buddhist Thought* (Washington, DC: Georgetown University Press, 1999), 44–45.

73. "On Vedanta Philosophy," *Complete Works*, vol. 5, www.ramakrishnavivekananda.info/vivekananda/volume_5/vol_5_frame.htm (accessed November 16, 2004). This too is a matter of intense debate. Both Ian Whicher and Georg Feuerstein

argue the *Yoga Sutras'* dualism is mostly pedagogical. See King, *Indian Philosophy,* 189–96, 210–12.

74. Feuerstein, *Yoga Tradition,* 311–31.

75. "Alluding to the huge manufacturing systems of Great Britain, her innumerable railroads and her ubiquitous marine, it was remarked by Emerson that steam is the half of an Englishman. If this be so, it may be said with equal truth that electricity is the half of an American, for while the earlier discoveries in electric science were made in other lands, no nation has displayed such aptness and ingenuity in adapting them to practical use." Bancroft, *Book of the Fair,* 399.

76. *Complete Works,* vol. 8, www.ramakrishnavivekananda.info/vivekananda/volume_8/vol_8_frame.htm (accessed May 15, 2009).

77. Jessica Glasscock, "Nineteenth-Century Silhouette and Support," Costume Institute, Metropolitan Museum of Art, www.metmuseum.org/toah/hd/19sil/hd_19sil.htm (accessed June 2, 2009).

78. *Complete Works,* vol. 8, www.ramakrishnavivekananda.info/vivekananda/volume_8/vol_8_frame.htm (accessed November 11, 2004).

79. *Complete Works,* vol. 7, www.ramakrishnavivekananda.info/vivekananda/volume_7/vol_7_frame.htm (accessed November 17, 2004).

80. Vivekananda also inserted elements of the later commentarial literature, which mentions Tantric concepts. Feuerstein, *Yoga Tradition,* 236.

81. *The Gospel of Sri Ramakrishna,* trans., and introduction by, Swami Nikhilananda (New York: Ramakrishna-Vivekananda Center, 1942), 244–45. "There are two kinds of yoga: hathayoga and rājayoga. . . . Of these two, rājayoga is the better." This statement is found in Nikhilananda's English translation of the multivolume Bengali text authored by Mahendranath Gupta, one of Ramakrishna's household disciples. Recent scholarship has undermined the accuracy of this translation.

82. Ibid., 245, 362–63.

83. Jeffrey J. Kripal, *Kali's Child: The Mystical and the Erotic in the Life and Teachings of Ramakrishna,* 2nd ed. (Chicago and London: University of Chicago Press, 1998), 56–58.

84. *Gospel,* 20–21. See also Kripal, *Kali's Child,* 29–33.

85. Kripal, *Kali's Child,* 112–21. *Gospel,* 20–22.

86. According to a review in *Udbodhana,* the Ramakrishna Mission's house organ, Müller's book successfully avoided "the Scylla of the Christian missionaries on the one hand, and the Charybdis of the tumultuous Brahmos on the other." (From the translation of a review of *Ramakrishna: His Life and Sayings* by Professor Max Müller, contributed to the *Udbodhana,* March 14, 1899.) *Complete Works,* vol. 4, online edition accessed November 29, 2004.

    Vivekananda had been instrumental in its production. In addition to the collection of sayings itself, he had supplied "biographical material," which the aged scholar presented faithfully. Müller didn't allow Vivekananda's portrait to go untested. To counteract the distortions inherent in any biography, and particularly one rendered by a disciple, Müller quotes others' accounts of "the Saint" and sides with Mozoomdar on one crucial point: Müller believed Ramakrishna had imbibed Vedanta as all Hindus do, but was himself no Vedantin.

    For all his sophistication about his subject, Müller makes some audacious and inaccurate statements about yoga in his introductory remarks. He equates Hatha-yogins and jugglers and mistakenly attributes a taxonomy of four different yogas—

Mantra, Laya, Raja, and Hatha—to Patanjali. (This list actually appears in the *Yoga-Tattva-Upanishad*.) More damning still, early in his explanation of the practice, Müller insists, "The idea that [yoga] meant originally union with the deity has long been given up." Müller's explanation of Vedanta is more lucid, betraying his own bias, but this information was never meant to do more than offer a better window on his subject. F. Max Müller, *Ramakrishna: His Life and Sayings* (New York: Charles Scribner's Sons, 1899), 8, 62, 96. Sumi Sakar, *An Exploration of the Ramakrishna Vivekananda Tradition* (Rashtrapati Nivas: Indian Institute of Advanced Study, 1993), 44–45.

87. Albanese, *Republic of Mind and Spirit*, 354–56.
88. Prabuddhaprana, *Saint Sara*, 119.
89. The Theosophist William Judge had put out his own version of the *Sutras* in 1889. Albanese, *Republic of Mind and Spirit*, 351–52. Elizabeth De Michelis, *A History of Modern Yoga: Patanjali and Western Esotericism* (London and New York: Continuum, 2004), 124–25.
90. Prabuddhaprana, *Saint Sara*, 216, 509.
91. Ibid., 139.
92. Ibid., 130–31.
93. Ibid., 207.
94. July 1896, Bull Curtis Papers.
95. Prabuddhaprana, *Saint Sara*, 190–91.
96. Program for Cambridge Conferences, Bull Curtis Papers.

4. SWAMI VIVEKANANDA'S LEGACY

1. Prabuddhaprana, *Saint Sara*, 256–58.
2. Vivekananda, *Yogas and Other Works*, 134.
3. Prabuddhaprana, *Saint Sara*, 247–69; Pravrajika Prabuddhaprana, *Tantine: The Life of Josephine Macleod, Friend of Swami Vivekananda* (Dakshineswar and Calcutta: Sri Sarada Math 1990, 1994), 31–32.
4. Robert S. Ellwood, Jr., *Alternative Altars: Unconventional and Eastern Spirituality in America* (Chicago: University of Chicago Press, 1979), 115.
5. Robert S. Ellwood, Jr., "The American Theosophical Synthesis," in *The Occult in America: New Historial Perspectives*, ed. Howard Kerr and Charles L. Crow (Urbana and Chicago: University of Illinois Press, 1983), 90–99, 104.
6. Ellwood, "Theosophical Synthesis," 116–19.
7. Ellwood, *Alternative Altars*, 120–21.
8. Ellwood, "Theosophical Synthesis," 117.
9. Helena P. Blavatsky, "A Hindu Professor's Views on Yoga," in *H. P. Blavatsky's Collected Writings, 1881–1882* (Wheaton, IL: The Theosophical Publishing House, 1968), 104–6. Blavatsky was careful to distinguish Patanjala Yoga from Hatha Yoga, which she disdained but didn't entirely dismiss in the early 1880s. See "Comments on a Treatise on the Yoga Philosophy," in *H. P. Blavatsky's Collected Writings, 1879–1880* (Wheaton, IL: The Theosophical Publishing House, 1968), 453.
10. Thomas A. Tweed, *The American Encounter with Buddhism, 1844–1912: Victorian Culture and the Limits of Dissent* (Chapel Hill: University of North Carolina Press, 1992), 30.

11. Tweed outlines four components of Victorian culture—theism, individualism, activism, and optimism—that "played a crucial role in the discussion about Buddhism." This negative view began to change in the early 1860s, when European scholars such as Max Müller defended the Buddha and his philosophy, arguing that both were essentially moral. Ibid., xxxii–xxxv, 14–15.

12. Prabuddhaprana, *Saint Sara*, 256–70.

13. Vivekananda, *Complete Works*, 9:312. Online edition accessed December 17, 2004.

14. Sil, *Vivekananda*, 65.

15. Vivekananda went so far as to proclaim "Renunciation and Service" national ideals, and this determination to improve life for his countrymen was one of the reasons Sara had traveled those many miles to his side in Belur. "Men of character" from the mission would deluge the country with spirituality, triggering social and political reform and, finally, the wholesale transformation of Indian society. "Reawakening of Hinduism on a National Basis," interview in *Prabuddha Bharata*, September 1898, *Complete Works*, vol. 5, www.ramakrishnavivekananda.info/vivekananda/volume_5/vol_5_frame.htm (accessed November 21, 2004); Carl T. Jackson, *Vedanta for the West: The Ramakrishna Movement in the United States* (Bloomington and Indianapolis: Indiana University Press, 1994), 31; Prabuddhaprana, *Saint Sara*, 272.

16. Mike Davis, *Late Victorian Holocausts: El Niño Famines and the Making of the Third World* (New York and London: Verso, 2001), 1–17, 143. Vivekananda faulted Indian selfishness and inertia for the "frequent ravages of famine"; however, he blamed the British. "Famine has come to be a constant quantity in our country, and now it is, as it were, a sort of blight upon us. Do you find in any other country such frequent ravages of famine? No, because there are *men* in other countries, while in ours, men have become akin to dead matter, quite inert." From conversation with Shri Priya Nath Sinha, translated from Bengali, *Complete Works*, vol. 5, *Conversations and Dialogues*. "The still more terrible famines that have become the inevitable consequence of British rule (there never is a famine in a native state)." Letter to Miss Mary Hale, October 30, 1899, *Complete Works*, vol. 8, online edition accessed December 13, 2004.

17. Cunningham, *The Atlantic Monthly* 84, no. 1 (July 1899): 3.

18. Davis, *Late Victorian Holocausts*, 7.

19. Ibid., 143–48, 163.

20. Prabuddhaprana, *Saint Sara*, 262.

21. Ibid., 304.

22. "I have found enough to make me hope that the coming months of this quiet life with nature will bring an inner strength that I needed." Ibid., 247–318.

23. Ibid.

24. Chattopadhyaya, *Swami Vivekananda in the West*, 29.

25. Prabuddhaprana, *Saint Sara*, 316; Vivekananda, *Yogas and Other Works*, 127.

26. In fact, this aspect of Vivekananda's work is most consistent with the Brahmoism, which recent scholarship has shown shaped his thinking as much if not more than Ramakrishna, despite his repudiation of the Brahmo Samaj. From "The Diary of a Disciple," *Complete Works*, vol. 5 (translated from Bengali): "The disciple is Sharatchandra Chakravarty, who published his records in a Bengali book, *Swami-Shishya-Samvâda*, in two parts. The present series of 'Conversations and Dialogues' is a revised translation from this book. Place: *Baghbazar, Calcutta.* Year: *1897.*"

Online edition accessed December 17, 2004; Kripal, *Kali's Child*, 279; De Michelis, *History of Modern Yoga*, 108–10.

27. See Kripal, *Kali's Child*, 109–10.

28. Nikhilananda, *Gospel*, 373–74.

29. Kripal, *Kali's Child*, 26. Moreover, recent scholarship has shown that Ramakrishna never formally initiated Vivekananda or any of the other direct disciples of the Ramakrishna Order. De Michelis, *History of Modern Yoga*, 105.

30. Ramakrishna himself recognized this soon after Narendra arrived at the Dakshineswar temple. "Look! In you is Shiva. In me is Shakti! And these two are One." The homoerotic overtones of this statement have not been lost on recent scholars. Sil, *Vivekananda*, 28, 37. Feuerstein, *Yoga Tradition*, 83–84.

31. Vivekananda studied at the Presidency College of Calcutta for a year, then entered "the General Assembly's Institution, founded by the Scottish General Missionary Board and later known as the Scottish Church College." Vivekananda, *Yogas and Other Works*, 6.

32. Ibid., 712; Kripal, *Kali's Child*, 172.

33. Kripal, *Kali's Child*, 172.

34. Prabuddhaprana, *Saint Sara*, 329–31.

35. *Cambridge Tribune*, undated, 1899, Bull Curtis Papers.

36. Prabuddhaprana, *Saint Sara*, 122; "Marie Louise a Monk," *New York Times*, March 20, 1896, ProQuest Historical Newspapers, p. 9.

37. "Boston of course is the great field for everything but the Boston people as quickly take hold of anything as give it up." Burke, *Vivekananda*, 2:166.

38. Swami Abhedananda, *How to Be a Yogi* (New York: Vedanta Society, 1902), 54–58.

39. Ibid., 41, 45–52.

40. Prabuddhaprana, *Saint Sara*, 371.

41. "Balm of the Orient Is Bliss-Inspiring Yoga," *New York Herald*, March 27, 1898.

42. Vivekananda, "Six Lessons on Raja Yoga: First Lesson," www.ramakrishnavivekananda .info/vivekananda/volume_8/vol_8_frame.htm (accessed October 5, 2009).

43. *The Yoga Sutras of Patanjali*, trans., and with commentary by, Edwin F. Bryant (New York: North Point Press, 2009), 10.

44. Around the time of the Parliament of Religions, a short story titled "A Western Yoga" had appeared in *The New York Times*. It gave a succinct description of the practice: you balanced on one foot and stared ad nauseam at the tip of your nose. The payoff for standing like a "barnyard animal" was an "Aladdin's lamp," which filled every wish, made "earth, fire, water, air, time and distance vassals at your feet." "A Western Yoga," *New York Times*, October 15, 1893, 22.

45. Burke, *Vivekananda*, 1:241–43. Vivekananda was less emphatic about the dangers of Tantra, which encompasses Hatha Yoga, when addressing Indian or Bengali audiences, which makes his private views on the matter hard to fathom. See Prabuddhaprana, *Tantine*, 146–47.

46. Bryant, *Yoga Sutras*, 360.

47. Feuerstein, *Encyclopedia*, 105, 121–22. "Just as a door is opened with a key," avers Yogi Swatmarama in the third chapter, "similarly the yogi opens the door to liberation with kundalini." *Hatha Yoga Pradipika*, commentary by Swami Muktibodhananda (Munger, Bihar: Yoga Publications Trust, 1993), 418. The third chapter is

emphatic on this point and opens with the sutra "As the serpent (Sheshnaga) upholds the earth and its mountains and woods, so kundalini is the support of all the yoga practices" (p. 279). Agehananda Bharati, *The Tantric Tradition* (New York: Samuel Weiser Inc., 1975), 238.

The most detailed descriptions of the subtle body appear in key Hatha Yoga texts written sometime between 800 and 1600 c.e. Of course, as with most aspects of yoga, iterations of the subtle body can be found in much earlier scriptures including the *Upanishads*.

And later commentaries on the *Yoga Sutras* incorporate the subtle body, including the injunction to raise Kundalini. Feuerstein, *Yoga Tradition*, 236.

48. Nikhilananda, *Gospel*, 245.
49. Sil, *Vivekananda*, 121, 157–58.
50. Vivekananda, *Vedânta Philosophy: Lectures by the Swâmi Vivekânanda, on Râja Yoga and Other Subjects* (New York: The Baker and Taylor Company, 1899), 19, 50.
51. Ibid., 19, 133; Feuerstein, *Yoga Tradition*, 236; Bryant, *Yoga Sutras*, 358.
52. Prabuddhaprana, *Saint Sara*, 318, 349, 372.
53. Ibid., 373.
54. Ibid.
55. Ibid., 416–18.
56. "American Women Victims of Hindu Mysticism," *Washington Post*, February 18, 1912.
57. In a strange twist of fate, Olea had died the day before, exactly six months after her mother. It was left to her lawyer, and lover, Ralph Bartlett, to administer Sara's estate, and he was now legally empowered to ignore the codicil, which would have left part of it to Sara's fellow Vedantins.
58. *New York Times*, May 24, 1911; *Washington Post*, May 27, 1911; *New York Times* May 31, 1911.
59. James Creelman, "A Mahatma in New York," *Pearson's Magazine* 18, no. 4 (October 1907): 345–62.
60. Mott, *History of American Magazines*, 5:145–53.
61. Daggett reports that Sewall "is suffering from ill health and is said to be a physical wreck through the practice of yoga and the study of occultism." Mabel Potter Daggett, "The Heathen Invasion," *Hampton-Columbian Magazine* 27, no. 4 (October 1911): 399–411.
62. "City Bulletins," *Washington Post*, February 24, 1911, 14.
63. Rajagopal Chattopadhyaya, *Swami Vivekananda in India: A Corrective Biography* (Delhi: Motilal Banarsidass Publishers, 1999), 359–64.
64. Paul S. Reinsch, "Energism in the Orient," *International Journal of Ethics* (University of Chicago Press) 21, no. 4 (July, 1911): 407–22, www.jstor.org/stable/2376566 (accessed February 5, 2009); William James, *The Varieties of Religious Experience* (New York: Touchstone, 1997), 314–15.

5. THE MAKING OF AN AMERICAN GURU

1. Cornelia F. Bedell, *Now and Then and Long Ago in Rockland County, New York* (New City, NY: Historical Society of Rockland County, 1968, 1992), 298.
2. Nancy Cacioppo, "Enticing Waves of Settlers for More Than 300 Years," *The Journal News Online*, June 17, 2003, www.thejournalnews.com/LivingHere/rockland/

features/history.html (accessed March 18, 2005); Edward Hopper House Art Center history page.

3. Wallace Bruce, *The Hudson: Three Centuries of History, Romance and Invention* (Bryant Union Company, 1907), 72.

4. LJ MS, 138–39; Grace Gordon was the archivist of the Pierre A. Bernard collection at HSRC and author of "Pierre Bernard and the Clarkstown Country Club," *South of the Mountains* (New City, NY: HSRC) 44, no. 1 (January–March 2000): 8–9.

5. Robert Love has written a biography of Pierre A. Bernard, *The Great Oom: The Improbable Birth of Yoga in America* (New York: Viking, 2010). His input, in e-mail correspondence and in one extended interview and several shorter ones, has been enormously helpful. Love interview, June 29, 2005; LJ MS, 142.

6. LJ MS, 130–47.

7. Undated statement, HSRC.

8. *Los Angeles Times*, November 28, 1919, 114.

9. Eckert Goodman, "The Guru of Nyack: The True Story of Father India, the Omnipotent Oom," *Town and Country*, April 1941, 93.

10. Bernard may have been born in 1876; records are not clear and he dissembled about the exact date and location of his birth. Love interview, June 29, 2005; Gordon, "Pierre Bernard," 3; VWB tr., August 3, 1987, 60, and June 25, 1991, 4; Love phone interview, May 29, 2009.

11. Bernard described Hamati as a mix of Syrian and Bengali; according to Robert Love, he described himself as the son of a French mother and Persian father and was raised in Palestine and trained in Bengali Tantric yoga traditions. Paul G. Hackett, "Barbarian Lands: Theos Bernard, Tibet, and American Religious Life," (Ph.D. diss., Columbia University, 2008), 192. One Elias Hamati, in Calcutta, appears in VWB's address book for her trip to India. VWB Papers, HSCU; Janet M. Davis, *The Circus Age: Culture and Society Under the American Big Top* (Chapel Hill and London: University of North Carolina Press, 2002), 215; Joan M. Jensen, *Passage from India* (New Haven and London: Yale University Press, 1988), 14.

12. Undated statement, HSRC.

13. Love interview, May 29, 2009; undated statement HSRC; Gordon, "Pierre Bernard," 4; Love interview, June 29, 2005.

14. "Harry Houdini," *St. James Encyclopedia of Popular Culture*, 5 vols. (St. James Press, 2000), reproduced in *Biography Resource Center* (Farmington Hills, MI: Gale, 2009), galenet.galegroup.com.ezproxy.cul.columbia.edu/servlet/BioRC (accessed October 16, 2009).

15. "Claude Bernard," *Encyclopedia of World Biography*, 2nd ed., 17 vols. (Gale Research, 1998), reproduced in *Biography Resource Center* (Farmington Hills, MI: Gale, 2009), galenet.galegroup.com.ezproxy.cul.columbia.edu/servlet/BioRC (accessed October 16, 2009).

16. Love interview, June 29, 2005.

17. Perry's education was informal. After his father left, he had lived with his grandparents for a while where his family schooled him in the basics as well as some natural history, philosophy, and science. Gordon, "Pierre Bernard," 3.

18. Undated legal statement, HSRC; Gordon, "Pierre Bernard," 5.

19. Tantrik Oath, undated, HSRC.

20. Undated Tantrik test, HRSC.
21. Quoted in Hugh B. Urban, "The Omnipotent Oom: Tantra and Its Impact on Modern Western Esotericism," *Esoterica: The Journal* 3 (2001), www.esoteric.msu.edu/VolumeIII/HTML/Oom.html (accessed June 30, 2005).
22. Ibid.
23. Bharati was a professor at Syracuse University for thirty years, first of anthropology and then of South Asian studies. Bharati, *Tantric Tradition*, 238; Feuerstein, *Encyclopedia*, 107–108. Bharati, who was Austrian by birth, was initiated into the Dasanami Sannyasi Order. "Obituaries: Agehananda Bharati (1923–1991)," *The Journal of Asian Studies* (Ann Arbor) 50, no. 4 (November 1991): 1017.
24. Bharati, *Tantric Tradition*, 244–48.
25. Ibid., 282–83.
26. Feuerstein, *Yoga Tradition*, 343; David Gordon White, "Transformations in the Art of Love: Kamakala Practices in Hindu Tantric and Kaula Traditions," *History of Religions* 38, no. 2 (November 1998): 172, links.jstor.org/sici?sici=0018-2710%28199811%2938%3A2%3C172%ATITAOL%3E2.0.CO%3B2-L.
27. The ceremony is exceedingly complex; I've given only a summary here. See Bharati, *Tantric Tradition*, 248–65, 286.
28. *Gospel of Sri Ramakrishna*, 123, quoted in Urban, *Tantra*, 151.
29. Bharati, *Tantric Tradition*, 284.
30. Love interview, October 20, 2009.
31. Urban, *Tantra*, 10–11, 216–17. Randolph, who was born of mixed race in 1825 and raised in New York City, also believed that if a man focused on a woman's sexual satisfaction, he and his partner could experience "depths of pleasure and spirituality" and strengthen the marriage bond. Sex magic was a source of inspiration for a number of Western occult groups including the H.B. of L. For more of Bernard's views on sex, see his lectures of May 1915. The first, on the ninth, "Sexual Perversion: Chemical and Anatomical Values," dispensed graphic information in the clinical language of physiology and perversion. A little more than a week later, Bernard gave a follow-up lecture—in the format of Q and A—that related some of his ideas about sex perversion to Tantra. What he had to say was fairly startling and may have prompted one woman to tell a reporter Bernard's goal was to teach "men and women to love, and make women feel like queens": "In Tantra, we believe that the burden should be put on the man. . . . He should always be ready to satisfy the woman's wishes, for a great many reasons." He defined *Yoni Mudra* as the "art of sex" and *sex congress* as the "art of all arts of the world." He closed by advising his listeners to "read the Kama Sutra." Seabrook, *Witchcraft*, 356–57, quoted in Urban, "Omnipotent Oom"; lecture notes, May 17, 1915, HSRC.
32. Love interview, October 20, 2009.
33. For a detailed discussion of Western esotericism and occultism in the nineteenth century, see Joscelyn Godwin, *The Theosophical Enlightenment* (Albany: State University of New York Press, 1994), and in particular pages 257–60. Love interview, May 29, 2009; Godwin, 262–67.
34. They'd don pins or badges, they'd proceed through elaborate and sometimes secretive rituals, and they'd socialize. Because most had complex hierarchies, with local, state, and national chapters, these groups afforded many Americans who lacked power—workingmen, white-collar employees, women—a taste of it. Love inter-

view, May 29, 2009; Theda Skocpol, *Diminished Democracy: From Membership to Management in American Civic Life* (Norman: University of Oklahoma Press, 2003), 74–105.

35. Abhedananda, *How to Be a Yogi*, 33. Elizabeth De Michelis cites the hermetic societies as one of the "two most influential esoteric schools" of the late nineteenth century and argues that these schools influenced Vivekananda as well. While true enough, Bernard's debt was far greater and more visible. *History of Modern Yoga*, 118.

36. "Chicago Followers of Strange Religions," *Chicago Daily*, April 16, 1899, ProQuest Historical Newspapers, *Chicago Tribune* (1849–86), 46. Secrecy was a particularly important feature of the European occult lodges. As chronicler of the occult Mitch Horowitz puts it, "Theosophy's Annie Besant never tired of creating elite offshoots of the organization: orders within orders and inner lodges, each with its own badges, seals, and ceremonies." Mitch Horowitz, *Occult America: The Secret History of How Mysticism Shaped the Nation* (New York: Bantam Books, 2009), 208.

37. Clever as it was, it's unlikely Bernard edited the journal as he maintained; his half brother Glen described him as merely the "front man" for the enterprise. Records show that Hamati contributed as much as half or even more of the contents of the first and only issue. For this, Bernard paid him a huge fee, more than five thousand dollars (about one hundred thousand in today's dollars!). Bill of sale, October 26, 1907, HSRC.

38. *International Journal of the Tantrik Order* (New York: 1906), HSRC.

39. In their effort to rehabilitate the Tantras, others argued that the difference between the left- and right-hand paths was not always so stark. In an unpublished introduction to the *Maha Nirvana Tantra* (considered the ur-text of revisionists) found amid Bernard's lecture notes, the author states, "The Tantrik worshippers of Bengal are generally Bamacharas [left-hand]," and then insists there really is no right-hand path at all; initiation turns a right-hand practitioner into a Bamachari, or left-hand one, forevermore. *Maha Nirvana Tantra* MS, HSRC.

40. The journal talks about sex as a sacrament in the most literal terms. "The whole world is embodied in the woman. Sex worship as a religion constitutes the basis of all that is sacred, holy and beautiful." "In Re Fifth Veda," *International Journal of the Tantric Order*, 35–36, HSRC, quoted in Urban, *Tantra*, 213.

41. *International Journal of the Tantric Order*, "Legacy of an Initiate," 49, HSRC.

42. Undated statement, HSRC; Love interview, June 29, 2005.

43. Bernard letter to Tantrik Order, HSRC, quoted in Love, *Great Oom*.

44. *Evening Herald News*, May 3, 1910; *Evening Mail*, May 3, 1910; HSRC. "Girl Describes Rites and 'Hindoo's' Oriental Séances" *New York Evening Telegram*, May 4, 1910; Robert Love, "Fear of Yoga," *Columbia Journalism Review*, November 2006, 84.

45. *The Encyclopedia of New York City*, 1st ed., ed. Kenneth T. Jackson (New Haven: Yale University Press, 1995).

46. Love interview, June 29, 2005.

47. *New York Times*, January 4, 1910, 5; *Chicago Daily Tribune*, April 30, 1910, 4.

48. *New York Evening Mail*, May 3, 1910, quote courtesy Robert Love.

49. *Evening Telegram*, May 4, 1910.

50. *New York American Journal*, May 3, 1910.

51. Love interview, October 20, 2009.

52. *New York Evening Mail*, May 3, 1910, quote courtesy Robert Love.

53. Gordon, "Pierre Bernard," 5; Love interview, June 29, 2005, and October 20, 2009; Goodman, "Guru of Nyack," 93.
54. Western Union telegram to Mrs. P. A. Bernard, October 31, 1941, HSRC; Love interview, June 2, 2009.
55. Dace was the youngest, following her brother, James, and sister, Frankie. Her father was a "ne'er-do-well" who left her mother, a creative and resourceful woman who raised her three children by herself. It's likely Frankie and De Vries were half sisters. See VWB tr., 175–76, VWB Papers, HSCU.
56. Her hometown paper promptly dubbed her "one of the most talented of Detroit's galaxy of theatrical performers." *Detroit Free Press*, October 1908, HSRC; VWB tr., August 27, 1987, 173, 181, VWB Papers, HSCU.
57. Not long before her death, she insisted that "nothing would ever be known about her, the story would never be told," and to this day, little is known about her personal life. VWB tr., August 27, 1987, 199, VWB Papers, HSCU.
58. Goodman, "Guru of Nyack," 93.
59. Lecture notes, "Tantrik Yoga," August 13, 1912, HSRC.
60. The description of Bernard comes from Goodman, "Guru of Nyack," 93.
61. Lecture dated August 13, 1912, HSRC. Put another way: "The body is the abode of God, O Goddess." Feuerstein, *Yoga Tradition*, 390.
62. *New York Times*, December 15, 1911, 22.
63. Ibid.
64. Undated statement, HSRC; *New York American*, May 3, 1910; Love interview, June 29, 2005; Charles Boswell, "The Great Fuss and Fume over the Omnipotent Oom," *True: The Man's Magazine*, January 1965, www.Vanderbilt.edu/~stringer/fuss.htm (accessed September 22, 2003).
65. Gordon, "Pierre Bernard," 6–7; Love interview, June 2, 2009, and program illustrations, e-mail correspondence, June 3, 2009.
66. LJ MS, 112–13, HSCU.
67. Clara Spring, "In Memoriam," VWB Papers, HSRC.
68. Goodman, "Guru of Nyack," 98.
69. Love interview, June 2, 2009, and program illustrations, e-mail correspondence, June 3, 2009.
70. Undated statement, 7–8, HSRC.
71. LJ MS, 127, VWB Papers, HSCU.
72. Even though Cheerie quickly mastered the poses, she wasn't immediately promoted. LJ MS, 127, VWB Papers, HSCU.
73. Ibid., 121.
74. Ibid., 128.
75. James, *Varieties of Religious Experience*, 90.
76. Horatio W. Dresser, *A History of the New Thought Movement* (New York: Thomas Y. Crowell Co., 1919), www.harvestfields.ca/etexts1/01/39/04.htm (accessed February 11, 2005).
77. This includes the meeting of the International Metaphysical League held at Madison Square Garden Concert Hall in the fall of 1900. *Washington Post*, November 19, 1900, 3.
78. *Chicago Daily Tribune*, March 19, 1902, 12.
79. Wendell Thomas, *Hinduism Invades America* (New York: The Beacon Press, 1930), 218.

80. Two books by Atkinson, *Mental Fascination* and *Thought-Force*, show up in the catalog of Bernard's library, as does a translation of the *Bhagavad-Gita* by Ramacharaka. For a good discussion of New Thought and the body, see Albanese, *Republic of Mind and Spirit*, 304.

81. August 1912 lecture on Tantrik Yoga, HSRC.

82. Mrs. Vanderbilt (Stanley) undated letter to De Vries, HSRC.

83. Marriage certificate, HSRC.

84. LJ MS, 127–29, VWB Papers, HSCU.

85. *Los Angeles Times*, November 28, 1919; Love interview, June 29, 2005.

86. Love interview, June 29, 2005; Goodman, "Guru of Nyack," 93.

87. LJ MS, 133, VWB Papers, HSCU.

88. James M. Mayo, *The American Country Club: Its Origins and Development* (New Brunswick, NJ: Rutgers University Press, 1998), 134; "Facts and Figures of the Automobile Industry, 1920–1930," National Automobile Chamber of Commerce, www.railsandtrails.com/AutoFacts/1927p39-100-8jpg (accessed July 10, 2009).

89. The club became famous for both its Open Forum lecture series, which featured experts in science, philosophy, Sanskrit, and many other fields, as well as travelers and artists, and its annual circus. First held in the fall of 1920, the circus was no amateur affair. The big top seated two thousand; Bernard hired professionals to train club members on the trapeze and in acrobatics. There were elephants and lions (a whole menagerie, including up to nine elephants, Bengali and Sumatra tigers, monkeys, Chinese geese, and a dwarf stallion, boarded on the grounds). Gordon, "Pierre Bernard," 14; *Rockland County Redbook*, 1927, 112–13, HSRC.

90. Club members performed and produced the entire event, with a few professional circus hands to train them. The results were spectacular. One observer, the Swedish actor and producer Ernst Rolf, recalled that he had expected "a nice polite little entertainment—a society circus. . . . I sat spellbound. . . . An acrobatic number—women and men stood on their heads and turned somersaults in designs; one woman high on a rope, head down,—and all were beautiful. Sir Paul Dukes took part, an acrobat as only God could make. Dancers à la Broadway, but so much more wonderful." Rolf might have exaggerated, but only slightly. *Life at the Clarkstown Country Club* (Nyack, NY): 1935, HSRC.

91. HSRC collection photograph; Love interview, June 29, 2005; *New York Times*, June 13, 1911, 9; *Life at the Clarkstown Country Club*, 11.

92. Jane Desmond, "Dancing Out the Difference: Cultural Imperialism and Ruth St. Denis's 'Radha' of 1906," *Signs* 17, no. 1 (Autumn 1991): 37–45.

93. Ibid., 31–33. Her interpretation of "Radha" afforded New Yorkers a guilty pleasure. "Every lascivious thought flees shy into the farthest corner," wrote one reviewer; "[St. Denis's] body is that of woman divinely planned," noted another, from the *Boston Herald*, adding, "There is no atmosphere of sex about her."

94. William Leach, *Land of Desire: Merchants, Power, and the Rise of the New American Culture* (New York: Pantheon Books, 1993), 144.

95. Gordon, "Pierre Bernard," 11.

96. Cyril Scott, typed excerpt of "Yoga and Health," in *Modern Mystic and Monthly Science Review*, 1937, HSRC; Love interview, October 20, 2009.

97. American Tantrik Order roster, HSRC.

98. Love interviews, June 2 and 29, 2009, and October 20, 2009; VWB tr., July 28, 1987, 41.
99. Love interview, May 29, 2009.
100. Outlines of Yoga, November 22, 1924, 5, HSRC.
101. Gordon, "Pierre Bernard," 16.
102. "Outlines of Yoga," November 22, 1924, HSRC.
103. Lecture notes, November 22, 1924, and March 25, 1928, 2, HSRC.
104. Lecture notes, October 17, 1920, HSRC.
105. *Principles of Tantra* is a translation of the *Tantratattva* of S'ri-yukta S'iva Candra Vidya-rnava Bhattaca-rya Mahodaya.
106. Love interview, June 2, 2009.
107. "There is nothing where there now is something when Ramakrishna came, nothing. And all that there is materially has been put up by one of his pupils. . . . This pupil is Abhedananda." Transcript dated October 17, 1920, HSRC.
108. Alphabetical lecture notes, HSRC.
109. Case #2, digital copy of HSRC catalog of Bernard's library, www.oldmom.com/catalog/case2.pdf (accessed May 5, 2005). "The thing to go after is character. It is akin to universal law, and thus you are getting closer and closer to the Divine in a specific and personal sense." Lecture notes, February 20, 1927, HSRC.
110. Vivekananda's works were well represented as were those of Swami Abhedananda, Swami Ram Tirtha, Max Müller, and Tantric scholar Sir John Woodroffe (who also published under the name Arthur Avalon), and even some of the Theosophists'.
111. VWB tr., August 11, 1987, 149, VWB Papers, HSCU.
112. Lecture notes, "On Character," July 25, 1924, 3–4, HSRC.
113. For instance, when Vivekananda described pranayama, he could readily explain its mechanical action on the spinal column, pituitary gland, and "nerve centers"—"This *Sushumnâ* is, in ordinary persons, closed up at the lower extremity. . . . The Yogi proposes a practice by which it can be opened and the nerve currents made to travel through it." But he had to resort to scientific *metaphors* to elucidate its *subtler* effects: Pranayama, he says, will produce "a tendency of all the molecules in the body to have the same direction. When mind changes into will, the currents change into a motion similar to electricity. . . . When all the motions of the body have become perfectly rhythmical the body has, as it were, become a gigantic battery of will." Vivekananda sounded convincingly technical, but on closer inspection, his use of electricity to elucidate pranayama is imprecise or figurative or both. Vivekananda, *Râja Yoga*, 49–51.
114. Chatterji lecture notes, September 4, 1927, HSRC; letter to Mr. L. V. Platten, November 21, 1927, HSRC.
115. Lecture notes, October 1920, HSRC.
116. Lecture notes, June 17, 1928, HSRC. This diverged even from his sources. For instance, Arthur Avalon, who was then the most famous Western exponent of Tantra and one of Bernard's key influences, accepted Indian metaphysics and its devaluation of worldly life. In one of the most read expositions of Tantra, Avalon repeated the truism that the Yogi's sole aim was "cessation from rebirth," and that through yoga "man exchanges his limited or worldly experience for that which is unlimited whole . . . or Perfect Bliss."
      Avalon, as it was later revealed, was a pseudonym for Sir John Woodroffe and his Bengali collaborator, Atal Behari Ghosh. Whether Woodroffe attempted to en-

act this or took Tantra to be more of a this-worldly enterprise, as many besides Bernard do, is a subject of some scholarly debate. Arthur Avalon, *The Serpent Power: The Secrets of Tantric and Shaktic Yoga* (1919, 1964; repr., New York: Dover Publications, 1974), 18, 24.

117. He may also have consulted his neighbor Bernarr Macfadden, a promoter of physical culture and a media mogul, who denounced processed food and advocated plenty of fresh fruit and vegetables, whole wheat, and frequent fasts. See Mary Macfadden and Emile Gauvreau, *Dumbbells and Carrot Strips* (New York: Henry Holt & Co., 1953), 239. However, the food at C.C.C. was universally praised.

118. Lecture notes, May 8, 1927, HSRC.

119. In another lecture, he spoke about techniques for prolonging lovemaking and the curative properties of certain yogic postures. "The sphinctor muscles of the vaginal vault can be developed to such an extent that they can grip a broom handle and retain it against a full strength pull from an individual," he explained in the fall of 1928. "Yoginas have developed such strength and tone of their Vaginas. It would be impossible to picture any female troubles with such a tone." Lecture notes, September 8, 1928, HSRC.

120. One year, some members stayed awake for two days straight, putting the finishing touches on an elaborate "Russian Party" that entailed high tea, dozens of performances, yogic asanas, and a midnight feast. After the show was over and early breakfast was served, they began dancing. When queried by a stunned guest, they explained, "We've had no sleep for forty-eight hours, but we know other ways of refreshing our bodies and minds besides sleeping." Charles Francis Potter, *The Preacher and I: An Autobiography* (New York: Crown Publishers, 1951), 338.

121. E. B. White, "Mammy India," *The New Yorker*, March 3, 1928, 19–20.

122. "Émile Coué," *Encyclopedia of Occultism and Parapsychology*, 5th ed. (Gale Group, 2001), reproduced in *Biography Resource Center* (Farmington Hills, MI: Gale, 2009), galenet.galegroup.com.monstera.cc.columbia.edu:2048/servlet/BioRC.

123. *East-West*, November-December 1928; *New York Times*, October 1, 1928, 33.

124. "My reputation is such that when young [Indian] men come to this country for the purpose of entering universities they are directed to see me in the belief that I can help them in many ways," Bernard explained in a legal statement he made sometime in the early 1920s. "At one time I rented a studio on Broadway . . . where lectures were given to the public by Baba Bahaerati, Dr. Khed Kar, Koli Phar, Dr. P.C.V. Shastri, Dr. Desai." Undated statement, 5, HSRC; Love interview, June 29, 2005. The letters tended to make two related points: Bernard was a scholar of the highest order, and he put his philosophy into action. "I was impressed with the idea that the lecturer had actually lived more philosophy than most [sic] of us will ever know," wrote Edmund Dana, a professor of philosophy at Harvard and the University of Minnesota who studied with Bernard in the early 1920s. "I believe him to be the most able and brilliant exponent of the theory and practice of the Veda in the English-speaking world." Undated document, HSRC; www.vanderbilt.edu/~stringer/welcome.htm (accessed April 29, 2005).

125. Incidentally, the prospectus makes only vague reference to the author of *Yoga: Its Theory and Practice*—"a distinguished educationist of India" and yoga practitioner. I suspect it was Swami Abhedananda who published a book by this title. However, his name may have attracted the wrong sort of attention, since at least one reporter

had singled him out some years before, when he was attracting a healthy following to his Connecticut retreat center.

126. Katherine Mayo, *Mother India* (New York: Harcourt Brace & Co., 1927), ix. Stephen Prothero pointed out Mayo's contribution to perceptions of Hinduism and Hindus in "On Hindu-Bashing in Early 20th Century USA: 'Mother India's Scandalous Swamis,'" *Religions of the United States in Practice*, vol. 2, ed. Colleen McDannell (Princeton, NJ: Princeton University Press, December 2001), www .infinityfoundation.com/mandala/h_es/h_es_proth_hindu.htm (accessed October 13, 2002).

127. Mayo, *Mother India*, 11–12.

128. The full text of Ghandi's review, "The Drain Inspector's Report," appeared in an Ahmadabad-based magazine, *Young India*). Prothero, "On Hindu-Bashing," 2.

129. "We have become used to understanding . . . that the art (perfected by the British) of government includes the harnessing of the secret services of men learned and reported to be honest and honorable for shadowing suspects and for writing up the virtues of the Government of the day as if the certificate had come from disinterested quarters. I hope that Miss Mayo will not take offense if she comes under the shadow of such suspicion." Gandhi, extract of "Drain Inspector's Report," *The Nation* 125, no. 3252 (November 2, 1927): 488; M. K. Gandhi and Rabindranath Tagore, "'Mother India': A Symposium," *The Living Age* 333, no. 4320 (December 15, 1927): 1084, APS online (accessed April 13, 2005).

130. The immediate cause of discord was the Indian Statutory Commission, charged with determining whether India was fit for complete autonomy. The commission was lily-white and so insulted Indians that the heretofore moderate National Congress joined the "extremists" in flouting it. *New York Times*, February 13, 1928, 5.

131. *New York Times*, October 1, 1928, 33; *East-West* 3–6 (November–December 1928); *The Nation* 127, no. 3304 (October 31, 1928): 439.

132. *East-West*, November–December 1928; *New York Times*, October 1, 1928, 33.

133. Extracts from letters to P. A. Bernard from G.C.O. Haas, HSRC.

134. *London Times Educational Supplement*, November 24, 1928, HSRC.

135. Letter, December 17, 1928, HSRC.

136. Thomas, *Hinduism Invades America*, 14, 197.

137. Letter to Dr. Potter, June 3, 1930, HSRC.

138. Joshi letter to Chatterji, June 9, 1930, HSRC.

139. *New York World Telegram*, May 7, 1931, HSRC; Potter, *Preacher and I*, 338.

6. THEOS BERNARD'S SPIRITUAL HEROISM

1. TCB letter to VWB, January 17, 1937; and TCB letter to VWB, one Saturday evening in February, VWB Papers, HSCU.

2. Lecture notes, September 29, 1941, BANC MSS 2005/161z.

3. Letters to VWB, February 16 and March 28, 1937, VWB Papers, HSCU.

4. Letters to VWB, one Saturday evening in February, and March 8, 1937, VWB Papers, HSCU.

5. Ibid.

6. Hackett, "Barbarian Lands," 190.

7. Typed copy of VWB journal, 13–16, HSCU.
8. Ibid., 31.
9. Ibid., 13.
10. Glen wanted none of the trappings of being a teacher or running a school; he was a chemist who kept his commitments in the States to a minimum so he could go to India when the mood struck. Viola also speculates that Hamati trained Glen. He may well be the "family guru" Theos refers to in *Heaven Lies Within Us* (London: Rider and Company, 1940, 1950), 19. See also VWB tr., June 25, 1991, 11–14, 18, HSCU.
11. Hackett, "Barbarian Lands," 248–57.
12. Joseph S. Alter, *Yoga in Modern India: The Body Between Science and Philosophy* (Princeton, NJ: Princeton University Press, 2004).
13. That said, another yoga researcher, Dr. Vasant Rele, impressed Viola, who was returning to the States to start her medical residency, with his physiological interpretations of Sanskrit scriptures such as the *Bhagavad-Gita* and his hypothesis that Kundalini was the vagus nerve. VWB journal, 20–23, VWB Papers, HSCU.
14. Ibid., 23–24, VWB Papers, HSCU.
15. TCB letter to VWB, January 10, 1937, quoted in Douglas Veenhof, *The White Lama: In Search of Theos Bernard* (New York: Doubleday, forthcoming), 104–105.
16. TCB letter to VWB, January 24, 1937, VWB Papers, HSCU.
17. Bernard, *Heaven Lies Within Us*, 126–30.
18. Theos debated which department to study in—philosophy or anthropology—and ultimately was the first Columbia University graduate to be awarded a doctorate in the Department of Religion.
19. TCB letter to VWB, April 7, 1937, VWB Papers, HSCU.
20. TCB letter to VWB, January 24, 1937, VWB Papers, HSCU.
21. See also *Time*, April 26, 1937.
22. Kovoor T. Behanan, *Yoga: A Scientific Evaluation* (New York: Macmillan Company, 1937), 234
23. *Time*, April 26, 1937.
24. Behanan, *Yoga*, xi.
25. Data was from Miller's Book Store and Davison-Paxon's Department Store. "Best Sellers of the Week Here and Elsewhere," *New York Times*, May 10, 1937, 16.
26. Series 2.1, folder 28, and Series 6, folders 31, 32, BANC MSS 2005/161z. Transcript of VWB's notes re letters from TCB from India and Tibet, July/August 1996, 34–35, VWB Papers, HSCU.
27. VWB tr., June 25, 1991, 18, VWB Papers, HSCU.
28. Hackett, "Barbarian Lands," 407.
29. "Secret Rites I Saw in Darkest Tibet, I Was a Lama," *Daily Mail* (U.K.), November 13, 1937, 13, 16, quoted in Hackett, "Barbarian Lands," 664–65.
30. See contracts from Bell Syndicates dated December 14, 1937, and from North American Newspaper Alliance dated December 8, 1937, and undated letter from William B. Chamberlain to John N. Wheeler, BANC MSS 2005/161z.
31. James Hilton, *Lost Horizon* (New York and London: Pocket Books, 1933, 1960), 138–39.
32. It goes almost without saying that Americans were still deeply ambivalent about the Orient and its intoxicating mysticism. Capra's Shangri-La is oppressively peaceful.

The Americans who believed in its existence flirted with madness. Those who tried to return flirted with death.

33. *New York Times*, December 26, 1937.
34. Quoted in Veenhof, *White Lama*, 471–72.
35. VWB tr., June 25, 1991, 28, VWB Papers, HSCU; Bernard, *Heaven Lies Within Us*, 14. See also Hackett, "Barbarian Lands," 213n547.
36. Apparently, Theos's mother, Aura Gordon, had suffered ill health for much of her life and had exhausted Theosophy, yoga, and other veins of Eastern religion in her quest for health, happiness, or at the very least solace. Glen left Aura when Theos was only two years old and so did little to shape Theos's earliest impressions of Indic thought.
37. Veenhof, *White Lama*, 25; Hackett, "Barbarian Lands," 195–96.
38. VWB tr., June 25, 1991, 29. See also letters to Mrs. Bernard from Raisbeck, June 6 and 9, 1938, VWB Papers, HSCU. "I was much impressed by the change of the heart size. I believe that the effect of his abdominal exercises and the . . . circulation may be a factor here."
39. Milton J. Raisbeck letter to TCB, August 28, 1938, VWB Papers, HSCU; Letter from TCB to VWB, May 29, 1938, quoted in Veenhof, *White Lama*, 493–94.
40. Transcript VWB's notes re letters from TCB from India and Tibet, July/August 1996, 11, VWB Papers, HSCU. See also letter from Charles A. Lindbergh to TCB, September 24, 1937, BANC MSS 2005/161z.
41. Hackett, "Barbarian Lands," 687–90.
42. NBC Artists Services Memo no. 38, January 1939, BANC MSS 2005/161z.
43. Veenhof, *White Lama*, 510.
44. Hackett, "Barbarian Lands," 672–75.
45. Ibid., 683–86; VWB tr., June 25, 1991, 17, VWB Papers, HSCU. "Divorce Decree Granted to Mme. Ganna Walska," *Los Angeles Times*, July 14, 1946.
46. Circulation and readership details are based on *Cleveland and the Family Circle Magazine: A Study of the Market Characteristics and the Magazine Reading Habits of Cleveland Housewives* (Newark, NJ: The Family Circle, 1942), 62; Veenhof, *White Lama*, 521.
47. Veenhof, *White Lama*, 510–11.
48. Bernard, *Heaven Lies Within Us*, 161, 191–95.
49. Ibid., 62–64.
50. N. E. Sjoman, *The Yoga Tradition of the Mysore Palace* (New Delhi: Abhinav Publications, 1999), 47.
51. Bernard, *Heaven Lies Within Us*, 243–52.
52. Hackett, "Barbarian Lands," 700n1880.
53. Veenhof, *White Lama*, 513.
54. Hackett, "Barbarian Lands," 898, 912–14.
55. Veenhof, *White Lama*, 515.
56. "Miscellaneous fan mail," Series 6, carton 4, folders 61, 62, BANC MSS 2005/161z. There was a ready model for this format: Paramahansa Yogananda, who had headquarters in Los Angeles, had had considerable success teaching yoga this way for years. Thomas, *Hinduism Invades America*, 170.
57. Horne letter, December 30, 1939, TCB reply, February 16, 1940, "Miscellaneous fan mail," Series 6, carton 4, folders 61, 62, BANC MSS 2005/161z.

58. Hankins letter, January 31, 1940, TCB reply, February 7, 1940, "Miscellaneous fan mail," Series 6, carton 4, folders 61, 62, BANC MSS 2005/161z.

59. Mary Wilkeson letter to TCB, August 7, 1939, "Miscellaneous fan mail," Series 6, carton 4, folders 61, 62, BANC MSS 2005/161z.

60. Lecture notes, May 11 and October 19, 1939, BANC MSS 2005/161z.

61. Marianne Lamonaca and Jonathan Mogul, eds., *Grand Hotels of the Jazz Age: The Architecture of Schultze & Weaver* (Miami: The Wolfsonian-Florida International University; New York: Princeton Architectural Press: 2005), 10–15, 30–31, 217–18.

62. *Wall Street Journal*, March 8, 1932; *New York Times*, October 27, 1938. Getty, it later came out, besides steadying the hotel's finances, was orchestrating elaborate and illegal transactions there—sending oil to Nazi Germany via Mexico—and had installed a number of spies and traitors. *Telegraph* (U.K.), August 24, 2003.

63. In 1939 the influx of new residents into the Hotel Pierre's soaring tower routinely made the papers. Top business executives—Raymond Rubicam, chairman of the ad firm Young & Rubicam; a vice president of Bethlehem Steel; the owner of the Red Sox; the treasurer of Warner Bros.—leased suites, as did actresses and diplomats (including the consul general of Iraq). Most had views of the park. Macy's ad in *The New York Times*, October 26, 1930, quoted in Lamonaca and Mogul, *Grand Hotels*, 31; *New York Times*: "Dr. Stuart Craig Takes Penthouse," September 27, 1939, 51; "East Side Duplex for L. W. Douglas," September 29, 1939, 45; "Music Notes," November 22, 1939, 16.

64. Hackett, "Barbarian Lands," 726, 728.

65. Ibid., 726.

66. Brochure drafts, Pierre Health Studios, 1938–41, BANC MSS 2005/161z.

67. *Family Circle* 15, no. 8 (August 25, 1939): 14–15, 18, 21; Hackett, "Barbarian Lands," 737–47; Veenhof, *White Lama*, 426; Ganna Walska, *Always Room at the Top* (New York: Richard R. Smith, 1943).

68. Take just his brief description of the chakras: "Study nature of body from abstract side, what the subtle forces are, known as the tattvas that control its every manifestation, how this law of fate is fulfilling itself, all the laws that pertain to the subtle and abstract side of human nature." Pierre Health Studios curriculum, n.d., BANC MSS 2005/161z.

69. Hackett, "Barbarian Lands," 730–31.

70. Vivekananda, "Six Lessons on Raja Yoga: Fourth Lesson," www.ramakrishna vivekananda.info/vivekananda/volume_8/vol_8_frame.htm (accessed June 9, 2009).

71. TCB lecture notes, "The Psychological Basis of Yoga," n.d., 11, BANC MSS 2005/161z.

72. Introduction to seminar "How to Live Yoga Today" and "The Psychological Basis of Yoga," c. 1939, BANC MSS 2005/161z. This lecture may have been delivered at De Vries's Living Arts Studio in Manhattan, where Theos had been lecturing just before establishing the American Institute of Yoga. Hackett, "Barbarian Lands," 720.

73. This lecture was given to private classes that were a forerunner to his Pierre Health Studios, May 10, 1939, BANC MSS 2005/161z.

74. Feuerstein, *Encyclopedia of Yoga*, 146, 339; Lecture notes, May 2, 1939, BANC MSS 2005/161z.

75. Lecture draft, "The Psychological Basis of Yoga," c. 1939, BANC MSS 2005/161z.

76. Lecture notes dated May 1, 1940, BANC MSS 2005/161z.

77. Lecture notes, May 10, 1939; the Pierre Health Studios' "Full Course in Yogic Physical Culture for an Average Man of Health" entailed ten postures, one mudra, one Bandha, two Kriyas, and two pranayamas. Translated into plain language, the student would perform back bends and forward bends, headstands, balance her whole body on her elbows (Mayurasana), among other poses, then tighten various sphincters to lock the breath in the body, before churning her abdominal muscles for about eight minutes and then attempting the breathing exercises. Theos included Kumbhaka, or breath retention, if the student was capable. BANC MSS 2005/161z.
78. Notes on physiological yoga, c. 1939, BANC MSS 2005/161z.
79. Lecture notes, May 17, 1939, BANC MSS 2005/161z.
80. *Daily News*, April 13, 1940, VWB Papers, HSCU.
81. Birrell & Dimmock correspondence, 1941, BANC MSS 2005/161z.
82. Hackett, "Barbarian Lands," 743–47.
83. *American Weekly*, December 12, 1943, quoted in Veenhof, *White Lama*, 463.
84. Hackett, "Barbarian Lands," 737–47; Veenhof, *White Lama*, 426; Walska, *Always Room at the Top*, 487–90.
85. Lecture notes, October 23, 1942, BANC MSS 2005/161z.
86. Ibid.
87. Hackett, "Barbarian Lands," 770–74.
88. Bernard, *Heaven Lies Within Us*, 52, 75, 129.
89. Lecture notes, May 8, 1939, BANC MSS 2005/161z; Bernard, *Heaven Lies Within Us*, 28–30. While the sequence of events Theos relates in *HLWU* is falsified and the identity of his real guru veiled, Theos did master advanced Hatha Yoga practices.
90. Lecture notes, October 15, 1942, BANC MSS 2005/161z.
91. Lecture notes, October 8, 1942, BANC MSS 2005/161z.
92. Lecture notes, October 15, 1942, BANC MSS 2005/161z.
93. *Family Circle* 15, no. 8 (August 25, 1939): 14–15, 18, 21.
94. Lecture notes, May 23, 1939, BANC MSS 2005/161z.
95. Claire Pricelondon, "Indian Magician Again Puzzles Scientists," *New York Times*, October 20, 1935, SM9.
96. Lecture notes, October 15, 1942, BANC MSS 2005/161z; *The New Yorker*, January 8, 1938, 32. Hatha Yoga was now spoofed ad nauseam; usually some naïf and frivolous female, taking some pose or proselytizing about yoga, produced raised eyebrows. Occasionally, an intrepid writer would attempt yoga on her own and report back the disappointing results. See *The New Yorker* cartoon, March 30, 1935; *New Yorker* cartoon by Richard Decker, January 8, 1938; Cornelia Otis Skinner, "Yoga Attempted," *New Yorker*, June 8, 1938.
97. The Teachers College and Columbia University professors in general had long been receptive to yoga; many professors affiliated with the university are listed in the ISVAR prospectus funded by Pierre Bernard.
98. See *Vanity Fair*, May 2007; "Art of Relaxation to Be Taught in Spring at Teachers College," *New York Times*, November 30, 1939, 23.
99. For every piece hailing Hatha Yoga as a complete system of self-culture, two reduced it to mere acrobatics. The boxer Lou Nova trained up at C.C.C. with Theos's half uncle, and sports reporters seemed to agree that yoga would help him. However, one reader felt compelled to point out that Nova was studying Hatha Yoga,

which, while powerful enough, dealt "purely with the physical and bodily functions." Letters to the sports editors, *New York Times*, August 30, 1941.

100. Lecture notes, October 15, 1942, BANC MSS 2005/161z.

101. *Gettysburg (PA) Times*, July 13, 1946, quoted in Hackett, "Barbarian Lands," 799.

7. MARGARET WOODROW WILSON "TURNS HINDU"

1. "Margaret Wilson Embraces Brahmin Faith; President's Daughter Joins Retreat in India," *New York Times*, June 17, 1940, 17.

2. The last time Margaret Wilson's name had prominently appeared in the papers had been almost fourteen years before, when she had refused to press charges against two boys who burglarized her Greenwich Village apartment, and then soon after, when she was sued for an unpaid loan. Ronald M. Johnson, "Journey to Pondicherry: Margaret Woodrow Wilson and the Aurobindo Ashram," *Indian Journal of American Studies* (Hyderabad: American Studies Research Center) 21, no. 2 (1991): 3.

3. *Washington Post*, June 17, 1940, 29.

4. Only two published biographical sketches of Margaret Woodrow Wilson deal with her years in Pondicherry, and both are by Georgetown historian Ronald M. Johnson. Besides his "Journey to Pondicherry," see his essay "The Ramakrishna Mission to America: An Intercultural Study," in *American Studies in Transition*, ed. David E. Nye and Christen Kold Thomsen (Odense, Denmark: Odense University Press, 1985), 79–96.

5. Eleanor Wilson McAdoo and Margaret Y. Gaffey, *The Woodrow Wilsons* (New York: Macmilllan Company, 1937), 41.

6. Johnson, "Journey to Pondicherry," 3; "Margaret Woodrow Wilson Finds Peace as Disciple of Yoga in India," *New York Times*, January 28, 1943, 21.

7. Sri Aurobindo, *The Integral Yoga: Sri Aurobindo's Teaching and Method of Practice* (Twin Lakes, WI: Lotus Press, 1993), 29. See Stephen Phillips, "Aurobindo's Philosophy of Brahman" (Leider, Netherlands: E. J. Brill, 1986), electronic edition, March 2001, 133.

8. McDermott, *Essential Aurobindo*, 64–82, 164–70. See also Phillips, "Aurobindo's Philosophy of Brahman," 125.

9. McDermott, *Essential Aurobindo*, 152–54.

10. This methodology came largely out of Aurobindo's own mystical experiences, which began not long after he started practicing pranayama and progressed over his lifetime. Phillips, "Aurobindo's Philosophy of Brahman," 74, 79. See also Feuerstein, *Yoga Tradition*, 55–58.

11. Excerpt of an undated fragment written by Margaret W. Wilson, Wilson-McAdoo Papers LOC.

12. "Margaret Woodrow Wilson Finds Peace," 21.

13. From a letter by Boyd Fisher to Margaret W. Wilson, February 21, 1924, Wilson-McAdoo Papers LOC.

14. Thomas J. Pritchett letter to Margaret W. Wilson, September 3, 1925, Wilson-McAdoo Papers LOC.

15. Letters from Thomas Pritchett, 1924–26, Wilson-McAdoo Papers LOC. Historian Ronald M. Johnson characterizes Pritchett as an acquaintance whose relationship to Margaret was partly business in nature. However, his correspondence with her

suggests a much more intimate relationship, one that was also somewhat secretive. Johnson, "Journey to Pondicherry," 3.

16. Letter to Margaret W. Wilson, December 30, 1940, Wilson-McAdoo Papers LOC.

17. Excerpt from Margaret W. Wilson letter to Eleanor Wilson-McAdoo as cited in Johnson, "Ramakrishna Mission," 88.

18. For Bodhananda's teaching see Display Ad 10, no title, *New York Times*, April 20, 1935, 9. The AEL drummed up support for its cause with parades and speeches. Riots often ensued. In Bellingham, Washington, in 1907, a mob of five hundred attacked two Indians and then destroyed their waterfront barracks. Indian workers feared for their lives. Local officials made mostly empty promises to protect them. Editorialists on the West Coast took up the AEL's cause. "The Hindu is not a good citizen," wrote the editor of the *Bellingham Herald*, no matter that most Indian laborers were Sikhs. "It would require centuries to assimilate him, and our country need not take the trouble." Joan M. Jensen, *Passage from India* (New Haven and London: Yale University Press, 1988), 44–52.

19. Jensen, *Passage from India*, 2–15, 139, 142–61.

20. McAdoo and Gaffey, *Woodrow Wilsons*, 118.

21. Undated letter, Wilson-McAdoo Collection UCSB.

22. Letter from Sri Aurobindo to Margaret W. Wilson, September 17 (or 7), 1936. Transcript of letter is available at the official Auroville (the name of the town surrounding the ashram) website, www.auroville.org/art&culture/theatre/nishtha.htm.

23. Letter from N. K. Gupta to Margaret W. Wilson, December 19, 1937, Wilson-McAdoo Collection UCSB.

24. The website Measuring Worth, www.measuringworth.com, offers a number of data points for comparison. In 2005, $2,500 from 1937 is worth:

      $34,000.70   using the Consumer Price Index
      $27,933.60   using the GDP deflator
      $77,451.60   using the value of consumer bundle
      $77,667.98   using the unskilled wage
      $147,468.22   using the nominal GDP per capita
      $338,841.13   using the relative share of GDP

Letter to the Mother, May 29, 1939, Wilson-McAdoo Collection UCSB; Letter from Gupta to Wilson, December 19, 1937.

25. Undated letter to Lois Roth Kellog, summer of 1936, Wilson-McAdoo Collection, UCSB.

26. Undated letter to Eliot Clark (c. early 1938), Wilson-McAdoo Collection UCSB.

27. Bernard, *Heaven Lies Within Us*, 250.

28. Undated letter to Eliot Clark, winter 1937–38, Wilson-McAdoo Collection UCSB.

29. Letter from N. K. Gupta, July 12, 1938, Wilson-McAdoo Collection UCSB.

30. Letter to Connie and unknown, c. summer 1938, Wilson-McAdoo Collection UCSB.

31. Johnson, "Journey to Pondicherry," 2.

32. *New York Herald Tribune*, February 14, 1944, BANC MSS 2005/161z. Nor had she limited herself to a single issue. Dr. Cowles's "healing cult," the community-center movement, Montessori Educational Association of America, and the women's rights movement were among the causes that crowded her curriculum vitae. See also Johnson, "Journey to Pondicherry," 4.

33. Johnson, "Journey to Pondicherry," 3.

34. Letter to Connie and unknown, c. summer 1938, Wilson-McAdoo Collection UCSB. Not long after Wilson left for Pondicherry, Brunton embarked on his third tour of the subcontinent, though the two never crossed paths. Annie Fung Cahn, "Paul Brunton: A Bridge Between India and the West," translated from "Paul Brunton: Un pont entre l'Inde et l'Occident," (Ph.D. diss., Department of Religious Anthropology, Université de Paris IV, Sorbonne, 1992), 39–40.

35. *Good Housekeeping*, "Who Is the Lady with the Mask?" November 1925, 67.

36. *Time*, "Passage to India," January 18, 1937.

37. Besides the collections of Margaret Woodrow Wilson's letters at the University of California at Santa Barbara and the Library of Congress, which had originally been a single set, some additional letters are in the Sri Aurobindo Ashram archives in Pondicherry, India. See Margaret W. Wilson letter to Mother Lalita, October 27, 1942, Wilson-McAdoo Papers, LOC.

38. Letter to Margaret W. Wilson by Swami Nikhilananda, September 20, 1938, Wilson-McAdoo Papers LOC.

39. Letter to Swami N., undated, c. fall of 1938; letter to Tantine, November 15, 1938. Letter to Eleanor McAdoo, November 1936, Wilson-McAdoo Collection UCSB, refers to her apartment and her "cute little closet kichenette." The stationery has a printed header that reads 134 West Fourth Street, which is crossed out on the first page, and Wilson wrote her new address, 1028 Park Avenue, below; presumably the Park Avenue apartment, on Manhattan's Upper East Side, is the one she is describing. Johnson, "Journey to Pondicherry," 4.

40. Letter to Mr. and Mrs. Gorham, undated, c. early January 1939, Wilson-McAdoo Collection UCSB.

41. Letter from Margaret W. Wilson, November 15, 1938, Wilson-McAdoo Collection UCSB; Linda Prugh, *Josephine Macleod and Vivekananda's Mission* (Mylapore, India: Sri Ramakrishna Math, 1999), 453.

42. Letter to Nell, January 6, 1939, Wilson-McAdoo Collection UCSB.

43. Letter to Elizabeth, undated, c. early 1939, Wilson-McAdoo Collection UCSB.

44. Letter to Nell, January 6, 1939, Wilson-McAdoo Collection UCSB.

45. Swami Nikhilananda, "Sri Aurobindo: The Silent Yogi," *Asia*, December 1938, 734.

46. McDermott, *Essential Aurobindo*, 43.

47. Feuerstein, *Encyclopedia*, 254. The former posits the unity of all existence but deems nature illusory, or maya; the latter divides reality into purusha, or pure consciousness, and prakriti, nature, the point of yoga being to disentangle the two. Aurobindo, *Integral Yoga*, 29.

48. See Phillips, "Aurobindo's Philosophy of Brahman," 82–84.

49. McDermott, *Essential Aurobindo*, 105.

50. From Romain Rolland, *Prophets of the New India*, as cited by Nikhilananda, "Sri Aurobindo," 733.

51. Ibid. The actual date is taken from the timeline of Aurobindo's life in McDermott, *Essential Aurobindo*, 42. See also, Stephen H. Phillips, "Yogic *ekagrata*: The Analogical Key to Aurobindo's Philosophy," link.lanic.utexas.edu/asnic/phillips/pages/yoga/ekagrataaurobindo.pdf; Phillips, "Aurobindo's Philosophy of Brahman," 56.

    Apparently Aurobindo was consulted in preparation of "Yoga: Its Theory and Practice," though as far as the record shows, the book was never completed or published. Interestingly, none of Aurobindo's books are listed in the catalog of Pierre Bernard's library.

52. McDermott, *Essential Aurobindo*, 26.

53. Letter to Lois Roth Kellog, June 8, 1939, Wilson-McAdoo Collection UCSB; undated writing, Wilson-McAdoo Papers LOC; letter to Elsie Walsh, May 1939, Wilson-McAdoo Collection UCSB.

54. "But I'm not going to worry about that any more for now that which is called my income is really yours and at all times at your disposal." Letter to the Mother, May 29, 1939, Wilson-McAdoo Collection UCSB.

55. The Congress resigned because the British demanded the nationalists' commitment to the war effort but refused to address the issue of independence. Sugata Bose and Ayesha Jalal, *Modern South Asia: History, Culture, Political Economy*, 2nd ed. (New York: Routledge, 2004), 128–34.

56. Undated letter to Elsie Weil, Wilson-McAdoo Collection UCSB.

57. "Hull Promises Refugee Ships for the Orient," *Chicago Daily Tribune* (1872–1963), October 13, 1940, ProQuest Historical Newspapers, *Chicago Tribune* (1849–1986), 6.

58. The swami privately effused about her work and, in his preface, thanks both Joseph Campbell and Margaret, for "her ungrudging help." Nikhilananda, *Gospel of Sri Ramakrishna*, viii.

59. Letter to Mr. and Mrs. Gorham, January 1939, Wilson-McAdoo Collection UCSB.

60. Swamis from the Ramakrishna Mission supplied lists of prominent American scholars of religion and philosophy who might be sympathetic. She knew some— her name had opened many doors, including those to academia—and friends such as Elsie Weil, an editor at *Asia* magazine, happily connected her to those thinkers, such as George Santayana, she wasn't already acquainted with.

61. In early 1942, Aldous Huxley received a copy of what is likely *The Life Divine*; he mentions "three vast tomes" sent directly from Pondicherry, of which he said, "It looks good, as I glance through it, but is intolerably too long and verbose." Seven years later his opinion seems to have changed somewhat. He offered to recommend Aurobindo for the Nobel Prize in literature and described *The Life Divine* as "a book not merely of the highest importance as regards its content, but remarkably fine as a piece of philosophic and religious literature." See letter 459, to Christopher Isherwood, and letter 554, to Dilip Kumar Roy, in *The Letters of Aldous Huxley*, ed. Grover Smith (New York: Harper & Row, 1969), 475, 585.

62. Letter from Nikhilananda, January 9, 1939, Wilson-McAdoo Papers LOC; letter to Swami Nikhilananda, May 24, 1940, Wilson-McAdoo Collection UCSB.

63. Margaret's diary, Wilson-McAdoo Collection UCSB.

64. Excerpts of letters to Lois Roth Kellog, quoted by Seyril Schochen, *Nistitha: The Strange Disappearance of Margaret Woodrow Wilson* (unpublished play).

65. Margaret's diary, October 5, 1940, Wilson-McAdoo Collection UCSB.

66. Letter from Tantine, December 30, 1940, Wilson-McAdoo Papers LOC.

67. Undated letter to Ellen Plautiff, Wilson-McAdoo Papers LOC.

68. Letter to Margaret W. Wilson, May 9, 1925, Wilson-McAdoo Papers LOC.

69. Letter to Elsie Weil, 1941, Wilson-McAdoo Papers LOC.

70. *New York Times*, February 14, 1944. Margaret's remains are memorialized by a simple inscription, written in French, which reads, "Here lie / The Mortal Remains / of Nishtha / Margaret Woodrow Wilson / 16 April 1886–12 February 1944. www .srichinmoylibrary.com/america-depths/8.html.

71. Ganna Walska letter to TCB, February 14, 1944, BANC MSS 2005/161z.

72. TCB letter to VWB, March 28, 1937, VWB Papers, HSCU.

8. UNCOVERING REALITY IN HOLLYWOOD

1. See Feuerstein, *Shambhala Encyclopedia*, 206.
2. Christopher Isherwood, *My Guru and His Disciple* (London: Eyre Methuen, 1980), 34–35.
3. See for example Swami Prabhavananda, "Sri Ramakrishna, Modern Spirit, and Religion," in *Vedanta for the Western World*, ed., with an introduction by, Christopher Isherwood (Vedanta Press, 1945; repr., New York: Viking Press, 1960), 250.
4. *Eight Limbs of Yoga: A Lecture by Swami Prabhavananda*, filmed in 1971 (Hollywood: Vedanta Press, 2005); Isherwood, *My Guru and His Disciple*, 48.
5. Wyckoff had been a disciple of Swami Turiyananda, also a direct disciple of Ramakrishna. Isherwood, *My Guru and His Disciple*, 22–23, 33–35. "Two streets over the cylindrical windows and round towers of 1897—melancholy antiques which sheltered swamis, yogis, fortune tellers, dressmakers, dancing teachers, art academics and chiropractors—looked down now upon brisk buses and trolleys" is how F. Scott Fitzgerald introduced his 1928 short story "Magnetism" in *The Saturday Evening Post*, ably conjuring shabbiness and irrelevance. *The Saturday Evening Post*, March 3, 1928.
6. Isherwood, *My Guru and His Disciple*, 34–35.
7. Kevin Starr, *Embattled Dreams: California in War and Peace, 1940–1950* (Oxford, UK: Oxford University Press, 2002), 3–11.
8. Gerald Heard, "My Discoveries in Vedanta," in Isherwood, *Vedanta for the Western World*, 59–63.
9. Alison Falby, "Heard, Henry Fitzgerald (1889–1971)," *Oxford Dictionary of National Biography* (Oxford, UK: Oxford University Press, 2004), www.oxforddnb.com/view/article/54040 (accessed December 13, 2007).
10. Isherwood, *My Guru and His Disciple*, 9–11. See William York Tindall, "Transcendentalism in Contemporary Literature," in *The Asian Legacy in American Life*, ed. Arthur E. Christy (1942; repr., New York: Greenwood Press, 1968), 189.
11. Gerald Heard, "Vedanta as the Scientific Approach to Religion," based on a lecture given in 1939, in Isherwood, *Vedanta for the Western World*, 54.
12. Isherwood, *My Guru and His Disciple*, 77.
13. Isherwood, *My Guru and His Disciple*, 49–50; *Letters of Aldous Huxley*, ed. Grover Smith (New York: Harper & Row, 1969), 569–70. There is no record of the exact date of Huxley's initiation. See Sybille Bedford, *Aldous Huxley: A Biography, Volume Two: 1939–1963* (London: Chatto & Windus, 1974), 206n.
14. Carey McWilliams, *Southern California Country: An Island on the Land* (New York: Duell, Sloan & Pearce, 1946), 270–71; "The Lee Side o' L.A.," *Los Angeles Times*, September 29, 1937; Arthur Miller, "Aldous Huxley—the Congenital Intellectual," *Los Angeles Times*, May 1, 1938, 7, 21.
15. David King Dunaway, *Huxley in Hollywood* (London: Bloomsbury, 1989), 14–17, 46.
16. "Books of the Times," Charles Poore, *New York Times*, November 19, 1937, 21.
17. *Selected Letters of Aldous Huxley*, ed., and introduction by, James Sexton (Chicago: Ivan R. Dee, 2007), 381–82.
18. See Hal Bridges, "Aldous Huxley: Exponent of Mysticism in America," *Journal of the American Academy of Religion* 37, no. 4 (December 1969): 344–45, links.jstor .org/sici?sici=0002-7189%28196912%2937%3A4%3C341%3AAHEOMI%3E2.0 .CO%3B2-B. See also Huxley's essay "The Minimum Working Hypothesis," in Isherwood, *Vedanta for the Western World*, 34.

19. See his letter to Robert Nichols, January 13, 1935, in Smith, *Letters of Aldous Huxley*, 389.
20. Adamic quoted by McWilliams, *Southern California Country*, 160.
21. John Yale (Swami Vidyatmananda), *The Making of a Devotee* (Gretz, France: Ramakrishna Order of India, Centre Vedantique Ramakrichna, 2003), world.std .com/~elayj/Chapter5.html.
22. Kevin Starr, *The Dream Endures: California Enters the 1940s* (New York: Oxford University Press, 1997), 342.
23. Peter Parker, *Isherwood: A Life* (London: Picador, 2004), 429.
24. This was first published as part of *Goodbye to Berlin* in 1939. Christopher Isherwood, *The Berlin Stories* (New York: New Directions, 1963), vi, 200.
25. Isherwood, *My Guru and His Disciple*, 4, 18–19.
26. Parker, *Isherwood*, 436.
27. Isherwood hewed to the Marxist view that religion was "the opium of the people," and God a coercive fiction who eased the gears of capitalism. But he admired Heard and was eager to meet Huxley, drawn to both in part because of their pacifism. (Huxley's 1937 book, *Ends and Means*, was considered by many a pacifist textbook at the time.) Isherwood, *My Guru and His Disciple*, 6, 11; Parker, *Isherwood*, 430–33.
28. Christopher Isherwood, *Diaries: Volume I, 1939–1960*, ed., and introduced by, Katherine Bucknell (Michael di Capua Books, HarperCollins, 1996), 43–44; Isherwood, *My Guru and His Disciple*, 23–24.
29. Isherwood, *My Guru and His Disciple*, 25–28.
30. Isherwood, *Diaries*, 45.
31. Ibid., 127–29; Feuerstein, *Yoga Tradition*, 132, 350.
32. Isherwood, *Diaries*, 156–57.
33. Ibid., 156, 159.
34. See correspondence from Lloyd Hartman to TCB, February 18, August 25, and September 22, 1941, and TCB's letter to Hartman, August 29, 1941, BANC MSS 2005/161z.
35. Still, Isherwood detected "unhappiness and strain . . . beneath the sleek disguise of her suppleness and charm." Isherwood, *Diaries*, 156.
36. Ibid., 156–57; Isherwood, *My Guru and His Disciple*, 85–87.
37. Ogden Nash, "Don't Shoot Los Angeles," *The New Yorker*, April 18, 1942, 24; quoted in McWilliams, *Southern California Country*, 249.
38. The population of L.A. nearly tripled between 1920 and 1940, when it topped 1.5 million residents, making it the fastest-growing metropolis in the nation's history. McWilliams, *Southern California Country*, 13–14. For census data see Campbell Gibson, "Population of the 100 Largest Cities and Other Urban Places in the United States: 1790 to 1990," Population Division Working Paper No. 27 (Washington, DC: Population Division, U.S. Bureau of the Census, June 1998), www.census .gov/population/www/documentation/twps0027.html, www.census.gov/population/ documentation/twps0027/tab15.txt, www.census.gov/population/documentation/twps 0027/tab16.txt.
39. McWilliams, *Southern California Country*, 240–72.
40. Ibid., 249–50.
41. Ibid., 110–11; Starr, *Dream Endures*, 3.
42. See McWilliams, *Southern California Country*, 10–14; Mike Davis, *City of Quartz: Excavating the Future in Los Angeles* (New York: Vintage Books, 1992), 30–35.

43. Demographics partly explain the unusually high number of health faddists. Among the first to heed the siren call of the Southland were the old and the infirm. They were drawn by early reports by enthusiastic tourists of its climate; one doctor believed it could cure nearly every major disease, tuberculosis, cirrhosis, and insomnia among them. The influx of invalids was so pronounced, out-of-state newspapers referred to the region as "the sanitarium and fruit country." However, the medical establishment was slow to come to L.A., so ill Americans who came were confronted with a shortage of doctors who might cure them. Under these conditions, otherwise conservative Iowans might find much to recommend the Chinese herbalists, osteopaths, chiropractors, and faith healers still highly visible into the 1920s. McWilliams, *Southern California Country*, 98–101, 258.

44. Ibid., 150–56, 343–44.

45. Carl T. Jackson, *Vedanta for the West* (Bloomington and Indianapolis: Indiana University Press, 1994), 32.

46. Tingley succeeded William Judge as head of the American Theosophical Society, which had seceded from the international organization. See Catherine L. Albanese, *Republic of Mind and Spirit*, 353.

47. McWilliams, *Southern California Country*, 252–53.

48. *Theosophical Path Magazine, January to June 1916*, ed. Katherine Tingley (Point Loma, CA: The Aryan Theosophical Press; repr., Kessinger Publishing, 2003), 185–86; Albanese, *Republic of Mind and Spirit*, 354.

49. Albanese, *Republic of Mind and Spirit*, 351–52. Annie Besant, who headed up the Theosophical Society's international wing, took a more extreme tack, at one point disavowing yoga in toto. See Robert Love, "Fear of Yoga," *Columbia Journalism Review*, November/December 2006, 80–90. Love conflates yoga and Hatha Yoga in his analysis. In the fall of 1909, Besant went on the record, insisting that "theosophy and Yogaism have nothing in common . . . the latter is, in fact, emphatically repudiated by the advanced thinkers." She defined yoga as "a development of psychic power." "Yoga Shocks Annie Besant," *Chicago Daily Tribune* (1872–1963), September 18, 1909, ProQuest Historical Newspapers, *Chicago Tribune* (1849–1986), 3; "'Yoga' Divides Theosophy Ranks," *Chicago Daily Tribune* (1872–1963), September 19, 1909, ProQuest Historical Newspapers, *Chicago Tribune* (1849–1986), 3; "'Yoga' Followers Shut Out of Hall," *Chicago Daily Tribune* (1872–1963), September 20, 1909, ProQuest Historical Newspapers, *Chicago Tribune* (1849–1986), 8.

50. "'Yoga' Divides Theosophy Ranks," 3.

51. Tingley, *Theosophical Path Magazine*, 185–86.

52. *Los Angeles Times*, August 7, 1901, 4; October 28, 1901, 7.

53. McWilliams, *Southern California Country*, 252–55.

54. Thomas, *Hinduism Invades America*, 104, 287.

55. "Native Lecturer of India Is Honored Guest at Dinner," *Los Angeles Times* (1886–Current File), January 4, 1925, 14; Alma Whitaker, "Swami Praises Spiritual Calm," *Los Angeles Times* (1886–Current File), January 19, 1925, A18.

56. *How to Know God: The Yoga Aphorisms of Patanjali*, trans., and with a commentary by, Swami Prabhavananda and Christopher Isherwood (Vedanta Press, 1953; repr., New York: New American Library, 1969), 47–48, 113–17; Yogananda, *Autobiography of a Yogi*, 264n.

57. The goal of yoga, as Yogananda formulated it, was to be "calmly active and actively calm." Thomas, *Hinduism Invades America*, 142. This was Yogananda's rendering of

Kriya Yoga, which is mentioned in the *Yoga Sutras*. It's considered by some to be Patanjali's only innovation, by others as simply a synonym for Karma Yoga. See Feuerstein, *Shambhala Encyclopedia*, 159. On Yogananda's Tantric roots, see Albanese, *Republic of Mind and Spirit*, 370.

58. See Prabhavananda and Isherwood, *How to Know God*, 104–105.

59. Yogananda, *Autobiography of a Yogi*, 289.

60. Ibid., 275–85; Albanese, *Republic of Mind and Spirit*, 370; "Make Yourself Venus," *Los Angeles Times* (1886–Current File), March 4, 1923, III13; "Émile Coué," *Encyclopedia of Occultism and Parapsychology*, 5th ed. (Gale Group, 2001), reproduced in *Biography Resource Center* (Farmington Hills, MI: Gale, 2009), galenet.gale group.com.monstera.cc.columbia.edu:2048/servlet/BioRC.

61. Here's an example of Yogananda's lecture schedule for January 10–17, 1932, in Kansas City:

Sunday	Everlasting Youth
Monday	How to Get What You Need (New Law of Success)
Tuesday	Developing Dynamic Power of Will for Lasting Success
Wednesday	Greatest Science of Healing
Thursday	Law of Attracting Abundance and Health Consciously
Friday	Highest Technique of Meditation
Saturday	Spiritual Marriage (How to scientifically attract your ideal life companion)
Sunday	Highest Science of Superconcentration and All Round Success—Yogoda

At ompage.net/SwamiYogananda/SwamiYogananda.htm (accessed July 15, 2009).

62. See Alma Whitaker, "Tete-à-tete," *Los Angeles Times* (1886–Current File), January 25, 1925, C18; Thomas, *Hinduism Invades America*, 148.

63. Yogananda, *Autobiography of a Yogi*, 345; Thomas, *Hinduism Invades America*, 148; "Swami Under Investigation," *Los Angeles Times* (1886–Current File), October 17, 1925, A1.

64. Thomas, *Hinduism Invades America*, 145–51.

65. Ibid., 148–73.

66. "Swami Under Investigation," A1.

67. "Swami Sued for $500,000," *Los Angeles Times* (1886–Current File), October 24, 1939, 5; "Swami Denies Profits Made by Hindu Philosophy School; Answer to $500,000 Suit Also Declares Petitioner Has No Interest in Enterprise," *Los Angeles Times*, April 8, 1940, 5; "Swami Fights $500,000 Aide's Demand in Court; Ex-Associate of Teacher of Hindu Philosophy Asks Accounting in Addition to Cash Plea," *Los Angeles Times*, December 4, 1940, A1; "Swami's Share Profits Pledge Told at Trial; Plaintiff Quotes Yogananda as Declaring Their Assets Valued at $1,000,000," *Los Angeles Times*, December 5, 1940, 2; "Swami Strikes Suit Contention; Letter Introduced Against Partnership Claim of Ex-Aide," *Los Angeles Times*, December 6, 1940, 11; "Absent Swami Wins in Court," *Los Angeles Times*, December 11, 1940, 2.

68. Isherwood, *My Guru and His Disciple*, 73–77, 100–103; Isherwood, *Diaries*, 143–44.

69. Isherwood, *Diaries*, 151.

70. Letter 469, to Swami Prabhavananda, in Smith, *Letters of Aldous Huxley*, 485. Isherwood was also well aware that some of his friends actively disapproved of his decision. This was precisely the problem. Isherwood felt caught between worlds—

Hollywood and its beau monde and Vedanta. As he put it, "If you'd . . . asked, 'What are you?' how could I have answered. 'A would-be monk?,' 'A writer at Paramount,' 'A celibate as from February 6,' 'A vegetarian, except on Christmas Day.'" Isherwood, *My Guru and His Disciple*, 99; Isherwood, *Diaries*, 261–62.

71. Isherwood, *Diaries*, 240, 261.

72. Isherwood, *My Guru and His Disciple*, 102, 112–15.

73. Swami Brahmananda was the head of the Ramakrishna Mission during the 1910s and early 1920s and Prabhavananda's own guru.

74. The shrine and its contents had been imported from India. Isherwood, *My Guru and His Disciple*, 57–59.

75. Ibid., 57–58.

76. Ibid., 121–23.

77. Ibid., 103–4; Isherwood, *Diaries*, 267–68.

78. *Contemporary Authors Online* (Gale, 2009), reproduced in *Biography Resource Center* (Farmington Hills, MI: Gale, 2009), galenet.galegroup.com.monstera.ccc .columbia.edu:2048/servlet/BioRC (accessed October 8, 2009); Tindall, "Transcendentalism in Contemporary Literature," 189–92.

79. Isherwood, *Diaries*, 252, 328–29; Isherwood, *My Guru and His Disciple*, 152.

80. Isherwood described the Viertels' house as a "haven of peace, after the tumults of monastic life." Berthold and Salka Viertel came to the States from Austria (though Salka was Polish by birth). Isherwood would also spend time away from the Vedanta Center altogether, taking weekends in Santa Monica and Long Beach. Isherwood, *Diaries*, 292, 1006–1008.

81. Ibid., 50, 119, 308. Isherwood promises to introduce his good friend Salka Viertel to Swami Prabhavananda. See also the Temple Archives when access becomes available.

82. Isherwood, *Diaries*, 308.

83. Yale, *Making of a Devotee*, world.std.com/~elayj/Chapter5.html.

84. Isherwood, *Diaries*, 974–75.

85. Robert Lawrence Balzer, *Beyond Conflict* (Indianapolis: Bobbs-Merrill Company, 1963), cover copy and 40–42; interview, June 11, 2007. See also Brandy Brent, "Carrousel," *Los Angeles Times*, January 19, 1950, ProQuest Historical Newspapers, *Los Angeles Times*, B2.

86. Isherwood moved out of the center right after the war and then almost immediately dove headlong into Hollywood and a series of love affairs, making only rare visits to see the swami. Isherwood, *Diaries*, 383–85; Isherwood, *Lost Years*, 81, 173, 181; *My Guru and His Disciple*, 194.

87. The Marcel Rodd edition came out in August 1944. Isherwood, *Diaries*, 348, 350, 354. Huxley was still in touch with Prabhavananda and still contributing to the society's magazine, *Vedanta and the West*. Smith, *Letters of Aldous Huxley*, 16–17, 574; "Universal Cult," *Time*, February 12, 1945. The issue featured an image of Himmler on the cover, with skull and crossbones on his hatband. Isherwood was humiliated, bemused, and offended by the *Time* piece, the latter in regard to its description of Prabhavananda, which Isherwood found condescending. Isherwood, *My Guru and His Disciple*, 182–84.

88. Until his death in 1952, Yogananda's organizational genius was undimmed. He had renamed his organization the Self-Realization Fellowship and, in the 1940s, had

added three temples, in Hollywood, San Diego, and Long Beach. In 1949, a student donated a lush ten-acre site in Pacific Palisades just half a mile from the ocean called the Lake Shrine. Yogananda, *Autobiography of a Yogi*, xvii–xix, 205–6, 317–18, 448–551. "Here Comes the Yogiman," *Time*, March 17, 1947.

89. "Church Members Total 1,000,000 in Los Angeles," *Los Angeles Times* (1886–Current File), October 6, 1946, ProQuest Historical Newspapers, *Los Angeles Times* (1881–1985) 3; Isherwood, *My Guru and His Disciple*, 180–83; Jackson, *Vedanta for the West*, 117. See Harry Hansen, "On the New York Literary Scene," *Chicago Daily Tribune* (1872–1963), February 7, 1954, ProQuest Historical Newspapers, *Chicago Tribune* (1849–1986), G13. The issue of whether later editions of *Autobiography of a Yogi* are valid became somewhat contentious after Yogananda's death. See "Why Read the First Edition of *Autobiography of a Yogi?*" www.ananda india.org/publications/books/autobiographyofayogi/yoganandas-lifetime.html (accessed October 8, 2009).

9. HATHA YOGA ON SUNSET BOULEVARD

1. There were so many murders that year that only half received more than a paragraph in most newspapers, and this at a time when five dailies were competing for Angelenos' attention. Starr, *Embattled Dreams*, 213–24.
2. Despite the new construction, the housing crisis was of such magnitude that detectives and real estate agents did a brisk trade. Detectives would call agents with the location of a corpse often before it had been removed, and the agents would have the apartment cleaned and rented sometimes within a day. Ibid., 208 and plate, 218, 221, 230–31.
3. Ibid., 288–89, 292–97.
4. Indra Devi, "Yoga for You: The Gentle Art of Being Healthy," *Health Movement Review* 1, no. 2 (November 1954): 3–7, Gloria Swanson Papers UTA. Also see poster from Magana Baptiste with photo of Magana and Devi.
5. Isherwood, *My Guru and His Disciple*, 55; Indra Devi, *Forever Young, Forever Healthy: Secrets of the Ancients Adapted for Modern Living* (New York: Prentice-Hall, 1953), 16, 135–53.
6. Devi, *Forever Young, Forever Healthy*, 25–27.
7. Ibid., 40–41, 131.
8. Mala Powers interview, May 28, 2005; Indra Devi, *Yoga for Americans: An Authentic Course for Home Practice*, LP (New York: Mace/Scepter Records, 1965).
9. Robert L. Balzer interview, June 11, 2007; Devi, *Yoga for Americans*, LP.
10. Gloria Swanson, *Swanson on Swanson* (New York: Random House, 1980), 485; Paul Buhle and Dave Wagner, "The Left and Popular Culture: Film and Television," *Monthly Review* (Platinum Periodicals) 54, no. 3 (July/August 2002): 51.
11. Devi, *Forever Young, Forever Healthy*, 3–4, 9.
12. Indian actresses were as a rule low-caste women, considered on par with prostitutes. Ibid., 9; Isherwood, *My Guru and His Disciple*, 186–87.
13. Devi, *Forever Young, Forever Healthy*, 8–9.
14. Ibid., 15.
15. Both Theos Bernard and his father, Glen, had made valiant, and unsuccessful, attempts to see Krishnamacharya perform this feat. Some footage of Krishnama-

charya's practice shot in 1938 captures him moving through a sequence of inverted postures with the greatest of ease. The fifty-year-old Yogi is dressed in only a loincloth, with the white markings on his forehead indicating his devotion to Vishnu. Though the film is grainy, his youthfulness is unmistakable. On Krishnamacharya's tours of India see Alter, *Yoga in Modern India*, and N. E. Sjoman, *Yoga Tradition*.

16. "Indra Devi, 102, Dies; Taught Yoga to Stars and Leaders," *New York Times*, April 30, 2002, C18; Devi, *Forever Young, Forever Healthy*, 10–22. For a more detailed discussion of Krishnamacharya, see chap. 8.

17. "Indra Devi, 102, Dies," C18.

18. Devi, *Forever Young, Forever Healthy*, 52.

19. Arden was so pleased with Devi's instruction, she invited her to join the staff, but Devi declined. "Indra Devi, 102, Dies," C18; Devi, *Forever Young, Forever Healthy*, 22.

20. Balzer believes that Bragg was instrumental in getting her a book deal in the first place. See Balzer, *Beyond Conflict*, 172.

21. In the late fall of 1948, Bragg had featured the seventy-year-old Ruth St. Denis, of the "Radha" Dance, in a recital. St. Denis—who was also a student of Devi's—illustrated Bragg's "new angle on health." Display ad 10, *Los Angeles Times*, October 5, 1948, 14.

22. Display ad 22, *Los Angeles Times*, February 1, 1949, A7.

23. Prabhavananda's instructions were to inhale through the left nostril and exhale through the right while visualizing the "Spirit" being drawn down the left side of your body and expelling purities up the other, then vice versa. Isherwood, *Diaries*, 124.

24. Karen Swenson, *Greta Garbo: A Life Apart* (New York: Scribner, 1997), 331n; Isherwood, *Diaries*, 50.

25. Hedda Hopper, "Looking at Hollywood," *Los Angeles Times* (1886–Current File), January 13, 1947, A2.

26. Swenson, *Greta Garbo*, 398.

27. Smith, *Letters of Aldous Huxley*, 482, 493; Isherwood, *Diaries*, 963. Huxley was also a devoted student of the Alexander technique, developed by an English actor, and the Bates method for retraining the eyes. "These two techniques," wrote Huxley in 1942, "have demonstrated the possibility, on the physiological plane, of a complete reconditioning, analogous to that which takes place through the techniques of mysticism on the psychological and spiritual plane." Although Huxley admitted the similarities of these new therapies to Eastern spiritual exercises, including "Hindu yoga," he preferred the Western methods. Smith, *Letters of Aldous Huxley*, 473, 525–26. Yet there seems to be some confusion about this. According to Heard, Huxley "set himself to test out and experiment with these traditional exercises." It's not clear to what extent this included Hatha Yoga. William York Tindall believes it did. My sense is that it might have—although it's just as likely, in my mind, that "exercises" referred to the meditation that Huxley had experimented with before he came to California. There's little evidence he engaged deeply, if at all, in Hatha Yoga. See Hal Bridges, "Aldous Huxley: Exponent of Mysticism in America," 341–52.

28. Feuerstein, *Yoga Tradition*, 390; Feuerstein, *Shambhala Encyclopedia*, 119–22.

29. Sri Yogendra's American Yoga Institute in Harriman, New York, had served as a branch of his Indian facility, then located in the suburbs of Bombay. Several schol-

ars, including Catherine Albanese, have recently located Yogendra's American Yoga Institute in Santa Cruz, California, rather than in Harriman, near Bear Mountain. I believe the confusion stems from the address of Yogendra's Indian headquarters. In 1918 he founded his Yoga Institute in Versova, a suburb of Bombay; in 1947, the institute found a permanent headquarters in Santa Cruz (East), which is part of the Bombay municipality. See Albanese, *Republic of Mind and Spirit*, 367, 577n71; Santan Rodrigues, *The Householder Yogi: Life of Shri Yogendra* (Bombay: The Yoga Institute, 1982), 187–92.

30. See *Los Angeles Times* (1923–Current File), February 16, 1929, A6; Mark Singleton, *Yoga Body: The Origins of Modern Posture Practice* (New York: Oxford University Press, 2010), 114, 140; Hackett, 195.

31. Letter to TCB from Dagobert D. Runes, president of the Philosophical Library, September 13, 1946, BANC MSS 2005/161z. Some devoted Hatha Yoga students had recently relocated to Los Angeles—notably Leopold Stokowski, who had been one of Garbo's lovers, and Hamish McLaurin, both members of Pierre Bernard's C.C.C. McLaurin was living on Ramos Drive in Pacific Palisades in 1937; VWB's address book, VWB Papers, HSCU.

32. Only Rishi Gherwal taught into the 1950s. See *Los Angeles Times* (1886–Current File), March 23, 1940, A2, and October 2, 1943, A2.

33. Devi, *Forever Young, Forever Healthy*, 23.

34. "Education: Exercise for Defense," *Time*, August 11, 1941. www.time.com/time/printout/0.8816.765900.00.html (accessed December 24, 2009); "Sweden Honors the Calisthenics King," *Life*, August 14, 1939, 21; "WAACS," *Life*, September 7, 1942, 78.

35. Ida Jean Kain, "Hollywood's Figure Aids Good for You," *Washington Post*, January 3, 1949, B4.

36. Ida Jean Kain, "Susan Hayward Good Example of How Mother Keeps Figure," *Washington Post*, July 17, 1946, 14; "Best Shape Ever," *Movie Stars Parade*, March 1949.

37. Joan Bennett, *How to Be Attractive* (New York: Alfred A. Knopf, 1942, 1951), 58.

38. Sjoman, *Yoga Tradition*, 53–61; Singleton, *Yoga Body*, 175–208.

39. Quoted in McWilliams, *Southern California Country*, 227.

40. "Recent Religious Books," *New York Times* (1857–Current File), April 18, 1953, ProQuest Historical Newspapers, *New York Times* (1851–2004), BR21; "Other Books of the Week," *New York Times* (1857–Current File), June 14, 1953, ProQuest Historical Newspapers, *New York Times* (1851–2004), 17; Isherwood, *My Guru and His Disciple*, 195–96.

41. Gerald Sykes, "The Song of the Gita," *New York Times*, March 28, 1954, BR11.

42. Mala Powers interview, May 28, 2005.

43. David Dempsey, "In and Out of Books," *New York Times* (1857–Current File), May 20, 1951, ProQuest Historical Newspapers, *The New York Times* (1851–2004), BR5.

44. Swanson, *Swanson on Swanson*, 259–60.

45. Jergen's ad, *Life*, February 12, 1951, 15.

46. Swanson, *Swanson on Swanson*, 504–10.

47. The photos are also testimony to the densely overlapping worlds of Hollywood and yoga. The pictures were taken at 13030 Mulholland Drive, the former home of Collier Young and his first wife, Ida Lupino, and then his second wife, Joan Fontaine,

whose sister, Olivia de Havilland, was a student of Devi's. In the spring of 1953, Robert Balzer was renting the house. Balzer had been a student of Vedanta for several years before his friends began raving about Devi and the rejuvenating effects of her classes. Swanson, who had been his lover since the late 1940s, may have been one of them. Balzer has fond memories of their sun-kissed sessions. But he understood, as clearly as any other observer at the time, that Swanson was more than a student and friend to Devi. She was a business asset. Balzer interview, June 11, 2007.

48. Letter from Gloria Swanson to Indra Devi, June 6, 1953, Swanson Papers UTA.

49. Devi, "Yoga for You," 5.

50. Instead, she makes vague mention of life pulsations, life forces, and their obstructions in a chapter on the endocrine glands. She also alludes to the spiritual value of pranayama and "certain esoteric teachings of Yoga," a reference to the subtle body, but goes on to say she won't discuss them and Westerners should avoid them unless they find a proper guru and the proper environment, which is clearly not a big city. In contrast, Prabhavananda talks about raising Kundalini through the six centers of consciousness in *How to Know God*. He calls this the "physiology of raja yoga." Devi, *Forever Young, Forever Healthy*, 37, 79–80. Prabhavananda and Isherwood, *How to Know God*, 112–17.

51. Devi, *Forever Young, Forever Healthy*, 10–14.

52. Devi, *Forever Young, Forever Healthy*, 36, 82, 95.

53. Devi alludes to the vast reaches of yoga beyond her discussion and rightly confesses she can't be much help there. (The curious pupil must find a real guru.)

54. "As Yoga* deals with the functions of life," she writes, "it has a very great influence on the endocrine glands because it is through them that life in us manifests itself in a grand way." The asterisked "Yoga" is explained in a brief footnote, which reads, "I am referring to Asanas, the first stage of Hatha Yoga." Devi, *Forever Young, Forever Healthy*, 25, 80. Hatha Yoga texts put forth a variety of limbs or stages; eight limbs are generally accepted, but some texts indicate a sevenfold path or even twenty limbs. Feuerstein, *Shambhala Encyclopedia*, 120.

55. "There is no word in the *Sanskreet* language that will bear so many interpretations as" the word *yoga*. Wilkins, *Bagavat-Geeta*, 138.

56. Devi wasn't the first to present Hatha Yoga in this way; Ramacharaka had given the discipline a similar treatment, and Devi was an avid reader of his books. Devi did so more skillfully than Atkinson (as Ramacharaka) had and had the good sense to address her book to women. Albanese, *Republic of Mind and Spirit*, 360.

57. This is real yoga: contorted postures by which the soul of an Indian Yogi seeks escape from its human body. *Life* 10 (February 24, 1941): 10–12.

58. Photographs of two young Yogis executing several difficult poses against a backdrop of desert dunes appeared in *Asia* magazine in 1931. Clad only in loincloths, both men have developed shoulders and biceps and look strong enough to pose for one of Macfadden's magazines. (They also bear white markings on their arms, torsos, and foreheads, signaling their devotion to Shiva.) But their impressive "exercises" were definitely not something you'd try at home. "Physical Exercises of the Ascetic," *Asia*, October 1931, 658. The plates in Behanan's book had also featured Indian Yogis, thin ones that to an American eye look half-starved.

59. Which is to say, Devi split Hatha Yoga into its constituent parts. One part was physical and good for ordinary people; the rest, including spiritual achievement,

was for the very few, and the very well prepared. Devi, *Forever Young, Forever Healthy*, 27.

60. Bennett, *How to Be Attractive*, 2–5, 31, 83.

61. Stephanie Guest, e-mail interview, December 23, 2007. Guest is one of Joan Bennett and Walter Wanger's children.

62. Devi, *Forever Young, Forever Healthy*, 126.

63. Indra Devi, *Yoga for Americans* (Englewood Cliffs, NJ: Prentice-Hall, 1959), 200.

64. *Los Angeles Times*, May 11, 1955; Display ad 18, *Los Angeles Times* (1886–Current File), March 17, 1954, 21.

65. Robert Love, "Fear of Yoga," 87; "The Needle's Eye—How's Your Back?" *Hartford Courant*, December 1, 1953, 12. Jack Zaiman was an unlikely advocate of Hatha Yoga. He was an everyman who spent a lot of time at the YMCA. For this reason he was given the review copy of *Forever Young, Forever Healthy* when it came across his editor's desk in the fall of 1953. Curious, he took the book to the YMCA, where he tried out some of the postures Devi recommends.

   These turn out to be useful mostly for comedic effect. The plow posture gives him a sore back, and when he's upside down in a headstand, a friend comes by. Puzzled, he asks Zaiman what he's doing. "I'm a Yoga," he answers, as he crashes to the floor. Something shifted for Zaiman in the ensuing months. By winter, he's relating how a friend from the Y, a lawyer and former state senator, has taken up Hatha Yoga and, after being observed by other Y members, is spreading the discipline to still other unsuspecting folks.

66. Devi, *Yoga for Americans*, 197–213.

67. "Lillian Gish Finds Imitating Cat Keeps Her Spine Limber," *Los Angeles Times*, November 7, 1954; "Joan Davis Slenderizes," *Los Angeles Times*, August 8, 1954.

68. "Southland Youngsters Turn Nudist as Heat Continues," *Los Angeles Times*, July 9, 1954, 3.

69. Devi, *Forever Young, Forever Healthy*, 39; "Carol Ohmart Tells How She Keeps Figure," *Chicago Tribune*, April 30, 1956, B9.

70. Walter Winchell, "Of New York," *Washington Post and Times-Herald* (1954–59), March 1, 1956, 47.

71. Lydia Lane, "Men: Look Younger," *Los Angeles Times* (1886–Current File), May 20, 1958, ProQuest Historical Newspapers, *Los Angeles Times* (1881–1986), A1.

72. "Yoga Held Way to Health," *Los Angeles Times*, August 12, 1957, 1.

73. Devi, *Forever Young, Forever Healthy*, 8–9.

74. Letter to Indra Devi, August 1, 1955, Swanson Papers UTA.

75. Devi, *Yoga for Americans*, 128–35.

76. To be fair, others had never covered over these dimensions of yoga. Theos had gone into far greater detail about the subtle body and his own (fabricated) spiritual ecstasies in *Heaven Lies Within Us*. But Devi was the first to popularize this information, and she had the advantage of a vastly bigger market and unprecedented prosperity.

10. PSYCHEDELIC SAGES

1. Lewis Lapham, "There Once Was a Guru from Rishikesh," pt. 2, *Saturday Evening Post* 241, no. 10 (May 18, 1968): 32.

2. Hal Bridges, *American Mysticism: From William James to Zen* (New York: Harper & Row, 1970), 148; "Year of the Guru," *Life*, February 9, 1968, 52–59; Fred Smithline interview, March 19, 2008.

3. Smithline interview, March 19, 2008.

4. This would be more than twenty-five hundred dollars today. To learn TM in the States, each devotee had to pay Mahesh's organization a week's salary, or $35 if you were a student. Mahesh maintained that when he first came West and offered his teaching for free, no one was interested. That peace of mind might be both readily had and cheap, in Mahesh's telling, didn't jibe with the Protestant work ethic, which, in 1959, had not yet given way to either Alan Watts's formulations—"the divine state simply IS here and now, and does not have to be attained"—or the "Now Trip," the righteous hedonism that Ken Kesey and his gang of Merry Pranksters shucked from their Day-Glo bus across the blessed land in 1964. Lapham, "There Once Was a Guru from Rishikesh," pt. 1, *Saturday Evening Post* 241, no. 9 (May 4, 1968): 24, and pt. 2, 31.

5. Lapham, "There Once Was a Guru," pt. 2, 32.

6. Lewis Lapham, *With the Beatles* (Hoboken, NJ: Melville House Publishing, 2005), 33–34.

7. Ibid., 106.

8. Lapham, "There Once Was a Guru," pt. 2, 30.

9. Ibid., 31.

10. Nancy Cooke de Herrera, *Beyond Gurus* (New Delhi, India: Rupa and Co., 1994), 224. Joseph Lelyveld, "Beatles' Guru Is Turning Them into Gurus with a Cram Course," *New York Times*, February 23, 1968, 13.

11. "Beatles Cut Ties to Maharishi," *Washington Post and Times-Herald*, May 17, 1968, D13. See also "Maharishi Yogi Turns Other Cheek to the Beatles' Slur," *Los Angeles Times*, May 17, 1968, D14.

12. Lapham, "There Once Was a Guru," pt. 2, 29; "Beatles Say They've Given Up Drugs," *Washington Post and Times-Herald*, August 28, 1967, A3. George Harrison was the first to groove on this idea. "The buzz of all buzzes which is the thing that is God—you've got to be straight to get it . . . if you really want to get it permanently," Harrison explained to an underground paper founded on the idea of psychedelics as a path to God. ". . . Be healthy, don't eat meat, keep away from those Night-Clubs and MEDITATE." From "The Way Out Is In," *Southern California Oracle*, May 27, 1967, 7, 21.

13. Paul Saltzman, *The Beatles in Rishikesh* (New York: Viking Studio, 2000), 102.

14. Lapham, "There Once Was a Guru," pt. 2, 33.

15. Maharishi Mahesh Yogi, *The Science of Being and Art of Living* (Fairfield, IA: Age of Enlightenment Press, 1966, 1992), 296–304; "India Mystic Delivers Peace—for a Price," *Los Angeles Times*, December 15, 1967, A1.

16. Lapham, "There Once Was a Guru," pt. 2, 29; Saltzman, *Beatles in Rishikesh*, 62.

17. Lapham left the same day. Lapham, "There Once Was a Guru," pt. 2, 88; Cooke de Herrera, *Beyond Gurus*, 259.

18. Transcribed by the Beatles Ultimate Experience Web site from an audio recording of the TV interview, www.geocities.com/~Beatleboy1/db1968.05ts.beatles.html. In June, George reaffirmed his own break with Mahesh, telling reporters in Los Angeles that he was "dissatisfied with the organization. It was too much of an organi-

zation." Pete Johnson, "Harrison Tells Why Beatles Gave Up on Maharishi Yogi," *Los Angeles Times*, June 15, 1968, B9.

19. Gerald Howard, ed., *The Sixties: The Art, Attitudes, Politics, and Media of Our Most Explosive Decade* (New York: Pocket Books, 1982), 5.

20. Alan Watts, *In My Own Way: An Autobiography, 1915–1965* (New York: Pantheon Books, 1972), 203–17; Monica Furlong, *Genuine Fake: A Biography of Alan Watts* (London: Heinemann, 1986), 88.

21. Watts, *In My Own Way*, 11; Walter Truett Anderson, *The Upstart Spring, Esalen and the Human Potential Movement: The First Twenty Years* (Lincoln, NE: Authors Guild Backinprint.com, 2004), 55; Nat Freedland interview with Alan Watts, *Southern California Oracle*, March 1967, 7.

22. Alan Watts, *Behold the Spirit: A Study in the Necessity of Mystical Religion* (New York: Pantheon, 1947, 1971), 92–93, 100.

23. Watts, *In My Own Way*, 237. Bernard Gunther was a young psychology student in the middle fifties. About the same time he took LSD he made a visit to Swami Prabhavananda at the Vedanta Temple. The swami told him he'd have to give up sex to become a monk, and after about a week of celibacy he decided it wasn't for him. He turned to Hatha Yoga and Zen. Gunther interview, March 4, 2008.

24. Augustus Owsley Stanley III, "the unofficial mayor of San Francisco" in the mid-1960s, sold his superpotent, superpure LSD for two dollars per dose and gave plenty away for free. Martin A. Lee and Bruce Shlain, *Acid Dreams: The CIA, LSD, and the Sixties Rebellion* (New York: Grove Press, 1985), 147.

25. Watts, *In My Own Way*, 237–40.

26. Ibid., 265.

27. Ibid., 247.

28. Ibid., 267–70.

29. In its early days, the AAAS was famous for its Friday-night colloquium, led by Spiegelberg, Watts, and Haridas Chaudhuri. "You had to get there about an hour early to get into the room," recalls Michael Murphy, an early student. "We used to have dinner at La Fontere up here about five in the afternoon, and there was this enormous excitement about coming in to the old academy . . . to get there early enough to sit in on those first meetings." From "The Early History of the California Institute of Integral Studies—CIIS," in *Commemoration of the Fiftieth Anniversary of the Opening of the American Academy of Asian Studies, 1951–2001*, www.well.com/~davidu/ciishistory.html.

30. Watts, *In My Own Way*, 247.

31. These included Esalen founders Michael Murphy and Richard Price. Jeffrey Kripal, *Esalen: America and the Religion of No Religion* (Chicago: University of Chicago Press, 2007), 59, 73–74; Anderson, *Upstart Spring*, 37.

32. Watts, *In My Own Way*, photograph, NY 1959, 312, 319.

33. Watts, *Beat Zen, Square Zen* (San Francisco: City Lights, 1959), foreword, pages are unnumbered.

34. Aldous Huxley, *The Doors of Perception* (New York: Harper & Brothers, 1954), 18. Since Huxley had been striving in this direction for most of his life, he was able to cull insight out of his chemical reverie. The experience convinced him that mescaline was a valid and indeed helpful method for "transfiguration."

In fact, he urged everyone "to take an occasional trip through some chemical Door in the Wall into the world of transcendental experience" and felt people should be "compelled" to do so if the prospect alone didn't tempt them. Ibid., 78.

35. John Yale, *A Yankee and the Swamis: A Westerner's View of the Ramakrishna Order* (Chennai, India: Sri Ramakrishna Math, 2001), 3.

36. Prabhavananda and Isherwood, *How to Know God*, 142.

37. The account of Huxley's inscription and the book's disappearance are from John Yale (Swami Vidyatmananda), *The Making of a Devotee*. The book has been published only online, world.std.com/~elayj/ and world.std.com/~elayj/Chapter5 .html.

38. Aldous Huxley, "Drugs That Shape Men's Minds," *Saturday Evening Post*, October 18, 1958, 28, 108, 110–11, 113. Huxley's essay appeared alongside articles on runaway inflation in the Soviet Union ("Silent Weapon of the Cold War"), sentimental short stories, and a meditation on college football (is it ". . . Worth Saving?"). The cover, by Thornton Utz, celebrated in loving detail suburban life: here's dad and the boys building a motorized box car, here's mom hauling bursting bagfuls of groceries from the car into the family split-level, here's baby sis playing by herself, parking toy cars in a neat line at the edge of the lawn.

39. This would have been the 1950 census, with results published in 1951, www .census.gov/population/censusdata/table-2.pdf. In less than a decade prescriptions increased substantially. According to David Farber, in 1965, doctors, with psychiatrists taking the lead, "wrote 123 million prescriptions for tranquilizers and 24 million prescriptions for amphetamines." From "The Intoxicated State," in *Imagine Nation: The American Counterculture of the 1960s and 1970s*, ed. Peter Braunstein and Michael William Doyle (New York: Routledge, 2002), 19.

40. "Zen: Beat & Square," *Time* 72, no. 3 (July 21, 1958). Watts had only a bit more hope than Huxley when it came to traditional mysticism. While Watts believed you really needn't bother with yoga as interpreted by most practitioners and scholars, which was just as joyless as a church sermon, he made at least one exception: Hatha Yoga as presented by his friend, colleague, and mentor Frederic Spiegelberg. See his introduction to Frederic Spiegelberg, *Spiritual Practices of India* (New York: Citadel Press, 1951), vii–xv.

41. Gay Talese, "Zen Selling Better Than Sodas, 'Village' Store Scraps Fountain," *New York Times*, September 12, 1959, 11.

42. Robert Greenfield, *Timothy Leary: A Biography* (Orlando, FL: Harcourt, 2006), 115–20.

43. Watts, *In My Own Way*, 347; Michael Schumacher, *Dharma Lion: A Critical Biography of Allen Ginsberg* (New York: St. Martin's Press, 1992), 343–44.

44. Lee and Shlain, *Acid Dreams*, 81.

45. Smith, *Letters of Aldous Huxley*, 928–29. Even *The New Yorker* (December 27, 1958, 67) was dazzled by Eliade's book, offering in its review, "Those who have succumbed to the fashionable preoccupation with Zen Buddhism will be particularly interested in the light the book throws on the origins of a number of Zen techniques and ideas," and that others, with more prurient interests, would find the passages that deal with Tantric Yoga especially rewarding.

46. Smith, *Letters of Aldous Huxley*, 928–29.

47. Mircea Eliade, *Yoga: Immortality and Freedom*, trans. Willard R. Trask (Princeton, NJ: Princeton University Press, 1958, 1990), 200–205.

48. Ibid., 205–206.

49. Swami Prabhavananda would have never permitted such a scene; as it was, the presiding swami split his time between the Boston and Providence Vedanta centers, making it difficult to monitor his flock as closely. This is the only way I can see to account for the temple's liberal stance toward psychedelics. Leary never mentions the swami. I have not been able to find any other mentions of this event.

50. The account of his time at the Boston Vedanta ashram is from Timothy Leary, *High Priest* (Oakland, CA: Ronin Publishing, 1968, 1995), 296–302.

51. Definition of *set* and *setting* from Richard Alpert, Sidney Cohen, and Lawrence Schiller, *LSD* (New York: New American Library, 1966), 29.

52. Alan W. Watts, *The Joyous Cosmology: Adventures in the Chemistry of Consciousness* (New York: Vintage Books, 1962), 30, 44–45.

53. Ibid., 40.

54. The part of this divine lila that really cracks Watts up is our skill at hiding the nature of reality from ourselves, and our likely response when informed. "How solemnly they would go through the act of not understanding me if I were to step up and say," remarks Watts, "'Well, who do you think you're kidding? Come off it, Shiva, you old rascal!' It's a great act but it doesn't fool me." Ibid., 61.

55. The problem was "this wisdom was simultaneously holy and disreputable," and so intolerable to minds steeped in Judeo-Christian binaries. Watts, *In My Own Way*, 344.

56. See *Joyous Cosmology*, Leary and Alpert introduction, xv.

57. Greenfield, *Timothy Leary*, 114.

58. Ibid.; Leary, *High Priest*, 12, 34.

59. Alpert was also a closeted bisexual man at the time. Obviously, being bisexual in the 1950s would put a premium on superficial conformity.

60. For biographical details see Andrew T. Weil, "The Strange Case of the Harvard Drug Scandal," *Look*, November 5, 1963, 38–48; Ram Dass, *Be Here Now* (Kingsport, TN: Kingsport Press, with permission from the Hanuman Foundation, 1978), unnumbered opening pages; recording made October 1968 Bucks County Seminar House in Pennsylvania, broadcast on WBAI as "Transformation of a Man."

61. Tom Wolfe, *Electric Kool-Aid Acid Test* (New York: Bantam Books, 1968, 1969, 1999), 52.

62. "How to Go out of Your Mind: A study of LSD and the Institute for Psychedelic Research at Millbrook," CBC broadcast, April 24, 1966, clip on YouTube: www.youtube.com/watch?v=cMdWWjTw4DA&feature=related.

63. Greenfield, *Timothy Leary*, 107–9.

64. They announced the formation of the International Federation of Internal Freedom, the beginning of a series of half-farcical organizations to "encourage, support and protect research on psychedelic [mind-manifesting] substances." Weil, "Strange Case of the Harvard Drug Scandal," 43, 46.

65. Leary, *High Priest*, 387; Greenfield, *Timothy Leary*, 192–93.

66. Lee and Shlain, *Acid Dreams*, 88.

67. "Timothy Leary's Press Conference at the Fairmont Hotel, San Francisco, December 12, 1966," *San Francisco Oracle* 1, no. 4 (December 16, 1966): 15/77 in fax edition.

68. Millbrook residents didn't take these retreats that seriously but needed them—the "fees" students paid went toward rent. Lee and Shlain, *Acid Dreams*, 103.

69. J. M. Flagler, "The Visions of 'Saint Tim,'" *Look*, August 8, 1967, 18; Watts, *In My Own Way*, 352.

70. See Flagler, "Visions of 'Saint Tim,'" 20; Ralph Blumenthal, "Leary Drug Cult Stirs Millbrook," *New York Times*, June 14, 1967, 49.

71. Greenfield, *Timothy Leary*, 226–29.

72. Here Leary is dressed against type, but true to his mid-1960s aesthetic, in chinos, a cable sweater, and white tennis shoes. The interview was taped in August 1965 but didn't air until April 1966. "How to Go Out of Your Mind," clip on YouTube, youtube.com/watch?v=CAgpAfNKLrQ.

73. Blumenthal, "Leary Drug Cult," 49.

74. By this point, Leary, Alpert, and Metzner had decided that if they were really going to shift consciousness, they had to have a way to shift it toward the things they believed in. They wanted trips to be spiritually productive. They wanted to find a way for people to stay in the luminous space they referred to as "the Clear Light Void."

   So together, Leary, Metzner, and Alpert wrote a guidebook for the voyager into inner space. Having been inspired by a comment Huxley made in *The Doors of Perception*, they adapted W. Y. Evans-Wentz's translation of *The Tibetan Book of the Dead* for their purposes.

   In 1964, University Books put out their manual, titled simply *The Psychedelic Experience*.

   As the authors themselves insisted, you can't really understand *The Psychedelic Experience* unless you are high. Whether the book was any good as a piece of literature or true to its original source was really irrelevant.

   The question was, did it work?

   By the fall of 1965, the *Free Press* reported that *The Psychedelic Experience* was sold out in every bookstore in San Francisco.

   Norman Hartweg, "Psychedelic Prophet Alpert to Speak in Los Angeles," *Los Angeles Free Press*, September 3, 1965, 3; Bernard Weinraub, "4-Level Bookshop Throws a Party," *New York Times*, February 22, 1965, 23.

75. Lee and Shlain, *Acid Dreams*, 104–5; Arthur Kleps, *Millbrook: A Narrative of the Early Years of American Psychedelianism* (Original Kleptonian Neo-American Church, 1975; ISBN: 0-9165-3405-7), 69–71, www.erowid.org/library/books_online/millbrook.pdf.

76. As he put it, "In Western terms, Kundilini Yoga can be understood as a biological statement couched in the language of poetic metaphor." John N. Bleibtreu, "LSD and the Third Eye," *Atlantic Monthly* 218, no. 3 (September 1966): 64.

77. They, in turn, returned the favor. "I really just dig the *Oracle*, the concept," says Alpert in a 1967 Q-and-A session, "and I really want it to make it and I want to help make it too because I like the struggly feeling out of which it's coming, you know, that we're really trying to be there and do it, and not make compromise because we're all . . . wow! we've got a big newspaper going." Interview "Ees Setisoppo" (See Opposites) with Dick Alpert, *San Francisco Oracle* 5 (January 1967): 10.

   The *Oracle* identified itself completely with Leary and Alpert. The paper's mission: "To get everyone to turn on, tune in, and drop out." By 1968, the *Oracle* had a nationwide circulation of more than one hundred thousand. Lee and Shlain, *Acid Dreams*, 149, 185.

78. Robert Simmons, "Yoga and the Psychedelic Mind," *San Francisco Oracle* 4 (December 16, 1966): 7/69 fax edition.

79. Theos said of Sivananda's Rishikesh ashram, "They practice all the various forms of Yoga and several of them can do all of the various mudras, bandhas and cleansing processes as well as Vajroli." He summed up, "It was the first time, that I had ever run on to a place where they had so much general information that seemed to be in order." Quoted in Veenhof, *White Lama*, 196; Robert (Azul) Simmons, e-mail correspondence, June 21, 2008.

80. Jackson, *Vedanta for the West*, 32, 114–16; Erik Davis, *The Visionary State: A Journey Through California's Spiritual Landscape* (San Francisco: Chronicle Books, 2006), 83.

81. Alpert, Cohen, and Schiller, *LSD*, 6–9.

82. And *Time* magazine predicted that these youngsters would soon constitute half the population! Robert S. Ellwood, *The 60s Spiritual Awakening: American Religion Moving from Modern to Postmodern* (New Brunswick, NJ: Rutgers University Press, 1994), 108–10; Warren Hinckle, "A Social History of the Sixties," *Ramparts*, March 1967, republished in Howard, *Sixties*, 209.

83. "LSD," *Encyclopædia Britannica*, search.eb.com/eb/article-9049184.

84. Greenfield, *Timothy Leary*, 300–302.

85. After the Civil War, victory tempered the magazine's factionalism, but this didn't stop later editors from taking unpopular positions on many issues. In 1881, for instance, the *Atlantic* published Henry Demarest Lloyd's explosive denunciation of Standard Oil and "Spencerian economics in general," as well as a piece on the Buddha and early Buddhism. Justin Kaplan, *Mr. Clemens and Mark Twain: A Biography* (New York: Simon & Schuster, 1996). See also L. Maria Child, "The Intermingling of Religions," *Atlantic Monthly* 28, no. 168 (October 1871): 385; Anonymous, "Buddha and early Buddhism," *Atlantic Monthly* 48, no. 290 (December 1881): 840; Percival Lowell, "The Soul of the Far East," *Atlantic Monthly* 60, no. 362 (December 1887): 835; William Davies, "The Teaching of the Upanishads," *Atlantic Monthly* 72, no. 430 (August 1893): 178; Jackson, *Vedanta for the West*, 187.

86. Satsvarūpa Dāsa Gosvāmī, *Srīla Prabhupāda-līlāmrta*, vol. 2, *Planting the Seed: New York City, 1965–1966* (Los Angeles, CA: Bhaktivedanta Book Trust, 1980), 21–27.

87. Robert (Azul) Simmons, e-mail correspondence, June 21, 2008.

88. The next morning, a teacher named Yarek gave a Hatha Yoga class to Millbrook residents. Yarek had studied for six years with Krishnamacharya in Madras. According to poet Diane Di Prima (a former ashram member), he taught with "great intuitive tact and understanding" and his class was quite long and "a little more complete than the others." See Diane Di Prima, Millbrook Journal, 1966–67, Series II, box 2, folder 27, Diane Di Prima Papers, Archives and Special Collections at the Thomas J. Dodd Research Center, University of Connecticut Libraries.

89. Hinckle, "A Social History," in Howard, *Sixties*, 222.

90. In Thompson's view, the genuine articles, those barefoot, ecstatically freaking souls, were few and far between. They'd come, sure, but only if they got in for free. Hunter S. Thompson, "The 'Hashbury' Is the Capital of the Hippies," *New York Times*, May 14, 1967, SM14.

91. James R. Sikes, "Swami's Flock Chants in Park to Find Ecstasy," *New York Times*, October 10, 1966, 24.

92. Gosvāmī, v. 3, 13–14. www.prabhupada1967.com/2004_01_25_sangalog_archive .html.

93. Feuerstein, *Yoga Tradition*, 364–65; Bharati, *Tantric Tradition*, 250–53; David Gordon White, *The Alchemical Body: Siddha Traditions in Medieval India* (Chicago: University of Chicago Press, 1996), 412n220.

94. Bernard, *Heaven Lies Within Us*, 245.

95. Sri Brahmarishi Narad may have been an Indian known simply as Narad, who was then living at Millbrook. He had the reputation for being intensely knowledgeable of yoga philosophy and physically strong, and also forgetful, horny, and in general a bit of a nuisance. (It was rumored that he had had an affair with Blanche De Vries.) Kleps, *Millbrook*, 130–31.

96. Timothy Miller, *The Hippies and American Values* (Knoxville: University of Tennessee Press, 1991), plates start p. 85.

97. Dass, *Be Here Now*, "The Journey," pages are unnumbered.

98. Richard Alpert, "Alpert Speaks on Meher Baba & LSD," *P.O. Frisco*, September 2, 1966, p. 5/7 in facsimile edition. (*P.O. Frisco* is considered the precursor to the *Oracle*, or issue #0.)

99. Ibid.

100. Bhagavan Das, *It's Here Now (Are You?): A Spiritual Memoir* (New York: Broadway Books, 1997), 149.

101. Wolfe. *Electric Kool-Aid*, 112.

102. In India, Leary wrote a book of poetry based on the *Tao Te Ching*, which was published as *Psychedelic Prayers* in 1966. Greenfield, *Timothy Leary*, 229–30.

103. Watts interview in *Southern California Oracle*, March 1967, 6.

104. See Di Prima, Millbrook Journal.

105. Di Prima, Millbrook Journal, 1966–67, Diane Di Prima Papers, Archives and Special Collections at the Thomas J. Dodd Research Center, University of Connecticut Libraries.

106. Gosvāmī, *Planting the Seed*, 199.

107. "Interview: Cinmayananda," *San Francisco Oracle* 10 (October 1967): 6/284 facsimile edition.

108. Emmett Lake, "Pop, Rock & Jelly," *East Village Other* 2, no. 22 (October 1–15, 1967): 13.

109. During his research, Lapham had cataloged two types of TM devotees—those older followers who saw Mahesh as a savior and his TM as a quick and sure path to God, and his younger followers, who saw TM as a way to "enlarge their perceptions." The youths were hip and mildly irreverent at times; their form of worship, besides the meditation itself, was to create centers that operated with the efficiency and urgency of campaign headquarters. Lapham, "There Once Was a Guru from Rishikesh," pt. 1, 25–26.

110. Das, *It's Here Now*, 154–55. Neem Karoli Baba kept things simple, advising his students only to "love, serve, and remember" God.

111. Dass, *Be Here Now*, "Ashtanga Yoga" section, unnumbered pages.

112. Ram Dass, *The Only Dance There Is: Talks at the Menninger Foundation, 1970 and Spring Grove Hospital, 1972* (Garden City, NY: Anchor Books, 1974), 17, 18.

113. "*Playboy* Panel February: The Drug Revolution," *Playboy*, February 1970, 53–74, 200–201. According to Dass, the roundtable was "phony." He, like all the other

participants, had been asked a series of questions, which he answered individually, then the magazine stitched together the discussion. Dass also claims this transpired in 1966, before he went to India, though the magazine allowed him to make corrections, at which point he added a little bit of information about his guru and yoga. Dass, *Only Dance There Is*, 15–16.

114. Peter Braunstein, "Forever Young: Insurgent Youth and the Sixties Culture of Rejuvenation," in Braunstein and Doyle, *Imagine Nation*, 250.

115. Dass, *Be Here Now*, 93.

116. Meher Baba admitted that for a few "LSD may have served as a means to arouse that spiritual longing." Meher Baba, "God in a Pill?" (Walnut Creek, CA: Sufism Reoriented, Inc., 1966), www.avatarmeherbaba.org/erics/godpill.html.

117. Robert S. Ellwood, "ISKCON and the Spirituality of the 1960s," in *Krishna Consciousness in the West*, ed. David G. Bromley and Larry D. Shinn (Lewisburg, PA: Bucknell University Press, 1989), 105.

118. A huge poster at Prabhupada's San Francisco Hare Krishna temple read, in part, "*Stay high forever.* No more coming down. Practice Krishna Consciousness. Expand your consciousness by practicing Transcendental Sound Vibrations. . . . *Turn on* through music, dance, philosophy . . . prasadam (spiritual food). *Tune in.* Awaken Your Transcendental Nature! Rejoice in the Ocean of Bliss! . . . *Drop out* of movements employing artificially induced states of self-realization and expanded consciousness." Gregory Johnson, "The Hare Krishna in San Francisco," in *The New Religious Consciousness*, ed. Charles Y. Glock and Robert N. Bellah (Berkeley: University of California Press, 1976), 36.

119. On the size of Mahesh's following, see Barney Lefferts, "Chief Guru of the Western World," *New York Times*, December 17, 1967, SM235; "3,600 Hear Guru Urge Meditation," *New York Times*, January 22, 1968, 24; Lapham, "There Once Was a Guru from Rishikesh," pt. 1, 26–27.

120. Dave Smith, "Despite Guru Fanfare: U.S. Hindu Philosophy Roots Strong, Deep," *Los Angeles Times*, February 25, 1968, J1.

121. Mahesh had banked on his celebrity students. He felt that the publicity he was receiving because of them would "create a big demand," for TM and TM teachers. Cooke de Herrera, *Beyond Gurus*, 244, 258. "The difference was, we'd give lectures to five, six hundred. And then the Beatles started and then we were giving lectures to one or two thousand. . . . It increased the interest immediately." Jerry Jarvis in *His Holiness Maharishi Mahesh Yogi*, pt. 3, History Channel International, November 28, 2007.

122. Dave Felton, "Mystic Stresses Deep Thought," *Los Angeles Times*, October 11, 1966, A1.

123. Linda Matthews, "U.S. Mystic Thinks Beatles' Yogi Is Religious Hypocrite," *Los Angeles Times*, February 19, 1968, 3. Vishnu-Devananda was so upset by Mahesh and his organization, he took out ads in national publications such as *Newsweek* denouncing TM.

124. Saltzman, *Beatles in Rishikesh*, 52.

125. Smithline interview, March 19, 2008.

126. "India Mystic Delivers Peace," A1.

127. Cooke de Herrera, *Beyond Gurus*, 245–46.

128. Cover of *Look*, February 6, 1968, ibid., 232. Jane Howard traveled up and down Manhattan to see for herself what all the fuss was about. She chanted, she did the

cobra and corpse poses, she meditated, she fasted. She was covering the "Swami Circuit" for *Life* (the second part of the "Year of the Guru" package). "The centers are cheery, busy places," Howard observed. "They range from slummy storefronts to chic brownstones, but they have one thing in common: none is big enough to handle the swelling crowds who drop by to exercise, chant or meditate and through these ancient disciplines of mind and body, reach the ultimate goal: bliss." Jane Howard, "Samadhi and Plaid Stamps on the Swami Circuit," *Life*, February 9, 1968, 57.

129. Monikers are from, respectively, Tom Buckley, "The Battle of Chicago: From the Yippies' Side," *New York Times Magazine*, September 15, 1968, SM134; William Buckley, *Firing Line*, 1968; Wolfe, *Electric Kool-Aid*, 173; Hinckle, "A Social History," in Howard, *Sixties*, 207.

130. Ginsberg quoted in Leary, *High Priest*, 111.

131. Tom Clark interview, mid-May 1965, published as "The Art of Poetry" (no. 8 in a series), *Paris Review*, Spring 1966, and reprinted in *Allen Ginsberg, Spontaneous Mind: Selected Interviews, 1958–1996*, ed. David Carter (New York: Harper-Collins, 2001), 46–48.

132. Ibid., 386–87.

133. Ibid., 46–48.

134. Peter Chowka interview, February 10 and 28, 1976, published as "This Is Allen Ginsberg," *New Age Journal*, April 1976, reprinted in Ginsberg, *Ginsberg*, 386.

135. Buried in one story, appearing in *The New York Times* on August 27, 1968, was this: Allen Ginsberg led some "300 Yippies in a gentle chanting of 'om'—a mystic Indian chant of peace and relaxation," in Lincoln Park. Sylvan Fox, "300 Police Use Tear Gas to Breach Young Militants' Barricade in Chicago Park," *New York Times*, August 27, 1968, 29.

136. Buckley, "Battle of Chicago," SM130.

137. Ginsberg's account starting with the note about how he was pronouncing "Om" is from his 1969 *Playboy* interview. In this interview Ginsberg claims this seven-hour session of chanting took place on Sunday night. In his trial testimony, Ginsberg refers to the session as having taken place Monday, though the transcript is a bit ambiguous. *Playboy* interview, *Playboy*, April 1969, 92; Ginsberg, *Ginsberg*, 225.

11. HOW TO BE A GURU WITHOUT REALLY TRYING

1. Four Kumbh Melas occur in any twelve-year cycle, and they cycle between four sites: Hardwar, Ujjain, Nasik, and Allahabad. "Kumbh Mela," *Encyclopædia Britannica*, search.eb.com/eb/article-9046410 (accessed December 11, 2008).

2. Jonathan Gould, *Can't Buy Me Love: The Beatles, Britain and America* (New York: Crown, 2007), 281. Besides the news cameras, the Woodstock festival was memorialized in a hugely popular documentary film. Edited by Martin Scorsese among others and released in 1970, *Woodstock* won an Academy Award for Best Documentary feature and grossed $13.3 million at the box office, more than any other documentary that year. Daniel F. Schowalter, "Remembering the Dangers of Rock and Roll: Toward a Historical Narrative of the Rock Festival," *Critical Studies in Media Communication* (Bell & Howell Information and Learning Company) 17, no. 1 (March 1, 2000): 86–102.

3. Footage included in *Living Yoga: The Life and Teachings of Swami Satchidananda* (Integral Yoga Multimedia, 2008). The text of his address has been published at www.swamisatchidananda.org/docs2/woodstock.htm (accessed December 11, 2008).

4. Display ad, *New York Times* (1857–Current File), February 13, 1969, ProQuest Historical Newspapers, *New York Times* (1851–2005), 41. Bernard Gunther recalls that the school was open for only a short while, between roughly six and twelve weeks. Interview with Bernard Gunther, December 22, 2008.

5. "*Playboy* Interview: Marshall McLuhan," *Playboy* 16, no. 3 (March 1969): 70.

6. Nora Sayre, "Film: Mysticism in the U.S.: The Program," *New York Times*, November 23, 1973. See Gregory Johnson, "The Hare Krishna in San Francisco," in Glock and Bellah, *New Religious Consciousness*, 34, for anecdotal evidence that this may have been the case.

7. Adam Smith, "Trying the Dance of Shiva," *Sports Illustrated*, August 13, 1973 (online archive accessed September 15, 2008).

8. Joan Mower and Peter Vandevanter, "Really Getting Away," *Washington Post*, September 28, 1975, 124.

9. "Beating the Blahs," *Time*, October 7, 1974.

10. For cast and plot summary see *Easy Come, Easy Go* at IMDb, www.imdb.com/title/tt0061610/ (accessed June 17, 2009).

11. The movie came and went. (Critics at the time called it "hokey," but to this day Elvis fans point to the movie and the song "Yoga Is as Yoga Does" as career low-points.) Kevin Thomas, "Elvis Stars in 'Easy Come, Go,'" *Los Angeles Times* (1886–Current File), March 24, 1967, D9.

12. *Enlighten Up!* directed by Kate Churchill, 2009.

13. www.babasfootsteps.com/meetbaba.htm (accessed June 18, 2009).

14. *Public Papers of the Presidents of the United States: Lyndon B. Johnson, 1965*, vol. 2, entry 546, pp. 1037–40 (Washington, DC: Government Printing Office, 1966), www.lbjlib.utexas.edu/Johnson/archives.hom/speeches.hom/651003.asp (accessed January 5, 2009); "Trek of Asians, Europeans to U.S. Increases," *Washington Post and Times-Herald* (1959–73), February 3, 1967, A4.

15. *Living Yoga: The Life and Teachings of Swami Satchidananda.*

16. Roslyn Locks, "Swami Satchidananda: 'I am the dangerous drug,'" *Village Voice*, December 10, 1970, 11, 54.

17. Pandit Rajmani Tigunait, *At the Eleventh Hour: The Biography of Swami Rama* (Honesdale, PA: Himalayan Institute Press, 2001), 238–41.

18. Katharine Webster, "The Case Against Swami Rama of the Himalayas," *Yoga Journal*, December 1990; "The Rediscovery of Human Nature," *Time*, April 2, 1973.

19. Marty Altschul, "Tense Housewives, Businessmen Try Relaxing Hindu Way—Yoga Lessons," *Los Angeles Times* (1886–Current File), June 22, 1969, SF-A1; Sara Davidson, "The Rush for Instant Enlightenment," *Harper's*, July 1971.

20. Sasthi Brata, "How to Be a Guru Without Really Trying," *Village Voice*, January 15, 1970, 13–14, 59.

21. Paul Zweig, *Three Journeys: An Automythology* (New York: Basic Books, 1976), 146–54.

22. Charles S. J. White, "Swami Muktananda and the Enlightenment Through Sakti-pat," *History of Religions* 13, no. 4 (May 1974): 306–22.

23. Zweig, *Three Journeys*, 170, 175.

24. Moses later became one of the team of seven directors who ran the Sivananda Yoga Vedanta Centers after Vishnu-Devananda's death.

25. Robert Moses interview, October 1, 2008; Gopala Krishna, *The Yogi: Portraits of Swami Vishnu-Devananda* (St. Paul, MN: Yes International Publishers, 1995), 8.

26. Some have questioned Muktananda's lineage. William Rodarmor, "The Secret Life of Swami Muktananda," *CoEvolution Quarterly*, Winter 1983.

27. Alan Tobey, "The Summer Solstice of the Healthy-Happy-Holy Organization," in Glock and Bellah, *New Religious Consciousness*, 5–25.

28. The founders brought two groups together, the Holistic Life Foundation, later renamed the Feathered Pipe Foundation, and the California Yoga Teachers Association. Those not named are Rose Garfinkle, Jean Girardot, and Janis Paulsen. See "The Yoga Journal Story," which simplifies this history, Yogajournal.com, www .yogajournal.com/global/34 (accessed January 8, 2009).

29. Lasater interview, September 24, 2008.

30. During the 1960s, the YMCA had expanded its concept of fitness to include "the spiritual and mental as well as the physical." Some chapters (of both the YMCA and the YWCA) began offering Hatha Yoga classes as early as 1962. By the time teachers such as Swami Rama arrived at the end of the decade, these were commonplace in big cities and even smaller towns such as Austin, Texas, and Ann Arbor, Michigan. Indeed the Y had so deftly inserted yoga into its physical fitness programs, Swami Rama had made it a point to introduce philosophy and meditation, lest his students "mistake yoga for a mere set of physical exercises." Nancy Hennig, "Ancient Yoga Calms the Way," *Chicago Daily Tribune*, December 13, 1962, N3; Elmer L. Johnson, *The History of the YMCA Physical Education* (Chicago: Association Press, Follett Publishing Company, 1979), 353; Tigunait, *At the Eleventh Hour*, 240. When Elsberry left Austin, Lasater took over teaching her class at the Y, though as she admits, she was learning as she went. Judith Lasater e-mail interview, November 23, 2008.

31. Judith Lasater e-mail interview, November 23, 2008. As the years went on, Lasater broadened her education in the discipline. She and her husband, Ike, honeymooned at the International Sivananda Yoga Ashram in the Bahamas so they could take Visnhu-Devananda's teacher-training course. Lasater interview, September 24, 2008.

32. Eventually, the CYTA shed its original teacher-training institute, which became the Iyengar Yoga Institute. Lasater interview, September 24, 2008.

33. Schocken books put out a revised edition in 1977.

34. *Yoga, Youth, and Reincarnation* continued to sell so well, Bantam Books reprinted it in 1976.

35. Jack Kerouac, *Road Novels, 1957–1960: On the Road/The Dharma Bums/The Subterraneans/Tristessa/Lonesome Traveler/From the Journals, 1949–1954*, introduction by Douglas Brinkley (Library of America, 2007), 307.

36. Fritz Machlup, *The Production and Distribution of Knowledge in the United States* (Princeton, NJ: Princeton University Press, 1973), 250; Harry Castleman and Walter J. Podrazik, *The TV Schedule Book: Four Decades of Network Programming from Sign-On to Sign-Off* (New York: McGraw-Hill Book Company, 1984), 122–26.

37. "Friday Television Programs," *Los Angeles Times* (1886–Current File), November 3,

1961, ProQuest Historical Newspapers, *Los Angeles Times* (1881–1986), A10. No episodes remain of the show partly because it was live TV—and considered to have little value once aired. Gary Browning of the Paley Center for Media, e-mail correspondence, March 21, 2008.

38. Yoga circles have always been intimate. Henry Denison had shown up at the Hollywood Vedanta Temple in 1949, a fiery-eyed seeker with Gregory Peck looks, who offered Prabhavananda $250 a week to live up on Ivar Avenue as a probationer monk. Isherwood remembers him, with the pique of the prodigal son, as being quite obviously wealthy and changing the place around by having a shed built in the garden. Isherwood, *Diaries*, 408.

    Denison was a consummate gardener of plants and of people, cultivating in particular those people, such as Watts and Huxley, who might get him closer to his own spiritual realization. Virginia was his first wife.

39. Hittleman also won over Beverly Wilson, a reporter who touted his work in articles syndicated in newspapers across the country. She wrote a twelve-part series on Hatha Yoga for the *Los Angeles Times* and relied on Hittleman for both insight and instruction in all twelve parts. Beverly Wilson, "Yoga for All: The First Lesson," *Los Angeles Times* (1886–Current File), January 9, 1961, ProQuest Historical Newspapers, *Los Angeles Times* (1881–1986), A4.

40. This was of course the Hatha Yoga Swami Prabhavananda had so disparaged and which, according to its most revered sources, made no less claim to bliss consciousness.

    The *Hatha Yoga Pradīpikā* is clear on this point. Master the techniques outlined and not only will you conquer death, you'll attain "the greatest bliss of Brahman." And it doesn't stop there. Yogis able to enter samadhi through nada anusandhana will experience a "plentitude of bliss" that defies all description. No matter how one enters samadhi, this state of being is so wondrously good, so beyond our concepts of goodness, the scriptures fall into near silence. The most complete description you'll find is a list of attributes *missing* from this type of consciousness. HYP, 467; *Gherand Samhitā*, 7:1–23.

41. Beverly Wilson, "Yoga for All," A4.

42. Interview with Bernard Gunther, March 4, 2008; Richard Hittleman, *Guide to Yoga Meditation: The Inner Source of Strength, Security, and Personal Peace* (New York: Bantam Books, 1969), 135.

43. Hittleman, *Guide to Yoga Meditation*, 12.

44. Ibid., 11–14; Joe Hyams, "Hittleman's Taking Yoga to the Ladies," *Los Angeles Times*, August 2, 1961; "Around Town with Joan Winchell," *Los Angeles Times* (1886–Current File), August 13, 1961, N2.

45. Hyams, "Hittleman's Taking Yoga to the Ladies." Off the air, Hittleman was friendly with the Denisons, who hosted parties at their home in the Hollywood hills that drew seekers of all types.

46. "Beating the Blahs."

47. Deena Brown, "A Conversation with Lilias Folan," *Yoga Journal*, July-August 1979, 7–11.

48. *Yoga Journal* also ran a calendar and classified ads. (In these sections, the magazine's eclecticism was most visible. You were as likely to find a listing for the class "Yoga and Childbirth" as you were for "Ecstasy in Christian Mysticism" or "The

Kabala and the Tarot" or "A Jung Teilhard Symposium on Human Energy and the Formation of the Future.")

49. Paul Copeland, "Yoga, Sexuality, Matter and Energy: An Integration," *Yoga Journal* 1, no. 6 (January-February 1976): 16.

50. Interview with Judith Lasater, September 24, 2008.

51. *Yoga Journal* 1, no. 3 (July–August 1975): 8.

52. "Swami Vishnu Chronology," www.sivananda.org/teachings/teachers/swamiji/swamijis_story_chronology.html (accessed December 12, 2008).

53. Tobey, "Summer Solstice," 5–25.

54. "Cutting Loose," *Esquire*, July 1970, 53–57.

55. Winifred Rosen, "Down the Up Staircase: Upside Down at the Arica Institute," *Harper's*, June 1973, 22, 30; Aileen Jacobson, "Arica! Salvation at $600 a Head—with the Big O Along the Network of Seekers," *Washington Post and Times-Herald*, April 8, 1973, PO14.

56. Sally Kempton, "Hanging Out with the Guru," *New York*, April 12, 1976.

57. William H. Deadwyler, III, "Patterns in ISKCON's Historical Self-Perception," in *Krishna Consciousness*, 58.

58. According to one judge, the Hare Krishnas used far less force to grow their ranks than Patrick did in his efforts to thin them. However, being in the news constantly helped fuel demand for Patrick's services. Murray Schumach, "Judge Rejects Charges of 'Brainwashing' Against Hare Krishna Aides," *New York Times* (1857–Current File), March 18, 1977, 24.

59. J. Gordon Melton, "The Attitude of Americans Toward Hinduism," in Bromley and Shinn, *Krishna Consciousness*, 93.

   The 1978 publication of *Snapping: America's Epidemic of Sudden Personality Change* further buttressed Patrick's view of religious conversion, if not his methodology for addressing it. Authors Conway and Siegelman argued that converts were not healthy individuals electing a new religion or lifestyle. They were mentally unstable to start, and their psychopathology (or phase of life) made them exceptionally vulnerable to the nefarious techniques of the cult. See Robbins and Anthony, "Deprogramming, Brainwashing and the Medicalization of Deviant Religious Groups," *Society for Study of Social Problems* 29, no. 3 (February 1982): 283–97.

60. Some groups went on the offensive. In May 1979, two Hare Krishnas debated Ted Patrick himself on national television. As was to be expected, there was no common ground and little real dialogue. The two sides offered mutually exclusive views of reality. (What's really striking is the class difference between the ISKCON leadership, here represented by Hridayananda Goswami, and Patrick. Hridayananda, née Howard Resnick, is well-educated, well-spoken, and, as he admits, from an affluent background. He talks circles around Patrick, who, in his own defense, says as much.)

   Their "debate" can be boiled down to a single exchange:

   Says Hridayananda, it's "the material society . . . which is misleading and cheating these gullible young people and dragging them down into a fruitless and frustrating life based on material sense gratification and giving them no understanding of God and no understanding of the actual purpose of life."

   Says Patrick, "Hare Krishna is one of the main ones. It's no different from

Guyana—Jim Jones—no different from Hitler. It's no different from any group in the world that uses this mind control." The show was produced by WTCC-CH17, in Atlanta, Georgia.

61. Curiously, few of the details about life as a Hare Krishna were new (the notable exception being the extent to which Sacks and Berner were prevented from having contact with their friends and family).

　　In fact, Sacks's and Berner's descriptions of their lives sound a lot like those of active, happy devotees. The difference lay not so much in Sacks's and Berner's experiences as members of ISKCON, but in how they made sense of this experience.

　　All the chanting made Berner feel "high," just as it made other ISKCON members feel high. One even told the *East Village Other*, "You can chant your way right into Eternity."

　　The problem was Berner didn't like the feeling of being high. Elaine Markoutsas, "Krishna Converts Who Fled the Cult," *Chicago Tribune*, August 11, 1975, B1. Ellwood, "ISKCON and the Spirituality of the 1960s," in Bromley and Shinn, *Krishna Consciousness*, 105.

62. Judith Lasater interview, September 24, 2008.

63. Judith Lasater e-mail interview, November 23, 2008.

64. And in the case of Sivananda and Vishnu-Devananda, revised into a five-point program: "Proper Exercise (Asanas) Proper Breathing (Pranayama) Proper Relaxation (Savasana) Proper Diet (vegetarian) Positive Thinking (Vedanta) and Meditation (Dhyana)."

65. Judith Lasater, "Hatha Yoga as Meditation," *Yoga Journal* 1, no. 1 (May 1975): 5.

12. MARSHMALLOW YOGA

1. "Poll Finds Meditation, Mysticism and Yoga Growing in Popularity," *New York Times* (1857–Current File), November 18, 1976, 24.

2. Christopher H. Sterling and Timothy R. Haight, *The Mass Media: Aspen Institute Guide to Communication Industry Trends* (New York: Praeger Publishers, 1978), 346.

3. Roszak agreed that America was witnessing a "religious renaissance." Kenneth Briggs, "New Religious Movements Considered Likely to Last," *New York Times*, June 22, 1977, 15. Meanwhile, lest anyone make the mistake that 5 million yoga practitioners and a lot of positive press translated into widespread acceptance by the "religious and cultural majority," Harvard theologian Harvey Cox assured observers that the four "myths" about all new religions in America, many of which were not new in any historical sense, nor particularly new to America, would be levied at Eastern disciplines such as yoga for years to come. They were, in no particular order, that new religious groups are subversive, dishonest, dupe followers, and encourage sexual perversion. Repetition of these myths by successive generations didn't seem in any way to diminish their potency.

4. *The Joy of Sex* was published in the United States in December 1972; by November 1976, the book had sold about 4.7 million copies—hardcover and paperback combined—here. Jon Nordheimer, "'Joy of Sex' Author Gains on Royalties," *New York Times*, November 25, 1976, 20.

5. It later came out that Joya was taking Hungrex diet pills, which contained phenylpropanolamine (now known to cause psychosis and stroke) and, in all likelihood, caffeine.

6. Dass first disavowed Joya Santayana by telephone. This caused quite a stir. No one could really accept his explanation for either his initial ardor or its abrupt cooling, which was that he had been taken in by "a web of grandiose lies." "Egg on My Beard" was an attempt at a fuller explanation that allowed for his own inadequacies. Cowlette Dowling, "Confessions of an American Guru," *New York Times Magazine*, December 4, 1977.

7. Stephen Diamond, "In the Garden of the Forking Paths," *New Age Journal*, December 1976, 36; Ram Dass, "Egg on My Beard," *Yoga Journal*, November 1976; Dowling, "Confessions of An American Guru," 143.

8. Agehananda Bharati, *The Ochre Robe* (Seattle: University of Washington Press, 1962), 255. The refrain goes "Gurur brahma / gurur Vishnu / gurur devo / maheshwara / gurur sakshaat / parabrahma / tasmayi shree / guruve namah." Joshua M. Greene, *Here Comes the Sun: The Spiritual Musical Journey of George Harrison* (Hoboken, NJ: John Wiley & Sons, 2006), 184.

9. Dass himself described the relationship with the guru as *intra*personal not *inter*personal. There's the man or woman part, who is just a man or woman, and then the guru part. Dass, *Only Dance*, 79.

10. "I am as you see me," an interview with Swami Muktananda, *New Age Journal* 3 (1976): 52.

11. Dass, "Egg on My Beard."

12. Hugh Sidey, "Nothing Wrong with Normalcy" and "Yogi Bhajan's Synthetic Sikhism," *Time*, September 5, 1977.

13. Eileen Barker, "Religious Movements: Cult and Anticult Since Jonestown," *Annual Review of Sociology* 12 (1986): 332.

14. Quoted in Lis Harris, "O Guru, Guru, Guru," *The New Yorker*, November 14, 1994.

15. Russell Chandler, "Brother-Sister Gurus Now Lead Yoga Movement," *Los Angeles Times*, October 1, 1983, B6.

16. Harris, "O Guru, Guru, Guru."

17. Judith Lasater interview, September 24, 2008; Judith Lasater e-mail correspondence, November 21–December 1, 2008.

18. James Hillman, *Re-visioning Psychology*, quoted in Harvey Cox, *Turning East: The Promise and Peril of the New Orientalism* (New York: Simon & Schuster, 1977), 78–79.

19. Sara Davidson, "The Rush for Instant Salvation," *Harper's*, July 1971; Yogananda, *Autobiography of a Yogi*, 418.

20. Esalen was founded by Michael Murphy and Richard Price in 1962. Murphy had had a life-changing experience at Aurobindo's Pondicherry ashram in the late 1950s, and both he and Price had studied at the American Academy of Asian Studies with Watts, Chaudhuri, and Spiegelberg.

    One of their institute's operating principles was that religion is psychological. As religious scholar Jeffrey Kripal puts it, "Religion and the psychology of religion had seldom, if ever, come closer" than they had at Esalen.

    This in no way checked Esalen's ambition: to create a new language of personal growth and self-fulfillment and new tools for achieving it. They were crafting Spiegelberg's elusive "religion of no religion," and they signed up a host of experts, many of whom were mavericks in the field of psychology—people such as Fritz Perls, who, with his wife, developed Gestalt therapy, Abraham Maslow, a father of humanistic psychology, and Stanislav Grof, a founder of transpersonal psychology, as well as Alan Watts, Ram Dass, and Richard Hittleman. Jeffrey Kripal, *Esalen*, 8, 99, 135.

21. Albanese, *Republic of Mind*, 371–72. A host of other consequences of this privatization of religious experience including yoga are aptly detailed in Jeremy Carrette and Richard King, *Selling Spirituality: The Silent Takeover of Religion* (London and New York: Routledge, 2005), 69–86.

22. Jane Fonda, *Jane Fonda's Workout Book* (New York: Simon & Schuster, 1981), 67–68.

23. Gail Collins, *America's Women: Four Hundred Years of Dolls, Drudges, Helpmates, and Heroines* (New York: William Morrow, 2003), 447.

24. Made by the producers of the movie *Flashdance*, *Yoga Moves* brought the best of motion graphics—spinning pyramid crystals, figures that morph into silhouettes that morph into rainbows—and the bouncy energy of aerobics to Hatha Yoga, but it didn't fundamentally alter your sense of what Hatha Yoga was or could be.

   The opening sequence spoofs Olivia Newton-John's "Physical" video. Beautiful, bare-legged women in high-cut leotards, lashes weighed down by mascara, and tan young men in high-cut shorts perform poses in unison, always smiling broadly.

25. "An early look at the Macintosh Plus with its whiz-bang 7.8–MHz Motorola processor and 1 MB of RAM," from "10 Years Ago in BYTE," www.byte.com/art/9606/sec5/art2.htm (accessed January 9, 2009).

26. Unmesh Kher, "July 27, 1982: A Name for the Plague," from the series "80 Days That Changed the World," *Time*, www.time.com/time/80days/820727.html (accessed November 2, 2009).

27. Deborah Blumenthal, "Posturing," *New York Times* (1857–Current File), August 24, 1986, SMA72.

13. THE NEW PENITENTS

1. There is a beginning and an advanced series, but each is fixed.

2. Emmy Cleaves interview, March 10, 2009.

3. Blair Sabol, "Yogi to the Stars and Everyman," *Los Angeles Times* (1886–Current File), November 29, 1974, G1; Katharine Lowrie, "Star Fat: The Celebrity Exercise Circuit," *Los Angeles Times* (1886–Current File), January 11, 1981, M1.

4. Sabol, "Yogi to the Stars and Everyman."

5. "Television," *New York Times* (1857–Current File), August 23, 1974, 59; "New from Two Hatha Teachers," *Yoga Journal* 26 (May 1979): 58–59.

6. Jack McCallum, "Everybody's Doin' It," *Sports Illustrated*, December 3, 1984. Television and movie stars, including Tom Smothers and Ruth Buzzi, had demonstrated poses in Bikram's 1978 book *Bikram's Beginning Yoga Class*. Alijean Harmetz, "Hollywood: This Way In," *New York Times*, late ed. (East Coast), March 13, 1983, A42.

7. Cleaves interview, March 10, 2009.

8. Hilary E. MacGregor, "Had Your McYoga Today?" *Los Angeles Times*, July 7, 2002.

9. Bikram owned twenty-five cars, including a maroon Rolls-Royce limousine formerly the property of Queen Elizabeth and valued at seventy-five thousand dollars. He also spent lavishly on the needy, supporting impoverished children in South

America and funding orphanages and hospitals around the world. Harmetz, "Hollywood"; Ronald S. Miller, "Bikram Choudhury: A Yogi Stars in Hollywood," *Yoga Journal*, January–February 1982, 30.

10. Miller, "A Yogi Stars," 30.

11. However, the Ghosh brothers taught very different types of yoga; in effect, they had specialized. At first, Yogananda had spoken of raising the "Pranic Current" through seven centers. To do so, vigorous yoga, including asana, was quite useful. In some of his earliest lectures, the swami sold his method to Americans by convincing them they could gain complete control over their muscles and perfect physical and mental development by exercising their will. ("We have combined the basic laws of ancient Yogis with modern physiological science," he explained to a large audience in Los Angeles in 1923. "With the will developed fully, you will have perfect specimens of humanity, physically, mentally and morally.") To prove it, the then young swami demonstrated lotus position, which probably looked as difficult then as grabbing your knees in a back bend does today, and then curled his crossed legs up so that he was balancing on his hands, lotus suspended above the floor. But by the late 1920s, Yogananda was downplaying Hatha Yoga (though he had never called it that) and Kundalini in his public lectures and correspondence courses. Instead, he emphasized the Karma Yoga of the *Gita* and a type of autosuggestion.

By repeating Yogananda's affirmations you could tap the Power of Cosmic Consciousness or reap health and wealth. "Make Yourself Venus," *Los Angeles Times* (1886–Current File), March 4, 1923, III13; Thomas, "Hinduism Invades America," 151–61; Yogananda, *Autobiography*, 289; "Sri Byayamacharyya Yogindra Bishnu Charan Ghosh," www.ghoshtrustfund.com (accessed February 5, 2009).

12. According to his official bio, Bikram was also given the name Yogiraj, or King of Yogis, by Swami Sivananda, www.ghoshtrustfund.com/.

13. Cleaves interview, March 10, 2009.

14. Eddie Stern and Deirdre Summerbell, "Sri K. Pattabhi Jois: A Tribute" (New York: Eddie Stern and Gwyneth Paltrow, 2002).

15. "It was quite a mind-blowing experience, really. It took me to a place that felt very familiar, very deep, peaceful, and it felt like something that perhaps I'd done before or something that I definitely wanted to be doing again." Guy Donahaye and Eddie Stern, *Guruji: A Portrait of Sri K. Pattabhi Jois Through the Eyes of His Students* (New York: North Point Press, 2010).

16. Sri K. Pattabhi Jois, *Yoga Mala* (New York: Patanjali Yoga Shala, 1999), 12.

17. Ibid., 16–17.

18. "Sri K. Pattabhi Jois: A Tribute"; display ad 368, *Los Angeles Times* (1886–Current File), November 12, 1972, SE8.

19. McCallum, "Everybody's Doin' It." Drexel Burnham was at 9560 Wilshire. James B. Stewart, *Den of Thieves* (New York: Simon & Schuster, 1991, 1992), 65, 222.

20. Linda Grant, "Drexel Burnham Finds Self in Heady Company," and Thomas B. Rosenstiel, "Drexel's Bond Traders Like Their Daily Grind," *Los Angeles Times* (1886–Current File), March 11, 1984, F1.

21. Miller, "A Yogi Stars," 28.

22. Rebecca Mead, "The Yoga Bums," *The New Yorker*, August 14, 2000, 42.

23. Ibid., 40.

24. Jois, *Yoga Mala*, 94–95.

25. Sabol, "Yogi to the Stars and Everyman."

26. Iyengar Yoga Institute of San Francisco, "Workshops" section, www.iyisf.org/ (accessed June 29, 2009).

27. Both Bikram and Jois and his successors modify certain poses if you are injured or pregnant; however, as a rule, they don't prescribe particular poses for specific illnesses or injuries.

28. "Yoga Goes Mainstream: A Class in Urban Yoga Will Really Get Your Heart Rate Up," *U.S. News & World Report*, May 16, 1994.

29. Alicia Lasek, "Superwoman's Dead: Fitness Craze Goes Softer; Walking and Gardening Blossom," *Ad Age Chicago* 65, no. 47 (November 7, 1994), referencing a recent *New York Times* article.

30. Ibid.

31. Adrian Maher, "Yogamania: Weary of Body-Pounding Workouts, Fitness Buffs Turn with Relief to the Ancient Healing Exercise," *Los Angeles Times*, home ed. (pre-1997 Fulltext), November 20, 1994, 13

32. "Yoga Goes Mainstream," 80.

33. Linda Dyett, "Latest ways to get a real workout . . . and move beyond the boring treadmill and step class," *Cosmopolitan* 221, no. 5 (November 1996): 157.

34. William McKibben, "Talk of the Town," *The New Yorker*, January 23, 1984, 32–33.

35. Apparently, Miller wasn't supposed to be in the video. "Dr. Ray, as we all called him, was the host in Santa Cruz and had put the whole video thing together. Guru–ji was a bit reluctant, seemed like he got surprised by the idea and the project, but went along with it. I was supposed to just be the driver. I drove Guru–ji and Ama around a lot back in those days. He liked my big black Dodge van and called the passenger seat "Simasana." Like a throne of some kind. We drove up to UCSC campus. When we got there, Guru–ji decided that I would also have to be in it. I had just had a fairly good-sized lunch and it was the last thing I wanted to do, but he was the boss, so what else could I do but go along with it? I was supposed to be the one who knew what to do. . . . As you can tell, if you watched the tape, it was pretty windy. The picture of the deity kept getting blown over. The ground was pretty lumpy. It was hot. Guru–ji got frustrated, it wasn't going well." E-mail correspondence with Chuck Miller, July 1, 2009.

36. "Trust Me It's Tough," *U.S. News & World Report*, May 16, 1994, 83.

37. Sharon Gannon and David Life, *Jivamukti Yoga: Practices for Liberating Body and Soul* (New York: Ballantine Books, 2002), 11–12.

38. Mark Jolly, "Yoga's Big Stretch," *New York*, January 26, 1998.

39. Ibid.; Penelope Green, "Modern Yoga: Om to the Beat," *New York Times* (1857–Current File), March 15, 1998, ST1.

40. Green "Modern Yoga," ST1.

41. One of Madonna's yoga teachers, Eddie Stern, and Sanskritist Vyaas Houston did the translation.

42. Steve Morse, "A Changed Madonna Takes a Walk on the Quiet Side," Five Star Lift ed., *Boston Globe*, 1998; *St. Louis Post–Dispatch*, March 31, 1998, D1.

43. Ibid.

44. David Browne, "Ethereal Girl," *Entertainment Weekly*, March 6, 1998.

45. The lower figure of 15 million is from *Yoga Journal*'s 2003 "Yoga in America" study, conducted by Harris Interactive; *U.S. News & World Report* estimated higher. Car-

olyn Kleiner, "Mind-body fitness: Yoga Booms in Popularity as a Way to Heighten Flexibility, Improve Breathing, and Gain Sanity," *U.S. News & World Report*, 132, no. 16 (May 13, 2002): 53; Russell Wild, "Yoga, Inc.," *Yoga Journal*, November 2002, 108–13, 157.

46. *The New Yorker*, October 14, 2002.

47. Kempton, "Hanging Out with the Guru," 46.

48. Lis Harris, "O Guru, Guru, Guru," *The New Yorker*, November 14, 1994, 92 and on.

49. Margaret H. Parkinson, "A Personal Story of SYDA Involvement," August 1996, www.leavingsiddhayoga.net/syda_inv.htm (accessed July 1, 2009).

50. Harris, "O Guru, Guru, Guru," 92 and on.

51. Ibid.; Russell Chandler, "Brother-Sister Gurus Now Lead Yoga Movement," *Los Angeles Times*, October 1, 1983, B6.

52. Ron Rosenbaum, "When Betsy Met Sally: Two 'It Girls' Face the Material World," *New York Observer*, October 27, 2002; Harris, "O Guru, Guru, Guru," 92 and on.

53. Nori Muster, *Betrayal of the Spirit: My Life Behind the Headlines of the Hare Krishna Movement* (Urbana and Chicago: University of Illinois Press, 1997), 67; Frank Bures, "Murder, Sex and Free Food: How the Portland Sect of Hare Krishnas Are Struggling to Overcome a Very Shady Past," *Portland Mercury*, June 21, 2001, www .portlandmercury.com/gyrobase/Content?category=34029&mode=print&oid=24810 (accessed July 1, 2009); "Krishna Group Named in a Child Abuse Case," *New York Times* (1857–Current File), March 3, 1988, A17. In 2000, a Dallas attorney sued ISKCON for $400 million on behalf of hundreds of children who claimed to have been abused. ISKCON, which had already admitted that the abuse occurred, settled the case out of court. E. Burke Rochford, Jr., with Jennifer Heinlein, "Child Abuse in the Hare Krishna Movement: 1971–1986," *ISKCON Communications Journal* 6, no. 1 (June 1998), www.iskcon.com/icj/6_1/6_1rochford.html (accessed July 1, 2009).

54. See Muster's book, *Betrayal of the Spirit*, for a detailed look at this aspect of ISKCON.

55. Melton, "Attitude of Americans Toward Hinduism," in Bromley and Shinn, *Krishna Consciousness*, 95–96.

56. Jyothi Sampat, "Hindu Culture Is Taking Root in Arizona Enclaves; Religion: Immigrants from India linked to jobs in the tech field are responding warmly to the temples that are sprouting up," *Los Angeles Times*, March 3, 2002, B7.

57. Bures, "Murder, Sex and Free Food."

58. Steven Ruddell, "A Personal Experience with Baba Muktananda," *Yoga Journal* 2, no. 3 (May–June 1976): 25; Jois, *Yoga Mala*, 33.

59. Joelle Hann, "Pattabhi Jois Memorial, NYC, June 14, 2009," June 17, 2009, joellehann.com/yoganation/?p=304 (accessed July 2, 2009).

60. John Campbell e-mail correspondence, July 14, 2009; Hann, "Pattabhi Jois Memorial, NYC."

61. Hann, "Pattabhi Jois Memorial, NYC." Donna Karan—in a loose crimson blouse, soft black jacket, and khaki pants, dark hair braided—welcomed guests. Karan, of course, is one of the country's most famous fashion designers and a longtime seeker and yoga student. She had opened up her West Village studio to the assembled because she believes in yoga's power to heal.

62. U.S. Census Bureau, "2007 American Community Survey."

63. "Yoga Reduces Asthma Attacks, Say Researchers," MailOnline, June 2, 2009; "Yoga

for Anxiety and Depression," *Harvard Mental Health Letter*, April 2009, www.health
.harvard.edu/newsletters/Harvard_Mental_Health_Letter/2009/April/Yoga
-for-anxiety-and-depression (accessed July 2, 2009); Molly O'Neill, "Unusual Heart
Therapy Wins Coverage from Large Insurer," *New York Times*, July 28, 1993, www
.nytimes.com/1993/07/28/health/unusual-heart-therapy-wins-coverage-from
-large-insurer.html?scp=15&sq=Dean%20Ornish&st=cse (accessed July 2, 2009).

64. Jois, *Yoga Mala*, 15.

SELECTED BIBLIOGRAPHY

Abhedananda, Swami. *How to Be a Yogi*. New York: Vedanta Society, 1902.

Albanese, Catherine L. *A Republic of Mind and Spirit: A Cultural History of American Metaphysical Religion*. New Haven: Yale University Press, 2007.

Alter, Joseph S. *Yoga in Modern India: The Body Between Science and Philosophy*. Princeton: Princeton University Press, 2004.

Aurobindo, Sri. *The Essential Aurobindo: Writings of Sri Aurobindo*. Edited by Robert McDermott. Great Barrington, MA: Lindisfame Books, 1987, 2001.

———. *The Integral Yoga: Sri Aurobindo's Teaching and Method of Practice*. Twin Lakes, WI: Lotus Press, 1993.

Avalon, Arthur. *The Serpent Power: The Secrets of Tantric and Shaktic Yoga*. London: Luzac and Co., 1919. Reprint, New York: Dover Publications, 1974.

Behanan, Kovoor T. *Yoga: A Scientific Evaluation*. New York: Macmillan Company, 1937.

Bernard, Theos. *Haṭha Yoga: The Report of a Personal Experience*. New York: Columbia University Press, 1944.

———. *Heaven Lies Within Us*. London: Rider and Company, 1940, 1950.

Bharati, Agehananda. "The Hindu Renaissance and Its Apologetic Patterns." *The Journal of Asian Studies* 29, no. 2 (February 1970): 267–87.

———. *The Tantric Tradition*. Rider and Co., 1965. Revised American paperback edition, New York: Samuel Weiser Inc., 1975.

Bridges, Hal. "Aldous Huxley: Exponent of Mysticism in America." *Journal of the American Academy of Religion* 37, no. 4 (December 1969): 341–52.

Bromley, David G., and Larry D. Shinn, eds. *Krishna Consciousness in the West*. Lewisburg, PA: Bucknell University Press, 1989.

Bryant, Edwin F., trans. *The Yoga Sutras of Patanjali*. New York: North Point Press, 2009.

Buell, Lawrence. *Emerson*. Cambridge, MA: Belknap Press of the Harvard University Press, 2003.

Burke, Marie Louise. *Swami Vivekananda in the West, New Discoveries: His Prophetic Mission*. 4th ed. 2 vols. Calcutta: Advaita Ashrama, 1992. First published by Vedanta Society of Northern California, 1958.

Carpenter, Frederic Ives. *Emerson and Asia*. 1930. Reprint, New York: Haskell House Publishers Ltd., 1968.

Carrette, Jeremy, and Richard King, *Selling Spirituality: The Silent Takeover of Religion*. London: Routledge, 2005.

Chattopadhyaya, Rajagopal. *Swami Vivekananda in India: A Corrective Biography*. Delhi: Motilal Banarsidass Publishers, 1999.

———. *Swami Vivvekananda in the West*. Houston, TX: self-published by the author, 1993.

Christy, Arthur. *The Orient in American Transcendentalism: A Study of Emerson, Thoreau, and Alcott*. New York: Columbia University Press, 1932.

Colebrooke, H. T. *Essays on the Religion and Philosophy of the Hindus*. London: Williams and Norgate, 1858.

Cox, Harvey. *Turning East: The Promise and Peril of the New Orientalism*. New York: Simon & Schuster, 1977.

Daggett, Mabel Potter. "The Heathen Invasion." *Hampton Columbian Magazine*, October 1911, 399–411.

Das, Bhagavan. *It's Here Now (Are You?): A Spiritual Memoir*. New York: Broadway Books, 1977.

Dass, Ram. *Be Here Now*. Kingsport, TN: Hanuman Foundation, 1978.

———. "Eggs on My Beard." *Yoga Journal*, November 1976, 6–11.

———. *The Only Dance There Is: Talks at the Menninger Foundation, 1970 and Spring Grove Hospital, 1972*. Garden City, NY: Anchor Books, 1974.

Davidson, Sara. "The Rush for Instant Salvation." *Harper's Magazine*, July 1971, 40–42, 46–49, 52–54.

Davis, Mike. *Late Victorian Holocausts: El Niño Famines and the Making of the Third World*. New York: Verso, 2001.

De Michelis, Elizabeth. *A History of Modern Yoga: Patanjali and Western Esotericism*. London and New York: Continuum, 2004.

Devi, Indra. *Forever Young, Forever Healthy: Secrets of the Ancients Adapted for Modern Living*. New York: Prentice-Hall, 1953.

———. *Yoga for Americans*. Englewood Cliffs, NJ: Prentice-Hall, 1959.

Eliade, Mircea. *Yoga: Immortality and Freedom*. 2nd ed. Translated by Willard R. Trask. Bollingen Series 56. Princeton: Princeton University Press, 1990. Originally published in French as *Le Yoga: Immortalité et liberté*. Paris: Librairie Payot, 1954.

Ellwood, Robert S., Jr. *Alternative Altars: Unconventional and Eastern Spirituality in America*. Chicago: University of Chicago Press, 1979.

———. "The American Theosophical Synthesis." In *The Occult in America: New Historical Perspectives*. Edited by Howard Kerr and Charles L. Crow. Urbana and Chicago: Universtiy of Illinois Press, 1983.

Feuerstein, Georg. *The Shambhala Encyclopedia of Yoga*. Boston and London: Shambhala, 2000.

———. *The Yoga Tradition: Its History, Literature, Philosophy, and Practice*. With a foreword by Ken Wilbur. Prescott, AZ: Hohm Press, 1998, 2001.

Fields, Rick. *How the Swans Came to the Lake: A Narrative History of Buddhism in America*. Boston: Shambhala, 1992.

Ginsberg, Allen. *Allen Ginsberg, Spontaneous Mind: Selected Interviews, 1958–1996*. With a preface by Václav Havel and an introduction by Edmund White. Edited by David Carter. New York: HarperCollins Publishers, 2001.

Glock, Charles Y., and Robert N. Bellah, eds. *The New Religious Consciousness*. Berkeley: University of California Press, 1976.

Godwin, Joscelyn. *The Theosophical Enlightment*. Albany: State University of New York Press, 1994.

Goodman, Eckert. "The Guru of Nyack." *Town and Country*, April 1941, 50, 53, 92, 93, 98, 99, 101.

Gosvāmī, Satsvarūpa Dāsa. *Srīla Prabhupāda-līlāmrta*. Vol. 2, *Planting the Seed: New York City, 1965–1996*. Los Angeles: Bhaktivedanta Book Trust, 1980.

Hackett, Paul G. "Barbarian Lands: Theos Bernard, Tibet, and American Religious Life." Ph.D. diss., Columbia University, 2008.

Halbfass, Wilhelm. *India and Europe: An Essay in Understanding*. Albany: State University of New York Press, 1988.

Harris, Lis. "O Guru, Guru, Guru." *The New Yorker*, November 14, 1994, 92–109.

Hittleman, Richard. *Guide to Yoga Meditation: The Inner Source of Strength, Security, and Personal Peace*. New York: Bantam Books, 1969.

Hodder, Alan D. *Thoreau's Ecstatic Witness*. New Haven: Yale University Press, 2001.

Howard, Gerald, ed. *The Sixties: The Art, Attitudes, Politics, and Media of Our Most Explosive Decade*. New York: Pocket Books, 1982.

Huxley, Aldous. *The Doors of Perception* and *Heaven and Hell*. New York: Harper Perennial, 2004. The essays were first published separately by Harper & Brothers in 1954 and 1956 respectively.

———. "Drugs That Shape Men's Minds." *Saturday Evening Post*, October 18, 1958, 28, 108, 110–11, 113.

Isherwood, Christopher. *My Guru and His Disciple*. London: Eyre Methuen, 1980.

———, ed. *Vedanta for the Western World*. New York: Viking Press, 1960. First published by Vedanta Press, 1945.

Jackson, Carl T. *The Oriental Religions and American Thought: Nineteenth Century Explorations*. Westport, CT: Greenwood Press, 1981.

———. *Vedanta for the West: The Ramakrishna Movement in the United States*. Bloomington: Indiana University Press, 1994.

James, William. *The Varieties of Religious Experience*. 1902. New York: Touchstone, 1997.

Johnson, Ronald M. "Journey to Pondicherry: Margaret Woodrow Wilson and the Aurobindo Ashram." *Indian Journal of American Studies* 21, no. 2 (1991): 1–7.

———. "The Ramakrishna Mission to America: An Intercultural Study." In *American Studies in Transition*. Edited by David E. Nye and Christen Kold Thomsen. Odense, Denmark: Odense University Press, 1985.

Jois, Sri K. Pattabhi. *Yoga Mala*. New York: Pantanjali Yoga Shala, 1999.

Kempton, Sally. "Hanging Out with the Guru." *New York*, April 12, 1976, 36–38, 41–42, 45–46.

King, Richard. *Indian Philosophy: An Introduction to Hindu and Buddhist Thought*. Washington, DC: Georgetown University Press, 1999.

———. *Orientalism and Religion: Postcolonial Theory, India, and "The Mystic East."* London: Routledge, 1999.

Kripal, Jeffrey J. *Esalen: America and the Religion of No Religion*. Chicago: University of Chicago Press, 2007.

———. *Kali's Child: The Mystical and the Erotic in the Life and Teachings of Ramakrishna*. 2nd ed. Chicago: University of Chicago Press, 1998.

Krishna, Gopala. *The Yogi: Portraits of Swami Vishnu-Devananda*. St. Paul, MN: Yes International Publishers, 1995.

Lapham, Lewis. "There Once Was a Guru from Rishikesh." Pts. 1 and 2. *Saturday Evening Post*, May 4, 1968, 23–29; May 18, 1968, 28–33, 88.

———. *With the Beatles*. Hoboken, NJ: Melville House Publishing, 2005.

Leary, Timothy. *High Priest*. Oakland, CA: Ronin Publishing, 1995.

Love, Robert. "Fear of Yoga." *Columbia Journalism Review*, November/December 2006, 80–90.

———. *The Great Oom: The Improbable Birth of Yoga in America*. New York: Viking, 2010.

Macshane, Frank. "Walden and Yoga." *The New England Quarterly* 37, no. 3 (September 1964): 322–42.

Mayo, Katherine. *Mother India*. New York: Harcourt Brace & Co., 1927.

McWilliams, Carey. *Southern California Country: An Island on the Land*. New York: Duell, Sloan, and Pearce, 1946.

Miller, Barbara Stoler, trans. *The Bhagavad-Gita: Krishna's Counsel in Time of War*. New York: Columbia University Press, 1986.

Miller, Timothy. *The Hippies and American Values*. Knoxville, TN: University of Tennessee Press, 1991.

Muktibodhananda, Swami, trans. *Hatha Yoga Pradipika*. Munger, India: Yoga Publications Trust, 1993.

Muster, Nori. *Betrayal of the Spirit: My Life Behind the Headlines of the Hare Krishna Movement*. Urbana and Chicago: University of Illinois Press, 1997.

Nikhilananda, Swami, trans. *The Gospel of Sri Ramakrishna*. New York: Ramakrishna-Vivekananda Center, 1942.

Olivelle, Patrick, trans. *Upanishads*. Oxford, UK: Oxford University Press, 1996.

Phillips, Stephen. "Aurobindo's Philosophy of Brahman." Leiden, Netherlands: E. J. Brill, 1986. Electronic edition, March 2001.

———. "Yogic *ekagrata* (one-pointed concentration): The Analogical Key to Aurobindo's Philosophy." Plenary presentation, Fifth International Congress of Vedanta, Miami, FL, August 1994.

Potter, Charles Francis. *The Preacher and I: An Autobiography*. New York: Crown Publishers, 1951.

Prabuddhaprana, Pravrajika. *Saint Sara: The Life of Sara Chapman Bull, the Mother of Swami Vivekananda*. Dakshineswar and Calcutta: Sri Sarada Math, 2002.

Prothero, Stephen. "Mother India's Scandalous Swamis." In *Religions of the United States in Practice*. Edited by Colleen McDannell. Vol. 2 Princeton: Princeton University Press, 2001.

Richardson, Robert D., Jr. *Emerson: The Mind on Fire*. Berkeley: University of California Press, 1995.

———. *Henry Thoreau: A Life of the Mind*. Berkeley: University of California Press, 1986.

Rodrigues, Santan. *The Householder Yogi: Life of Shri Yogendra*. Bombay: The Yoga Institute, 1982.

Rosen, Winifred. "Down the Up Staircase: Upside Down at the Arica Institute." *Harper's Magazine*, June 1973, 28–32, 34, 36.

Roy, Rammohun, trans. *Translation of Several Principal Books, Passages, and Texts of the Veds, and of Some Controversial Works on Brahmunical Theology*. London: Parbury, Allen, and Co., 1832.

Saltzman, Paul. *The Beatles in Rishikesh*. New York: Viking Studio, 2000.

Sil, Narasingha P. *Swami Vivekananda: A Reassessment*. London: Associated University Press, 1997.

Simmons, Robert. "Yoga and the Psychedelic Mind." *San Francisco Oracle* 4 (December 16, 1966): 7–8, 23.

Sjoman, N. E. *The Yoga Tradition of the Mysore Palace.* New Delhi: Abhinav Publications, 1999.

Starr, Kevin. *The Dream Endures: California Enters the 1940s.* New York: Oxford University Press, 1997.

———. *Embattled Dreams: California in War and Peace, 1940–1950.* Oxford, UK: Oxford University Press, 2002.

Stein, William Bysshe, ed. *Two Brahmin Sources of Emerson and Thoreau.* Gainsville, FL: Scholars' Facsimiles and Reprints, 1967.

Stern, Eddie, and Deirdre Summerbell. *Sri K. Pattabhi Jois: A Tribute.* New York: Eddie Stern and Gwyneth Paltrow, 2002.

Tapasyananda, Swami, trans. *Srimad Bhagavad Gita: The Scripture of Mankind.* Mylapore, Madras: Sri Ramakrishna Math, 1984.

Thoreau, Henry David. *Letters to a Spiritual Seeker.* Edited by Bradley P. Dean. New York: W. W. Norton and Company, 2004.

———, trans. *The Transmigration of the Seven Brahmans: A Translation from the Harivansa of Langlois.* With an introduction by Arthur Christy. New York: William Edwin Rudge, 1931.

Tweed, Thomas A. *The American Encounter with Buddhism, 1844–1212: Victorian Culture and the Limits of Dissent.* Chapel Hill: University of North Carolina Press, 1992.

Urban, Hugh B. "The Omnipotent Oom: Tantra and Its Impact on Modern Western Esotericism." *Esoterica: The Journal* 3 (2001). www.esoteric.msu.edu/VolumeIII/HTML/Oom.html.

———. *Tantra: Sex, Secrecy, Politics, and Power in the Study of Religion.* Berkeley: University of California Press, 2005.

Vivekananda, Swami. *The Complete Works of Swami Vivekananda.* 1956. Reprint, Mayavati Memorial Edition. Calcutta: Advaita Ashrama, 1989. Online edition, www.ramakrishnavivekananda.info/vivekananda/complete_works.htm.

———. *Vedânta Philosophy Lectures by Swâmi Vivekânanda on Râja Yoga and Other Subjects.* New York: The Baker and Taylor Company, 1899.

———. *The Yogas and Other Works.* Chosen and with a biography by Swami Nikhilananda. New York: Ramakrishna Vedanta Center, 1953.

Wadleigh, Michael. *Woodstock: Three Days of Peace and Music.* Director's cut. Produced by Bob Maurice. Burbank, CA: Warner Home Video, 1999. Original documentary released 1970.

Ward, William. *A View of the History, Literature, and Mythology of the Hindoos.* 3rd ed. London: Black, Parbury, and Allen, 1817.

Watts, Alan. *In My Own Way: An Autobiography, 1915–1965.* New York: Pantheon Books, 1972.

———. *The Joyous Cosmology: Adventures in the Chemistry of Consciousness.* New York: Vintage Books, 1962.

White, David Gordon. *The Alchemical Body: Siddha Traditions in Medieval India.* Chicago: University of Chicago Press, 1996.

Wilkins, Charles, trans. *The Bhagavat-Geeta.* 1785. A facsimile reproduction with an introduction by George Hendrick. Delmar, NY: Scholars' Facsimiles and Reprints, 1959.

Wilson, H. H.. *Religious Sects of the Hindus.* Edited by Ernst R. Rost. Calcutta: Susil Gupta, 1958. This essay was first published in two parts in *Asiatic Researches* 16 (1828) and 17 (1832).

Wolfe, Tom. *The Electric Kool-Aid Acid Test.* New York: Bantam Books, 1999. First published by Farrar, Straus and Giroux, 1968.

Wright, Caleb, and J. A. Brainerd. *Historic Incidents and Life in India.* Chicago: J. A. Brainerd, 1869.

Yale, John. *The Making of a Devotee.* Gretz, France: 2003. world.std.com/~elayj/.

———. *A Yankee and the Swamis: A Westerner's View of the Ramakrishna Order.* Chennai, India: Sri Ramakrishna Math, 2001.

Yogananda, Paramahansa. *Autobiography of a Yogi.* 13th ed. Los Angeles, CA: Self-Realization Fellowship, 1946. Reprinted in 2001.

Ziolkowski, Eric J. *A Museum of Faiths: Histories and Legacies of the 1893 World's Parliament of Religions.* Atlanta: Scholars Press, 1993.

Zweig, Paul. *Three Journeys: An Automythology.* New York: Basic Books, 1976.

ACKNOWLEDGMENTS

This book was more than seven years in the making. Along the way, dozens of people have helped me. I cannot possibly thank them all enough for their insight, advice, and time.

Without Paul Elie's vision this book would have never found a home, nor would it have been half as good had I not had to meet his exacting standards. Jeff Seroy was an early and ardent advocate for this project. I thank them both as well as Laurel Cook and Georgia Cool at FSG for their support, enthusiasm, and most of all patience. Lydia Wills, my able agent, has stood by this book, through bad drafts and all. I thank her and Alyssa Reuben at Paradigm.

My family—Gary and Azita, Sharon, Kim and J.B., Hill, and Sandy Colony have all been fans and supporters from the beginning. I especially appreciate Hill and Kim for reading very early drafts and convincing me that, even then, the book was readable.

Eddie Stern deserves special mention for fielding my queries about yoga over the years, the countless leads he supplied, and his teaching of Ashtanga Yoga.

Professors Jack Hawley, Robert Thurman, and Stephen Prothero all supplied valuable information and advice at various stages of this project.

Michelle Legro and Liza Monroy were efficient and adaptable research assistants. Zoe Slatoff, Stephanie Guest, Paul Hackett, Robert Love, Krishna Das, Erik Davis, Erin Flynn, Steven Johnson, Stacey Platt, and Spiros Antonopoulos have all made crucial contributions, small and large.

I found invaluable resources in Columbia University Library, the Bancroft Library at the University of California, Berkeley, and the Historical Society of Rockland County. Over the course of this project, many of my primary sources were digitized and made more readily available via Pro-Quest and Google Books. Given other demands on my time, I would not have been able to complete this book without this enhanced access.

Robert Moses, Judith Lasater, Matzy Ezraty, Chuck Miller, and Patricia Walden spoke to me at length on record about their experiences as yoga teachers and students. They helped make this story come alive. I'm also grateful for the passion and dedication of the broader community of yoga teachers, practitioners, and sympathizers. Those I've spoken with over the past seven years have all greeted this book with enthusiasm and curiosity, and have helped me in whatever way they could.

But it is my husband, Christopher Kelley, and my daughters, Phoebe and Mavis, to whom I owe the greatest debt. To Phoebe and Mavis, thank you for letting me focus on this when you so wanted my undivided attention. And most of all, thank you, Chris, for putting me up to writing this book in the first place and challenging me to write the best one I could, and for taking on more than your share of the demands of family life as I did so.

INDEX